GUIDE TO
HEALTH INFORMATICS

Third edition

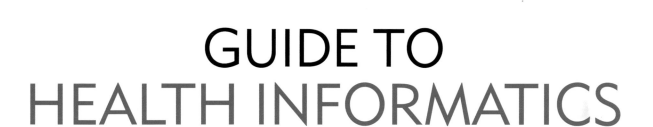

GUIDE TO HEALTH INFORMATICS

Third edition

ENRICO COIERA

Professor and Director
Centre for Health Informatics
Australian Institute of Health Innovation
Macquarie University
Sydney, Australia

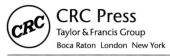

CRC Press
Taylor & Francis Group
Boca Raton London New York

CRC Press is an imprint of the
Taylor & Francis Group, an **informa** business

Cover art: A data visualisation of how often clinical trials directly compare different drugs. Arcs above and below the centre line show the differences between trials with or without industry funding. Colours reflect groups in the Anatomical Therapeutic Chemical Classification. Adam Dunn 2014 with permission.

CRC Press
Taylor & Francis Group
6000 Broken Sound Parkway NW, Suite 300
Boca Raton, FL 33487-2742

© 2015 by Enrico Coiera
CRC Press is an imprint of Taylor & Francis Group, an Informa business

No claim to original U.S. Government works

Printed in the UK by Severn, Gloucester on responsibly sourced paper

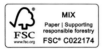

Version Date: 20150128

International Standard Book Number-13: 978-1-4441-7049-8 (Pack - Book and Ebook)

Library of Congress Cataloging-in-Publication Data

Coiera, Enrico, author.
  [Guide to medical informatics, the internet, and telemedicine]
  Guide to health informatics / Enrico Coiera. -- Third edition.
  p. ; cm.
  Includes bibliographical references and index.
  ISBN 978-1-4441-7049-8 (pbk. : alk. paper)
  I. Title.
  [DNLM: 1. Medical Informatics. 2. Computer Communication Networks. 3. Medical Informatics Applications. 4. Telemedicine. W 26.5]

  R858
  362.10285--dc23   2015002492

Visit the Taylor & Francis Web site at
http://www.taylorandfrancis.com

and the CRC Press Web site at
http://www.crcpress.com

In memory of Bob Palese

Contents

Part 4 Guideline- and protocol-based systems

Part 5 Communication systems in healthcare

Part 6 Language, coding and classification

Part 7 Clinical decision support and analytics

Part 8 Specialized applications for health informatics

Note

Healthcare is an ever-changing science. As new research and clinical experience broaden our knowledge, changes in treatment and drug therapy are required. The author and the publisher of this work have checked with sources believed to be reliable in their efforts to provide information that is complete and generally in accord with the standards accepted at the time of publication. However, in view of the possibility of human error or changes in medical sciences, neither the author nor the publisher or any other party who has been involved in the preparation or publication of this work warrants that the information contained herein is in every respect accurate or complete, and they are not responsible for any errors or omissions or for the results obtained from the use of such information. Readers are encouraged to confirm the information contained herein with other sources.

Preface

This book is written for healthcare professionals who wish to understand the principles and applications of information and communication methods and technologies in healthcare. The text is presented in a way that should make it accessible to anyone, independent of prior technology knowledge. It is suitable as a textbook for undergraduate and postgraduate training in the clinical aspects of informatics and as an introductory textbook for those pursuing a postgraduate career in health and biomedical informatics.

The text is designed to be used by *all* healthcare professionals, including nurses and allied health professionals, and not just medical practitioners. When I use the term 'clinician' in this book I am referring to any healthcare practitioner directly involved in patient care. Those with a background in information and communication technology should find the book a valuable introduction to the diverse applications of technology in health, as well as summarizing the unique challenges in this domain.

With the third edition of the Guide, I have kept the essential backbone of the informatics story the same as in previous editions. Part 1 contains foundational chapters that explain simply the abstract concepts that are core to informatics. Subsequent chapters then build upon those foundations. Part 2 contains a set of chapters that explore all the main themes of the book from the perspective of informatics skills. Practising clinicians must understand how to communicate effectively, structure information, ask questions, search for answers and make robust decisions. Informatics is as much about doing as it is about the tools we use, and these chapters make clear why the study of health informatics is the foundation of all other clinical activities.

We return to each of these information and communication system themes in later chapters, where we take a more technological focus. The book has a strong emphasis on demonstrating what works and what does not work in informatics. I have created a new evaluative framework based on the value of information that runs through the book, to help understand why some classes of intervention appear to work so much better than others. Each chapter ends with questions intended to test the reader's understanding of the chapter or stimulate discussion of the material. Not all the answers to the questions are easy or obvious, and some are specifically designed to challenge.

Health informatics has undergone many changes since the appearance of the second edition in 2003. New themes have emerged, and new methods and technologies have been adopted. Old ideas have fallen by the wayside. The third edition is thus significantly longer than earlier editions and contains six major new chapters. The chapters cover implementation, information system safety, social networks and social media interventions, model building for decision support, data analysis and scientific discovery, clinical bioinformatics and personalized medicine and consumer informatics. The new chapters are extensive and focus as much as possible on basic concepts and principles, rather than on simple narrative descriptions of the topics. All the old chapters have been overhauled, most of them significantly restructured, updated and extended. There are very many new sections within the updated chapters, covering diverse topics including health information exchanges, m-health, patient consent models, natural language processing and even augmented reality. Several old chapters have been deleted or merged.

It seemed a foolhardy mission for a single author to write a comprehensive text on health informatics in 1996 or even 2003. In 2014, the task took on Quixotic proportion as I debated which material should appear in an introductory text and what should be excluded. My rule of thumb was to include wherever possible basic principles and organizing structures as a priority and include only information that was likely to have a long half-life. The research base of our discipline grows rapidly, and it is very easy to create chapters that date quickly.

As always, the balance is between creating an introductory work that has some longevity and explores the core concepts needed to understand our discipline with a single and unified voice or writing an encyclopedic multi-author work that tries to do everything, but has too many voices, becomes out of date quickly and overwhelms students. At least for this edition I think we have still managed to keep the book to a 'single voice' overview – although I have had many expert colleagues help me with sourcing, writing and structuring the material and checking what has been written. I hope that the clarity of this text makes up for any limitations in its comprehensiveness.

EC
Sydney, Australia
November, 2014

Acknowledgements

I have been greatly helped, supported and influenced by many people as I wrote this book. To all of you, named and unnamed, I give my thanks.

Health informatics is now old enough as a discipline that we are beginning to lose the first great generation of informaticians. Since the last edition, Branko Cesnik, a pioneer of informatics in Australia, and Mario Stefanelli, a pioneer of artificial intelligence in medicine, have passed away and are both greatly missed by me. For those of you who are starting your careers, the next decade offers you a chance to meet and learn from many of the founding 'greats', and you should not lose that opportunity.

I have spent the last 15 years at the Centre for Health Informatics (CHI). Many of my past research staff and students are now leaders in their own right, and many are distributed across the globe. Others have stayed in Australia and still work closely with me as we investigate the edges of our discipline. You all are a daily inspiration to me and teach me far more than I teach you, I am sure. Denise Tsiros hovers over us all to make sure we are a family and never just an institution. I am also lucky to work with some outstanding senior colleagues who run sister centres to my own within the Australian Institute of Health Innovation – Jeffrey Braithwaite, Johanna Westbrook and Ken Hillman – all wise heads and supporting shoulders.

I have many wonderful international research partners, and their names appear on the many papers we all write together. Thank you for working with me. I spent several productive months on sabbatical in Harvard over 2010 and experienced the gracious hospitality of Ken Mandl at the Children's Hospital Informatics Program. Although this book was not written there, it was the necessary 'pre-contemplation' period I needed to start the project.

This book is based on a rich research tradition, and research cannot flourish without its backers. I am in particular much indebted to Shaun Larkin, without whose support the resources for many of our projects would not have been forthcoming, especially in consumer informatics.

I have a small cheer squad of people who keep me motivated, and you all pop up at different times, but just when I need you. Thank you, Terry Hannan and Louise Schaper. Thank you (again) Bill Caldicott. My cousin Dr Francesco Coiera needs a special thank you because I had to choose between finishing this book and visiting him in beautiful Italy, and the book won.

The ever-patient team at Taylor and Francis needs my thanks as they watched one deadline slip after another, but still believed in this project. I would specifically like to thank Jo Koster for being both delightful to work with and patient and understanding in adversity.

Back in 1999, Bruce Dowton, now the Vice-Chancellor of Macquarie University in Sydney, championed the creation of CHI and created the first Chair in Medical Informatics in Australia at the University of New South Wales. Without his faith and vision, I doubt we would have started or prevailed. Now, many years later, the circle has closed, and I have been gifted to again work with Bruce at Macquarie University and see where we can take this discipline over the next 10 years.

My biggest North American fans have always been my in-laws, Bob and Aline Palese. For this edition, we will deeply miss Bob's efforts to personally increase my sales by door knocking every physician he knew. Rest in peace, Bob.

As it was with the earlier editions but even more so with this one, writing has been a long and sometimes lonely marathon. I have finished only because I have been sustained by the love of my parents and, most of all, my pillars Blair and Lucca.

Contributors

I would like specifically to acknowledge and personally thank the following individuals who have each assisted me in creating this new edition:

Dr Vitali Sintchenko, from the University of Sydney, co-authored Chapters 29, 30 and 31.

Dr Farah Magrabi, from Macquarie University, co-authored Chapter 13.

Dr Annie Lau, from Macquarie University, co-authored Chapter 32.

Dr Zac Kohane, from Harvard University, provided material for the bioinformatics chapter as it appeared in the second edition, and we have retained some of this material in Chapters 30 and 31 of the current edition. The text and illustrations are drawn with permission from Kohane, Kho and Butte's *Microarrays for an Integrative Genomics*, published by MIT press.

Dr Guy Tsafnat and **Dr Blanca Gallego-Luxan** provided me with valuable material that helped in the creation of Chapter 27.

Both Farah and Vitali are dear colleagues, and they worked very closely with me in the early stages of writing this book. They helped me to think through the structure of this edition and specific details of the revisions. Their expertise, assistance and support are very much appreciated, and the book is far better for their many contributions.

Several other individuals with specialized expertise helped me by reading and providing feedback on specific chapters, including Grahame Grieve (Chapter 19), Dr Adam Dunn (Chapter 20) and Dr Guy Tsafnat (Chapter 24).

Margaret Jackson read and checked every chapter as it was finished, in the process becoming an instant health informatics expert. If there are any remaining grammatical disasters, logical inconsistencies or typographic blunders, they rest upon my shoulders.

Illustrations

Several illustrations in this book are either adapted or reproduced from other sources, and we have made our best effort to acknowledge the creators of these images appropriately as the images appear in the text. Many of these illustrations come from open access journals, which generously permit illustration reproduction as long as attribution is clear. Several illustrations appeared in the second edition with permission, and these have again been used. Figure 4.1 is taken from *BMJ* 1999; **318:**1527–1531 and appears with permission. Figure 16.1 is taken from Fox *et al.* (1996) and appears with kind permission of the copyright holder John Fox. Figures 28.6, 28.9, 28.10 and 28.11 appear with permission of W. B. Saunders Company Ltd., London. Figure 15.2 appears with permission of the World Health Organization and Figure 31.5 with permission of *Nature*.

Introduction to health informatics – the systems science of healthcare

Of what value, it may be urged, will be all the theorizing and speculation through which it would profess to guide us, when we come to practise at the bedside? Who has not heard so-called practical men say that medicine is a purely empirical science; that everything depends upon facts and correct experience; or, perhaps, that the power to cure is the main point? All arguments and theories, they say, do not enable the physician to treat his patients more correctly; in an art like medicine they rather do harm, or, at best, no positive good. It is there we are in need of experience - facts, and above all, remedies and their correct employment. All the rest is evil.

F. Oesterlen, Medical Logic, 1855, p 8

If physiology literally means 'the logic of life', and pathology is 'the logic of disease', then health informatics is the logic of healthcare. It is the study of how clinical knowledge is created, shaped, shared and applied. It is the rational study of the way we think about healthcare and the way that treatments are defined, selected and evolved. Ultimately, it is the study of how we organize ourselves, both patients and professionals, to create and run healthcare organizations. With such a pivotal role, the study of informatics is as fundamental to the practice of medicine and the delivery of healthcare in this century as anatomy or pathology was in the last.

Health informatics is thus as much about computers as cardiology is about stethoscopes (Coiera, 1995). Rather than drugs, x-ray machines or surgical instruments, the tools of informatics are more likely to be clinical guidelines, decision support systems, formal health languages, electronic records or communication systems such as social media. These tools, however, are only a means to an end, which is the delivery of the best possible healthcare.

Although the name 'health informatics' came into use only around 1973 (Protti, 1995), it is a study that is as old as healthcare itself. It was born the day that a clinician first wrote down some impressions about a patient's illness and used these to learn how to treat the next patient. Informatics has grown considerably as a clinical discipline in recent years fuelled, in part no doubt, by the advances in computer technology. What has fundamentally changed now is our ability to describe and manipulate health knowledge at a highly abstract level and to store vast quantities of raw data. We now also have access to rich communication systems to support the process of healthcare.

We can formally say that health informatics is the study of information and communication processes and systems in healthcare. Health informatics is particularly focussed on

1. Understanding the fundamental nature of these information and communication processes and describing the principles that shape them.
2. Developing interventions that can improve upon existing information and communication processes.
3. Developing methods and principles that allow such interventions to be designed.
4. Evaluating the impact of these interventions on the way individuals or organizations work or on the outcome of the work.

Specific subspecialties of health informatics include clinical informatics, which focusses on the use of information in support of patient care, and bioinformatics, which focusses on the use of genomic and other biological information.

The rise of health informatics

Perhaps the greatest change in clinical thinking over the last 2 centuries has been the ascendancy of the scientific method. Since its acceptance, it has become the lens through which we see the world, and it governs everything from the way we view disease to the way we battle it.

It is now hard to imagine just how controversial the introduction of theory and experimental method into medicine once was. Then, it was strongly opposed by empiricists, who believed that observation, rather than theoretical conjecture, was the only basis for rational practice.

With this perspective, it is almost uncanny to hear again the old empiricists' argument that 'healthcare is an art', and not a place for unnecessary speculation or formalization. This time, the empiricists are fighting against those who wish to develop formal theoretical methods to regulate the communal practice of healthcare. Words such as quality and safety, clinical audit, clinical guidelines, indicators, outcome measures, healthcare rationing and evidence-based practice now define the new intellectual battleground.

While the advance of science pushes clinical knowledge down to a fine-grained molecular and genetic level, it is events at the other end of the scale that are forcing us to change the most. First, the enterprise of healthcare has become so large that it now consumes more national resource than any country is willing to bear. Despite sometimes heroic efforts to control this growth in resource consumption, healthcare budgets continue to expand. There is thus a social and economic imperative to transform healthcare and minimize its drain on social resources.

The structure of clinical practice is also coming under pressure from within. The scientific method, long the backbone of medicine, is now in some ways under threat. The reason for this is not that experimental science is unable to answer our questions about the nature of disease and its treatment. Rather, it is almost too good at its job. As clinical research ploughs ahead in laboratories and clinics across the world, like some great information-generating machine, health practitioners are being swamped by its results. So much research is now published each week that it can literally take decades for the results of clinical trials to translate into changes in clinical practice.

So, healthcare workers find themselves practising with ever-restricting resources and unable, even if they had the time, to keep abreast of the knowledge of best practice hidden in the literature. As a consequence, the scientific basis of clinical practice trails far behind that of clinical research. Consumers struggle even more and have to contend with conflicting messages and information they find online, such as in social media.

Two hundred years ago, enlightened physicians understood that empiricism needed to be replaced by a more formal and testable way of characterizing disease and its treatment. The tool they used then was the scientific method. Today we are in analogous situation. Now the demand is that we replace the organizational processes and structures that force the arbitrary selection among treatments with ones that can be formalized, tested and applied rationally.

Modern healthcare has also moved away from seeing disease in isolation to understanding that illness occurs at a complex system level. Infection is not simply the result of the invasion of a pathogenic organism, but the complex interaction of an individual's immune system, bacterial flora, nutritional status and our social, environmental and genetic endowments. By seeing things at a system level, we come ever closer to understanding what it really means to be diseased, and how that state can be reversed.

We now need to make the same conceptual leap and begin to see the great systems of knowledge that enmesh the delivery of healthcare. These systems produce our knowledge, tools, languages and methods. Thus, a new treatment is never created and tested in intellectual isolation. It gains significance as part of a greater system of knowledge because it occurs in the context of previous treatments and insights, as well as the context of a society's resources and needs. Further, our work does not finish when we scientifically prove that a treatment works. We must try to disseminate this new knowledge and help others to understand, apply and adapt it.

These then are the challenges for healthcare. Can we put together rational structures for the way clinical evidence is pooled, communicated and applied to routine care? Can we develop organizational processes and structures that minimize the resources we use and the harms we create and maximize the benefits delivered? And finally, what tools and methods need to be developed to help achieve these aims in a manner that is practicable, testable and in keeping with the fundamental goal of healthcare – the relief from disease? The role of health informatics is to develop a systems science for healthcare that provides a rational basis to answer these questions, as well as to create the tools to achieve these goals.

The scope of informatics is thus enormous. It finds application in the design of clinical decision support systems for practitioners, consumer decision aids and online health services, in the development of computer tools for research and in the study of the very essence of healthcare – its corpus of knowledge. Yet the modern discipline of health informatics is still relatively young. Many other groups within healthcare are also addressing the issues raised here and not always in a co-ordinated fashion. Indeed, these groups are not always even aware that their efforts are connected or that their concerns are also concerns of informatics.

The science of what works

I want to let you in on a secret. There are really only three questions that matter in informatics. At the beginning of any new informatics endeavor, you just need to ask:

1. *What is the problem that we are trying to solve?*
2. *How will we know when we have succeeded?*
3. *Is technology the best solution, or are there simpler alternatives?*

If you make sure these questions are asked, then you will be thought of as wise indeed. If you know enough to answer them, you could be held up as an informatics guru.

Reading this at the very beginning of your informatics journey, you may be surprised by the triviality of these questions. Re-reading them at the end of your journey through this book, you may now understand why little else matters and may also understand how rare it is for these questions to be asked in the real world – and what the almost inevitable consequences of not asking them are.

With this framing, we need to understand three things about any informatics intervention – its *possibility,* its *practicability* and its *desirability.* Possibility reflects the science of informatics – what in theory can be achieved? Practicability addresses the potential for successfully engineering a system or introducing a new process – what can actually be done given the constraints of the real world? Desirability looks at the fundamental motivation for using a given process or technology.

These criteria are suggested because we need to evolve a framework to judge the claims made for new technologies and those who seek to profit from them. Just as there is a long-standing, sometimes uneasy, symbiosis between the pharmaceutical industry and medicine, there is a newer and consequently less examined relationship between healthcare and the computing and telecommunication industries. Clinicians should judge the claims of these newcomers in the same cautious way that they examine claims about a new drug and perhaps more so, given that clinicians are far more knowledgeable about pharmacology than they are about informatics and telecommunications.

Overview of the book

The first goal of this book is to present a unifying set of basic informatics principles that influence everything from the delivery of care to an individual patient through to the design of whole healthcare systems. The book is organized into a number of parts that revolve around the two distinct but interwoven strands of information and communication systems. Although the unique character of each strand is explored individually, there is also an emphasis on understanding the rich way in which they can interact and complement each other.

Part 1 – Basic concepts in informatics

This first part of the book offers an intuitive understanding of the basic theoretical concepts needed to understand informatics – the notions of what constitutes a model, what one means by information, and what defines a system. Each concept is used to develop an understanding of the basic nature of information and communication systems. A recurring theme of the book, first articulated here, is the need to understand the limitations imposed upon us whenever we create a model of the world or use it to design a technology. Understanding these limitations defines the ultimate limits of possibility for informatics, irrespective of whichever technology one may wish to apply in its service.

Part 2 – Informatics skills

Building upon the concepts in Part 1, the second part of the book looks at the practical lessons that can be drawn from informatics to guide everyday clinical activity. Every clinical action, every treatment choice and investigation, is shaped by the available information and how effectively that information is communicated. Five basic clinical informatics skills are explored, each with its own individual chapter:

1. *Communicating* effectively is based upon understanding cognitive models of information processing and is constantly challenged by the limits of human attention and the imperfection of models.
2. *Structuring information,* with a particular focus on the patient record, is shown to be dependent upon the task at hand, the channel used to communicate the message and the agent who will receive the message.
3. *Questioning* others to find information is essential in clinical practice to fill the ever present gaps in every individual's knowledge.
4. *Searching for knowledge* describes the broader strategic process of knowing where to ask questions, evaluating answers and refining questions in the light of previous actions, and it occurs in many different settings, from when patients are interviewed and examined through to when treatment options are canvassed.
5. *Making decisions* requires a clear problem formulation, followed by the assembly of the best scientific evidence, and an unbiased analysis that incorporates the wishes and needs of individuals.

Part 3 – Information systems in healthcare

The chapters in this part provide the technical core upon which all other parts depend. We introduce clinical information systems and their role in supporting the model, measure and manage cycle. Second, it is shown that it is not always necessary to formalize this cycle completely, especially when flexibility in decision-making is needed. Consequently, many information processes are left in an unstructured or informal state and are more likely to be supported by communication processes.

The electronic health record is introduced next and is the first major technical system discussed in the book. The benefits and limitations of existing paper-based systems are compared with their electronic counterparts. Because the electronic patient record feeds so many different clinical systems, later topics including decision support, protocol-based care, population surveillance and clinical audit are all also introduced here.

The next two chapters cover the foundational informatics topics of how to design, evaluate and then implement working technological systems into complex sociotechnical organizations. It is often a conundrum that well-designed systems do not deliver the benefits expected. The evaluation chapter introduces the concept of the *value of information* and uses it to explain the value chain that starts with information creation and extends to ultimate benefit from its use. Understanding where a system is meant to deliver value along this chain becomes a recurrent motif in later chapters. This theme is expanded in the chapter on implementation, which looks at system implementation as a process of fitting technologies into complex adaptive organizations. The unexpected outcomes of technology sometimes can be explained only by stepping back and taking such a wider system view.

System safety is deeply linked to design and implementation decisions, and the potential downsides of information and communication technologies are explored next, given how closely related the concepts are in these chapters. The final chapter in this section takes another systemic perspective on clinical systems and the value of information, this time coming from economics. Although evaluation methods tell us much about the value of information, economics brings its own equally valid insights.

Having completed this part, one should be able to move on to any of the other parts in any order because each explores a more specialized topic area.

Part 4 – Guideline- and protocol-based systems

In this part, the various forms and uses of clinical guidelines, care plans and protocols are introduced. The different roles that computer-based protocol systems can play in clinical practice are outlined in the second chapter. These cover both traditional 'passive' support where protocols are kept as a reference and active systems in which the computer uses the protocol to assist in the delivery of care. For example, protocols incorporated into the electronic record can generate clinical alerts or make treatment recommendations. The growing evidence base for the benefit of such technologies is also summarized, emphasizing that benefits are more likely to be easily demonstrated in process rather than clinical outcome improvements. The third chapter reviews the process of protocol creation, dissemination and application and explores how informatics can create tools to assist at each of these stages.

Part 5 – Communication systems in healthcare

Although interpersonal communication skills are fundamental to patient care, the process of communication has, for a long time, not been well supported technologically. Now, with the widespread availability of communication systems supporting mobility, voice mail, electronic mail and social media, new possibilities arise. The chapters in this section introduce the basic types of communication services and explain the different benefits of each.

The second chapter in this part is probably the most technical of the book, covering information and communication networks and healthcare-specific networks such as health information exchanges. It is the place in this text where interoperability standards are covered in detail, as well as topics that relate to how information is accessed across networks, including privacy and consent.

Social media comprise a different class of communication system, and their importance is underlined with a discrete chapter devoted to them. The chapter introduces basic concepts from social networking theory and the social determination of health and then explores how social media are being harnessed across the spectrum of healthcare services.

The final chapter in this part examines clinical communication from the perspective of telemedicine and m-health technologies. The potential of such systems for different areas of healthcare is described, along with the accumulating evidence base for their success, again using the value chain as one way of understanding sometimes unexpected negative results.

Part 6 – Language, coding and classification

If the data contained in electronic patient record systems are to be analyzed, then they need to be accessible in some regular way. This is usually thwarted by the variations in health terminology used by different individuals, institutions and nations. To remedy the problem, large dictionaries of standardized clinical terms have been created.

The chapters in this part introduce the basic ideas of clinical concepts, terms, codes and classifications and demonstrate their various uses. The inherent advantages and limitations of using different terms and codes are discussed in the second chapter. The last chapter looks at some more advanced issues in coding and describes the theoretical limitations to coding. It introduces natural language processing and text mining methods and explains how the statistical approach to language management is complementary, and sometimes preferred, to the more formal semantic approaches used in clinical terminologies and ontologies.

Part 7 – Clinical decision support and analytics

Clinical decision support systems (CDSSs) are historically among the most powerful classes of informatics intervention we have at our disposal. These computer programs range from systems that simply present data to help a human make a decision to those that generate prompts or alerts when a clinician's decision appears problematic, through to systems with the capability of making decisions entirely on their own. In the first chapter, the focus is on the different applications for CDSSs, particularly to see where clear successes can be identified. The next chapter takes a more technological focus and looks at the computational reasoning processes that underpin CDSSs. The final chapter in this part looks at how CDSS knowledge is created, through machine learning, data analytic and computational discovery methods.

Part 8 – Specialized applications for health informatics

The final chapters in this book explore some of the specialized ways that decision technologies are applied in clinical practice. These technologies find application in creating intelligent patient monitors or autonomous therapeutic devices such as self-adjusting patient ventilators. Along with communication technologies, CDSSs are essential components of public health and biosurveillance systems. In the field of bioinformatics, human genomic and metabolic knowledge is harnessed using computer techniques and reframes many classes of clinical decision as questions of genetics. When such bioinformatics knowledge is used in clinical practice, it is often described as personalized or precision medicine, and this topic is covered in its own chapter. The book concludes, not on a minor topic, but on one of the most transformational ones both for informatics and for healthcare delivery – the rise of consumer ownership and involvement in the process of care and the role that informatics has to play in making this necessity a reality.

References

Coiera, E. (1995). Medical informatics. *BMJ* **310**(6991): 1381.
Protti, D. (1995). The synergism of health/medical informatics revisited. *Methods of Information in Medicine* **34**(5): 441–445.

PART 1

Basic concepts in informatics

CHAPTER 1

Models

> A message to mapmakers: highways are not painted red, rivers don't have county lines running down the middle, and you don't see contour lines on a mountain.
>
> *Kent, 1978*
>
> Man tries to make for himself in the way that suits him best a simplified and intelligible picture of the world and thus to overcome the world of experience, for which he tries to some extent to substitute this cosmos of his. This is what the painter, the poet, the speculative philosopher and the natural scientist do, each in his own fashion … one might suppose that there were any number of possible systems … all with an equal amount to be said for them; and this opinion is no doubt correct, theoretically. But evolution has shown that at any given moment out of all conceivable constructions one has always proved itself absolutely superior to all the rest.
>
> *Einstein, 1935*

The study of human health is based upon a few foundational concepts such as the cell or the notion of disease. Informatics is similarly built upon the basic concepts of data, models, systems and information. Unlike the study of health, in which core ideas are usually grounded in observations of the physical world, these informatics concepts are abstract ideas. For those used to the study of healthcare, informatics concepts often seem detached from the physical realities of the clinical workplace.

This issue is further complicated because we use the same words that describe informatics concepts in everyday language. It is common to ask for more information about a patient, or to question what data support a particular conclusion. In informatics these intuitive ideas need to be more precisely defined.

In this first chapter, we begin our study of informatics by exploring the pivotal concept of a *model*. Whether diagnosing a patient's illness, writing into a patient's record, designing an information system or trying to create a more efficient health service, we use models to shape and direct our actions. Models define the way we learn about the world, interpret what we see and apply our knowledge to effect change, whether that is through our own actions or through the use of technology such as a computer.

A map is not the territory it represents, but, if correct, it has a similar structure to the territory, which accounts for its usefulness.… If we reflect upon our languages, we find that at best they must be considered only as maps. A word is not the object it represents … the disregard of these complexities is tragically disastrous in daily life and science (Korzybski, 1948).

Box 1.1
Therac-25

Between June 1985 and January 1987, Therac-25 linear accelerators operating in the United States and Canada famously delivered massive radiation overdoses to at least six patients, causing death or serious radiation injury. Patients received doses of up to 20 000 rads where a dose of 200 rads was a typical therapeutic dose, and a 500-rad whole-body dose will cause death in 50 per cent of cases. At the time, these overdoses were arguably the worst radiation incidents in the history of radiotherapy.

Medical linear accelerators operate by creating a high-energy electron beam. The beam is focussed onto a patient to destroy tumour tissue and leaves healthy tissue outside the beam focus relatively unaffected. The high-energy beam produced by these devices is focussed by a collimator, usually made of tungsten. This 'flattens' the beam to therapeutic levels and acts like a lens to focus the beam to a tissue depth appropriate for a given patient.

In the Therac-25 accidents, the tungsten shield was not in place when the radiation dose was delivered. As a result, patients received a full dose of the raw 25-MeV electron beam. There were a number of different causes of the various overdoses, but each overdose essentially resulted from modelling errors in the system's software and hardware (Leveson and Turner, 1993).

One critical error resulted from the reuse of some software from a previous machine, the Therac-20. This software worked acceptably in the Therac-20, but when reused in the Therac-25, it permitted an overdose to be given. This was because although the Therac-20 had a physical backup safety system, this had been removed in the design of the Therac-25. The Therac-20 software was thus reused in the Therac-25 on the assumption that the change in machines would not affect the way the software operated. Therefore, software modelled to one machine's environment was used in a second context in which that model was not valid.

Another problem lay in the measurement system that reported the radiation dose given to patients. The system was designed to work with doses in the therapeutic range, but when exposed to full beam strength, it became saturated and gave a low reading. As a result, several patients were overdosed repeatedly because technicians believed the machine was delivering low doses. Thus, the measurement system was built upon an assumption that it would never have to detect high radiation levels.

All these failures occurred because of the poor way models were used by the designers of the Therac-25. They did not understand that many of the assumptions that were left implicit in the specifications of the device would quickly become invalid in slightly changed circumstances and would lead to catastrophic failure.

The motto for this chapter is 'A map is not the territory'. Humans are naturally adept at developing mental models of the world and manage to use them robustly, despite the inherent weaknesses of the models themselves. When these flexible mental models are transferred into a fixed technological system such as a computer, the effects of modelling error can be amplified significantly, with sometimes disastrous consequences (Box 1.1). This is because much of the knowledge used in creating the model has not been transferred along with it. As a consequence, the technological system is unable to define the limits of its knowledge. The 'map' in the computer is not the same as the territory of the workplace in which it is placed. One of the major ideas to be explored in this chapter is that the implicit and explicit assumptions we make at the time a model is created ultimately define the limits of a model's usefulness.

1.1 Models are abstractions of the real world

What then is a model? People are familiar with the idea of building model aeroplanes or looking at a small-scale model of a building to imagine what it will look like when completed. In health, models underlie all our clinical activities. For example, whenever we interact with patients, we use internalized models of disease to guide the process of diagnosis and treatment.

Models actually serve two quite distinct purposes. The first use of a model is as a copy of the world. The modelling process takes some aspect of the world and creates a description of it. Imagine a camera taking a photograph. The image captured upon the camera's film is a model of the world:

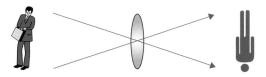

We can generalize from the way a camera records a physical object to the way that all models are created. The process of creating a model of the real world is called *abstraction*:

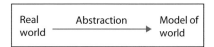

The effects of abstraction are directly analogous to the effects of using a camera. In particular, the image captured by camera has four important features characteristic of all models.

- First, an image is simpler than the real thing. There are always more features in the real world than can be captured in an image. One could, for example, always use a more powerful lens to capture finer detail. Similarly, models are always less detailed than the real world from which they are drawn. A city map will thus not contain every feature of the streets it describes. Because models are always less detailed than the things they describe, data are lost in the abstraction process.
- Second, an image is a caricature or distortion of the real world. The three dimensions of the photographed object are typically transformed into a two-dimensional image. Through the use of different filters or lenses, very different pictures of the observed world are obtained. None of them is the 'true' image of the object. Indeed, there is no such thing. The camera just records a particular point of view. Similarly, abstraction imposes a point of view upon the real world, and the resulting model is inevitably distorted in some way. Thus, a map looks very little like the terrain it models. Some land features are emphasized, and others are de-emphasized or ignored. In physiology, one view of the heart is as a mechanical pump. This model emphasizes one particular aspect of the organ, but it is clearly much more than this. It also has a complex set of functions to do with the regulation of blood pressure, blood volume and organ perfusion.
- Third, as a consequence of distortion and data loss, many possible images can be created of the same object. Different images emphasize different aspects of the object or show different levels of detail. Similarly, because we can model a variety of aspects of any physical object, in variable detail, many models can be created. Indeed, the number of possible models is infinite. As we all carry different 'lenses' when we see the world, it is no surprise that different people see the world so differently. Some psychiatrists, for

Abstraction: the process of identifying a few elements of a physical object and then using these to create a model of the object. The model is then used as a proxy representation of the physical object.

example, may consider the brain from a Freudian or Jungian perspective. Neurologists may model it as a collection of neurones, each with different functions. Psychologists may model the function of a brain on that of a computer. When a clinician meets a patient, do they see a person, an interruption, a client, a task, a disease, a problem, a friend or a billing opportunity?

- Finally, a camera records a particular moment in time. As the real world objects in an image change with time, their image is frozen at the moment the picture was taken. The difference between you and your photograph increases as you get older. The similarity between any model and the physical objects it represents also degrades with time. A map of a city becomes increasingly inaccurate as time passes because of changes to the city's roads and buildings. Computer programs that 'map' particular work processes slowly become less useful and need to be upgraded as work practices change around them.

As a consequence of these four characteristics of models, a final and central idea now becomes evident. All models are built for a reason. When we create a model, we actively choose among the many possible models that could be created, to try to build the one that best suits our particular purposes. For example, a driver's map emphasizes streets and highways. A hiker's map emphasizes terrain and altitude. Thus, one actively excludes or distorts aspects of the world to satisfy a particular purpose. There is no such thing as a truly 'general purpose' model. This last point is crucial to much of what follows in later chapters because it explains much about the challenges faced when trying to build computer systems that must model real world practices.

So just as a camera cannot capture a 'true' image of an object, one cannot ever build a 'true' model of an object. In philosophy, the argument against models ever being inherently correct is equivalent to arguing against the Platonic ideal. This is the idea that pure forms of physical objects exist outside the realms of the physical world. Although a physical sphere may always have an imperfection, Plato believed there existed an 'ideal' mathematical spherical form. The counterargument is that there is no such thing as ideal or objective truth in the world. There can only ever be our subjective and local point of view, shaped by the input of our senses.

Even in 'pure' geometry, there is no ideal sphere, just an infinite family of possible shapes that vary depending on the rules of the geometric system you choose. We cannot say that only one of these geometries is correct. Rather, they are different explanations of space, based upon different assumptions. We use the one that gives the most satisfactory explanation of the phenomenon we are interested in. For example, Riemann geometry works best for Einstein's relativity theory, rather than classic Euclidean geometry, because it handles the notion of curved space (Figure 1.1).

This philosophical argument continues into the debate about the basis of scientific enquiry and the nature of experimental evidence. A scientific hypothesis is nothing more than a model of some aspect of the world that is to be tested by an experiment. However, if a model can never be correct and objective truth can never be known, then our experiments can never actually *prove* anything to be true. We are never sure that we are right. The best that experiments can do is show us when our models of the world are wrong (Popper, 1976). What remain are theories that have best survived the tests set of them and are in some way more useful than others in interacting with the world.

Karl Popper would ask his students to 'observe and describe'. They would be puzzled, and eventually ask 'observe what?' That was his point. We always have to observe something in order to describe something. The notion of pure observation, independent of direction, is a myth (Skolimowski, 1977).

And though the truth will not be discovered by such means – never can that stage be reached – yet they throw light on some of the profounder ramifications of falsehood (Kafka, 1931).

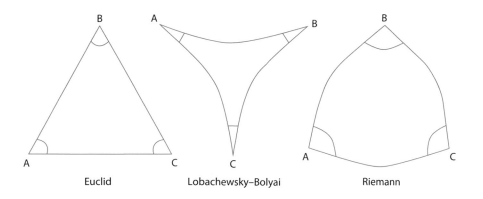

Euclid   Lobachewsky–Bolyai   Riemann

Figure 1.1
There is no 'correct' geometric shape, just an infinite number of possible geometries. The angles in classic Euclidian triangles always add up to 180°, but in Riemann geometry they always add to greater than 180°, and with Lobachewsky-Bolyai always less than 180°.

1.2 Models can be used as templates

So far, we have considered models as copies of the world. There is a second way in which we use models. Some models, rather than being copies of existing things, are used as templates from which new things will be created or that show how things are to be done. An architect creates a set of drawings that will be translated into a building. Economists build mathematical models of a country's economy and then use these to predict the effects of changes in monetary policy. A clinical protocol provides a template for the way a patient is to be managed.

Again, a simple example will make this second use of models clearer. Consider what happens when an image is projected onto a screen:

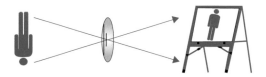

The stored image is a model of the real world. The projection process uses this model to create a second, slightly altered, display image. We can generalize from this to understand how models can act as templates. The process begins with the creation of a model. This could be a design, perhaps recorded as a set of blueprints or specifications. This is followed by a process of construction or model *instantiation*. A projected image is thus an instance of a stored image. In mathematics and logic, we instantiate the variables in an equation with data values. The equation is a template, and it interacts with supplied data values to arrive at a result. Instantiation uses a model as a template to build an artefact or process that is an instance of the model in the physical world:

Instantiation: the process of building an example or instance of a model, using the model as a template to guide the process.

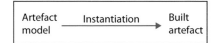

Many of the consequences of the instantiation process are similar to those of abstraction:

- Although abstraction loses data to create a model, the process of instantiation adds data to create an instance. The image you see from a projector varies depending upon whether it is projected on a white screen, a wall or the side of a building. The physical surface adds in its own features to shape the final result. The image is the result of the interaction of the projected image and the physical surface it strikes. This explains why implementing the same process in two different organizations yields different results. The local features of each organization uniquely shapes the way the process eventually works. Thus, an artefact is always more complex than the model that it came from because it is situated in the physical world.

- The constructed artefact is a distortion of the original template because the process of instantiation can transform it in many ways. A projected image can be shaped by the use of different filters and lenses to produce a variety of images.
- No two projected images are ever exactly the same because of variations introduced by the physical process of construction. No two physical artefacts are similar even if they are instances of the same template. Even mass-produced objects such as light bulbs, syringes or clay pots have minor imperfections introduced during manufacture that distinguish one instance of an object from another. In contrast, in digital or 'virtual' worlds, we can typically guarantee that the conditions for creating instance copies are identical.
- The effect of the captured image changes with the passage of time as the physical world changes. A movie usually has a greater impact on release than many years afterward as audiences change. A treatment guideline becomes increasingly inappropriate as time passes and new knowledge indicates that other methods are better treatment options.

Thus, the process of creating an instance has a variable outcome, and the impact of any instance of a model in the real world also varies. Two examples will help reinforce these ideas. Despite having identical DNA, two individual biological organisms are never truly identical. If DNA is a model (see Box 2.1), then the process of DNA transcription results in the 'manufacture' of an instance of an individual organism. Even if we take identical DNA as the starting point, local variations in the process of protein manufacture will introduce minor changes that at some level distinguish the clones.

Similarly, although two patients may be treated according to the same guideline, which is a template for treatment, no two actual episodes of treatment are ever exactly the same. Variations in the timing of treatments, availability of resources and the occurrence of other events all can conspire to change the way a treatment is given. Equally, a patient's physical and genetic variations may result in variations to the results of a treatment. The features of the specific situation in which a treatment is given thus result in variations in the way the treatment proceeds and in its final effects upon a patient.

A more general principle follows from these four characteristics of templates. Because the process of creating an instance from a template has a variable result, and the process of doing things in the real world is uncertain because we can never know all the variations that are 'added in' as we follow a template, there is no such thing as a general purpose template. All we can have are templates or designs that are better or worse suited to our particular circumstances and are better or worse at meeting the needs of the task at hand.

As we will see in later chapters, this means that there can be no 'correct' way to treat an illness, no 'right' way to describe a diagnosis and no 'right' way to build an information or communication system. There can never be an absolutely 'correct' design for a treatment protocol or a 'pure' set of terms to describe activities in healthcare. This principle explains why clinical protocols will always have varying effectiveness based upon local conditions and why medical languages can never be truly general purpose. What we do have are treatments, protocols, languages, information and communication systems that are better or worse suited to our specific purpose than others at a moment in time.

1.3 The way we model the world influences the way we affect the world

So far we have seen how models act either as copies of things in the world or as templates upon which new things are created. These two processes are deeply interrelated.

In photography, decisions about form and content at the moment an image is created ultimately influence the way it can be used and how useful it will be. Thus, if a picture is intended to be of print quality, it may require a higher-definition image to be taken than one intended for display on a computer screen.

When artefacts are created, it is assumed that they will be used for a particular purpose. If the purpose changes, then a design becomes less effective. Thus, the physical design of the waiting room and treatment areas for a general practice clinic will assume that a certain number of patients are seen during a day and that certain kinds of therapy will be given. If the clinic was bought by radiologists, they would have to remodel the clinic's design to incorporate imaging equipment and to reflect a different throughput of patients.

If a disease is based upon assumptions about the incidence of a disease in a given population, then it may not work well in a different setting. Treating infant diarrhoea in a developed nation is not the same task as in underdeveloped nations, where poorer resources, malnutrition and different infecting organisms change the context of treatment. Before a model is used, one therefore has to be clear about what has been assumed.

Similarly, a set of rules and procedures may be developed in one hospital and may be spectacularly successful at improving the way the hospital functions. One would have to be very cautious before imposing those procedures on other hospitals, given that they implicitly model many aspects of the original institution. Very small differences in the level of resources, type of patients seen or experience of the staff may make what was successful in one context unhelpful in another.

More generally, any designed artefact, whether it is a car, a drug or a computer system, has to be designed with the world within which it will operate in mind. In other words, it has to contain in its design a model of the environment within which it will be used. These specifications constitute its *design assumptions*. Thus, there are direct connections among the process of model creation, the construction of artefacts based upon such models and their eventual effectiveness in satisfying some purpose (see Figure 1.2).

A few examples should make the cycle of model abstraction and instantiation clearer. First, consider a car. The design blueprints of a car reflect both its purpose and the environment within which it will operate. The car's engine is built based upon the not unreasonable assumption that it will operate in an atmosphere with oxygen. The wheels and suspension

Before the work of the famous physician Galen, it was assumed that the arteries contained air. This was because arteries were observed to be empty after death (Schafer and Thane, 1891). The physicians making these observations had thought they had created a model of arterial function in living humans, but all they had created was a model valid in cadavers. Therefore, the context in which a model is created affects its validity for any other context within which it may be used.

There are no side effects – only effects. Those we thought of in advance, the ones we like, we call the main, or intended, effects, and take credit for them. The ones we did not anticipate, the ones that came around and bit us in the rear – those are the 'side effects' (Sterman, 2002).

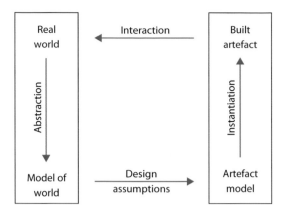

Figure 1.2
Models of the world
are used as a
template to define
how artefacts such
as devices or
processes will be
constructed.

may be designed with the assumption that they will operate on a highway or urban street. If the car was put into another physical environment such as a desert or the lunar surface, it probably would not work very well. Sometimes such design assumptions are left implicit, and they become obvious only when a device is used in a way in which it was not intended, sometimes with catastrophic results (see Box 1.1).

The human body also makes assumptions about its environment. The haemopoietic system adjusts the number of red blood cells needed for normal function based upon the available oxygen in the atmosphere. As a consequence, individuals living at sea level have calibrated their oxygen carrying system differently from those living in high altitudes. An athlete training at sea level will not perform well if moved quickly to a high altitude because these 'working assumptions' are no longer met.

Finally, consider an artificial heart (Figure 1.3). Such a device must model the biological heart in some way because it will replace that organ within the cardiovascular system. The artificial heart thus is based upon a model of the heart as a mechanical pump and is designed with the assumption that supporting the pump mechanisms will be beneficial. The better it models all the functions of a true heart, the better a replacement it will be. It is also designed on the assumption that it will need to be implanted, and as a consequence it is crafted to survive the corrosive nature of that environment and to minimize any immune reaction that could be mounted against it.

Figure 1.3
An artificial heart is
based upon two
kinds of model. First,
the cardiovascular
system has to be
modelled, and
second, a
mechanical blueprint
is used to model the
way the artificial
heart will be
constructed.

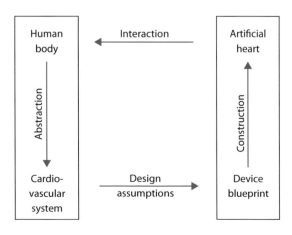

Conclusions

In this chapter, the foundational concept of a model is explored in some detail. Models underpin the way we understand the world we live in, and as a consequence they guide the way we interact with the world. We should never forget that the map is not the territory and the blueprint is not the building.

In the next chapter, a second basic concept of information is introduced. These two ideas are then brought together, as we begin to see that knowledge is a special kind of model and is subject to the same principles and limitations that are associated with all other models.

Discussion points

1. 'The map is not the territory'. Why not?

2. Observe and describe. Compare. Why?

3. Biologists have argued whether nature, expressed in an organism's DNA, or 'nurture', via the physical world, is most important in shaping development. If 'nature' is the template and 'nurture' creates instances of an organism, which is more important in shaping an organism based upon the first principles of modelling?

4. In what ways could the limitations of models result in errors in the diagnosis or treatment of patients? Use Figure 1.2 as a template to guide your thinking, if it helps.

Chapter summary

1. Models are the basis of the way we learn about, and interact with, the physical world.

2. Models can act either as copies of the world like maps or as templates that serve as the blueprints for constructing physical objects or processes.

3. Models that copy the world are abstractions of the real world.

   a. Models are always less detailed than the real world from which they are drawn.

   b. Models ignore aspects of the world that are not considered essential. Thus abstraction imposes a point of view upon the observed world.

   c. Many models can be created of any given physical object, depending upon the level of detail and point of view selected.

   d. The similarity between models and the physical objects they represent degrades over time.

   e. There is no such thing as a truly general purpose model. There is no such thing as the most 'correct' model. Models are simply better or worse suited to accomplishing a particular task.

4. Models can be used as templates and be instantiated to create objects or processes that are used in the world.

   a. Templates are less detailed than the artefacts that are created from them.

   b. An artefact is a distortion of the original template.

c. No two physical artefacts are similar even if they are instances of the same template.

d. The effect of an artefact may change while the original template stays the same.

e. The process of creating an instance has a variable outcome, and the impact of the instance of an artefact in the real world also varies. As a consequence, there is no such thing as a general purpose template. All we can have are templates or designs that are better or worse suited to our particular circumstances and tasks.

5. The assumptions used in a model's creation, whether implicit or explicit, define the limits of a model's usefulness.

a. When models are created, they assume that they are to accomplish a particular purpose.

b. When models are created, they assume a context of use. When objects or processes are built from a model, this context forms a set of design assumptions.

6. We should never forget that the map is not the territory and the blueprint is not the building.

CHAPTER 2

Information

The plural of datum is not information.

Anon

To act in the world we need to make decisions, and to make decisions we must have information that distinguishes one course of action over another. In this chapter, a basic framework is presented that defines what is meant by such information. Whether delivered in conversation, captured in a set of hand-written notes or stored in the memory of a computer, the same basic principles govern the way all information is structured or used. The ideas presented here build upon the concept of models developed in Chapter 1. The simple ways that models, data and information interrelate are then unfolded. It then becomes apparent that models and information underpin not just the specialized study of informatics, but also every aspect of the delivery of healthcare.

2.1 Information is inferred from data and knowledge

Informally we know that we have received information when what we know has changed. In some sense this new information must be measurable because intuitively some sources of information are better than others. One newspaper may generally be more informative than others. A patient's medical record may be full of new data, but to the clinician who sees the patient every day it may contain little new information.

Formally, information can indeed be linked to concepts of *orderliness* and *novelty*. The more order in a document, the more 'information' it contains. For example, a patient's record that is broken up into different sections such as past history and allergies is more informative than an unstructured narrative that jumbles the patient's details. Equally, if a patient's record contains nothing new, then it conveys no new information. Statistical measures for the amount of such 'information' communicated by a source are the basis of *information theory* (see Box 4.1). However, these statistical measures of information can only partly help us to understand the computational meaning of information, which underpins informatics.

Terms such as data, information and knowledge are often used interchangeably in common speech. Each of these terms has a quite precise and distinct definition in the information sciences.

Data consist of facts. Facts are observations or measurements about the world. For example, 'today is Tuesday', the 'blood pressure is 125/70 mm Hg' or 'this drug is penicillin'.

Knowledge defines relationships between data. The statement 'penicillin is an antibiotic' relates two data elements. The rules 'tobacco smoking causes lung cancer' and 'if a patient's blood pressure is greater than 135/95 mm Hg on three separate occasions, then the patient has high blood pressure' are more complex examples of knowledge. Knowledge is created by identifying recurring patterns in data, for example across many different patients. We learn that events occur in a certain sequence or that an action typically has a specific effect. Through the process of model abstraction, these observations are codified into general rules about how the world is and works.

> Information is constructed by people in a process of perception; it is not selected, noticed, detected, chosen or filtered from a set of given, static, pre-existing things. Each perception is a new generalization, a new construction (Clancey in Steels and Brooks, 1995).

As well as learning generalized 'truths' about the world, knowledge can be specific to a particular circumstance. For example, *patient-specific knowledge* comes from observing a patient's state over time. By abstracting observed patterns, one can arrive at specific knowledge such as 'following treatment with antihypertensive medication, there has been no decrease in the patient's blood pressure over the last 2 months'.

Information is the meaning obtained by the application of knowledge to data. Thus, the datum that 'blood pressure is 125/70 mm Hg' provides information only if it tells us something new. In the context of managing a patient's high blood pressure, by using general knowledge of medicine and patient-specific knowledge, the datum may lead to the inference that the patient's previously high blood pressure is now under control, which is indeed new information.

We can now see how these three concepts are related. By using a piece of knowledge, in a given context, data are interpreted to produce information. The data stored in DNA are interpreted by cellular molecules to create proteins (Box 2.1). Another example may make this even clearer. Imagine someone is speaking to you in a language that you do not

Box 2.1
DNA is just data

Conceptualizing an information system into model, data and interpretation components has a certain universality. In biology, there is a strong information paradigm arising out of our understanding of the role of DNA.

Since its structure and function began to be unfolded, DNA has been seen as some form of master molecule, dictating the development of individual organisms. The doctrine of DNA has perhaps reached its most extreme position in the notion of the selfish gene (Dawkins, 1982). DNA is characterized as clothing itself in cells, which allow DNA to survive and reproduce from generation to generation. DNA, in this view, creates and dictates the development and activity of organisms. The organism is merely the survival machine used by the genetic sequence.

Another view sees DNA as part of a far more complex system. DNA is among the most non-reactive and chemically inert molecules in biology. It thus is perfectly designed for its role, which is to store instructions, much like the memory in a computer. DNA is a kind of database and nothing more.

Thus, although DNA stores the models used to create proteins, it is of itself incapable of making or doing anything. That is the role of the cellular machinery (see Box 30.2). Whereas it is often said that DNA produces proteins, in fact proteins produce DNA (Lewontin, 1993).

The symbolic language of DNA and thus the ability to interpret DNA reside in the surrounding cellular structures. Without these molecules, there would be no way that we could decode the symbolic meaning of DNA – the data stored in the DNA would be uninterpretable. In other words, an organism's DNA has no meaning outside the context of the cellular structures that contain it.

We can thus regard a complex organism as being the result of a cell's interpretation of the data stored in the DNA database, by using a language encoded within its proteins and within the context of the data provided by the intra-cellular and extra-cellular environment.

understand. You have received a large amount of data during that conversation, but because you have no knowledge of the language, it is meaningless to you. You cannot say that you have received any information. For the same reason, when two people with different life experiences and knowledge read the same book, they can come up with very different interpretations of its meaning.

2.2 Models are built from symbols

Knowledge is the set of models we use to understand and interact with the world. Sometimes these models are stored as physical analogues of the real thing. A scale model of a township may display planned developments alongside existing structures. The pattern that iron filings make on a piece of paper models the magnetic field created when a magnet is placed underneath. Knowledge is also stored in the heads of people. With the development of language and writing, it became possible for these models to be shared and to evolve from being purely mental constructions to something we can examine and manipulate in the physical world.

A weather map, for example, describes processes that look nothing like its diagrammatic representation. In the realms of science and mathematics, it is common to create models in the form of diagrams or equations. These models are created from a set of symbols which are markings that are used to represent something else. When people talk about knowledge, they usually refer to symbolic models, and that is the sense in which knowledge is used here.

A fundamental characteristic of all symbolic models is that, on their own, they have no intrinsic meaning. The equation $e = mc^2$ is meaningless unless each of the letters in the equation is named and the concepts the letters stand for are explained. Mathematical operations such as equality and multiplication also must be understood. A weather map is equally mysterious without such definitions.

Symbolic models thus gain their meaning when we associate concepts with individual symbols. Specifically, symbolic models are built using a recognized *terminology* and a set of relationships or *grammar* that connects the terms (Figure 2.1). Together the terminology and these grammatical relationships constitute a *language*. In the information sciences, the languages used to create models are usually based upon logic or mathematics.

A terminology contains all the symbols that can be used in building a model, and it maps these symbols to particular concepts, just like a dictionary. For example, in healthcare we have

Terminology: a standard set of symbols or words used to describe the concepts, processes and objects of a given field of study.

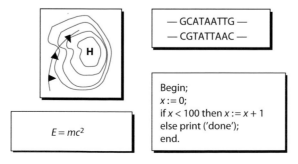

Figure 2.1
Symbolic models cannot be understood unless the symbol language and the possible relationships among the symbols are also understood.

used to make inferences (see Chapter 8). There are many different methods of inference beyond classical logic. Health epidemiologists make inferences using the rules of statistics. Lawyers have rules based upon precedent established in prior case law.

Together, a data model and ontology provide the grammar or *syntax* that defines relationships among data. The rules of inference are then used to interpret the meaning or *semantics* of the data.

2.4 Assumptions in a model define the limits to knowledge

In Chapter 1, we saw that assumptions made at the time a model is created affect the way it is used. The way a model is constructed, the context within which it is defined, what is included in it and the purpose for which is intended all affect its ultimate usefulness.

This is also the case for the models that define our knowledge of the world. The implication then is that the inferences we draw from a model are strongly influenced by the assumptions made when the knowledge in the model was first created.

For example, it is common for clinical protocols to define a standard way in which a particular illness is to be treated. Such a protocol is a kind of template model that drives the treatment delivered to a patient. When a protocol is created, its designers make many assumptions, not all of which are obvious at the time. For example, protocol designers may make an implicit assumption that the drugs or equipment they include in the protocol will actually be available and affordable.

What they are actually doing when they make such assumptions is to model the environment within which the designers expect the protocol to operate. This model usually matches their own local environment, and it is only when a designer is forced to check with others facing different circumstances that such implicit environmental assumptions are unearthed.

Thus, a protocol created for a well-equipped modern hospital may not be useful in a primary care clinic, where staff expertise and resources are very different. Equally, a protocol may assume that a patient has no other significant illnesses. This implicit assumption may be exposed when the treatment specified cannot be used because it interacts with a patient's other medications.

With these examples in mind, we can cast the creation and application of knowledge into the same form as the cycle of model creation and application developed in the Chapter 1 (Figure 2.4). First, the process of model abstraction is equivalent to the knowledge acquisition process. Observations made of the world are generalized into a model that describes how different parts of the world interrelate. Recall that such models are always limited, and they emphasize certain observations and omit others. Next, the knowledge model is applied to data. We can view this process as the construction of an inference, based upon a template model that represents our knowledge and a set of data. As we have just seen, design assumptions at the time a model is created affect how it can be used.

One special design assumption associated with a symbolic model is its language. Just as a photographic image cannot be used unless the right display software is available, a symbolic model cannot be used unless the right language and modelling relationships are also available. In other words, the modelling language becomes a design assumption, which needs to be explicitly catered for when the model is used.

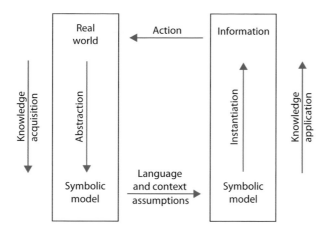

Figure 2.4
Knowledge is acquired through the construction of models, and these models are then applied to data, to draw interpretations of the meaning of the data.

Thus, a treatment protocol designer must assume that the people who read the protocol will be capable of understanding its language and form. If a clinician does not recognize the terms used in a protocol and is not familiar with the concepts and principles it is based upon, then they will be unlikely to understand the intentions of those who wrote the protocol.

2.5 Computational models permit the automation of data interpretation

If the knowledge and data components of a decision problem can be written down, then this problem can in principle be solved using a computer. At other times the task of data interpretation is shared between human and computer. For example, the computer may organize and consolidate data into a graphical presentation, and the human then examines the processed data to make a final interpretation. The proportion in which models are stored either in the computer or as mental models in the head of a human determines where the interpretation takes place. Computer systems thus form a spectrum, ranging from those that have no ability to assist in the interpretation of data to those that are able to carry out a complete interpretation, within the bounds of a given task (Figure 2.5).

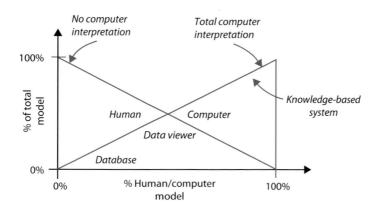

Figure 2.5
Humans and computers can share the burden of data interpretation. The amount of interpretation delegated to the computer depends upon how much of the interpretative model is shared between human and computer.

Computers can act as data stores

If a computer is used solely as a repository for data, it acts as a database. Data are organized according to a data model, so that the origin of each datum is recognizable. Medical data often consist of images or physiological signals taken from monitoring devices. As a consequence, the databases that store complex data from patients can be huge.

Computers can generate data views that assist interpretation

In contrast to passive databases, a computer can carry out some degree of interpretation by generating a view of the data. The computer system shows a user only that portion of data that is of immediate interest and in a way that is best suited to the task at hand.

Consider a database such as Medline, which holds publication data and abstracts of articles from research journals. Given the thousands of papers published weekly, there would be little value for a researcher simply to inspect each record in the database. It would be practically impossible to locate an article within it. What is required is a way of viewing a relevant subset of the data that matches the researcher's question.

For a computer system to provide such 'views' of stored data, a model of the user's needs has to be conveyed to the computer. This communication between the database and the human may be provided by what is known as a *query language*. This is a method commonly used to search library catalogues. Using special words such as 'and', 'or' and 'not', the user constructs a question for the query system about the things that should be displayed (see Box 6.1). Because it recognizes these special words and their meanings, the query system is able to retrieve those records from the database that match the terms provided by the user.

A patient's physiological monitor is also a kind of viewer. If a clinician looked at the raw data stream coming from a measurement device such as an electrocardiogram (ECG), then he or she would be confronted with streams of rapidly changing digits that would be completely unusable in a clinical setting. It is the monitor's role to present sensor data as a set of waveforms for a measurement such as the ECG, or as averaged numeric values for a measurement such as blood pressure. To do this, the computer must have models of the signals and of the kinds of noise and artefact that may corrupt the signals. It also needs a model of the preferred ways of displaying signals to allow humans to carry out the interpretation.

The same process occurs with computer-generated images. Computed tomography and magnetic resonance imaging, for example, both depend on complex models that reconstruct raw data into images that can be interpreted by clinicians. By varying the model parameters applied to the data, the imaging systems can produce different views, or 'slices' through the raw image data.

In general, the degree of division of responsibility for data interpretation between human and computer varies for a number of reasons. It may be that it is inherently difficult to formalize all the knowledge used in the interpretation of data, or it may simply be that the effort involved in modelling is greater than the reward. This is often the case when problems are rare or highly variable.

Computers can be responsible for all data interpretation

As the understanding of how knowledge could be represented in a computer developed, it soon became clear that computers could be used to perform quite powerful forms of reasoning on their own.

Computers are often used as a backup on reasoning tasks that are typically performed by humans. For example, in safety-critical situations such as the operation of a nuclear power plant, the computer watching over the complex system provides a second pair of 'eyes' looking over the operator's shoulder. Computers are also used to interpret data when the task is routine but frequent enough that automation would help. The interpretation of laboratory test results is a common example of this, although typically a human audits the results of such interpretation. Biomedical devices are also often capable of autonomous interpretation. A pacemaker may analyze cardiac activity to look for the development of an arrhythmia.

In all these cases, the interpreting computer does not just possess data and the knowledge that will be used to interpret the data. It also needs a model of the way the computer should 'think' about the problem (i.e. the rules of interpretation discussed earlier). For example, a computer's 'inference engine' may use rules of formal logic – most *knowledge-based systems* are built in this way. Sometimes the systems reason with rules of mathematics, probabilities or other more modern techniques such as fuzzy reasoning or neural networks.

Conclusions

In this chapter, we use the idea of a model to define data, information and knowledge and arrive at a rich understanding of everything from the way people draw conclusions to the role that DNA plays in the cell.

Chapters 1 and 2 are a prelude to introducing a third fundamental informatics concept – the notion of a system. In Chapter 3, the discussion introduces the concept of systems and leads to an exploration of what it means to create an information system. In this way, one can begin to understand the ways in which information systems can be forces for good, as well as understand some of their inherent limitations.

Discussion points

1. Take a patient's laboratory result sheet. Rewrite the information there into a database of facts and show the data model. If the results have been flagged or interpreted in some way, write out what you think was in the knowledge base that was used to make the interpretation. What rules of inference were applied?

2. Compare your answer to the previous question with someone else's answer. Why may there be differences in your answers? (Think back to Chapter 1).

3. Explain how an individual who reads the same patient's record on two different occasions can find the first reading full of information and on the second reading find no information at all.

4. There are many ways in which we can model the world, and it is not surprising that there are many different ways that data can be represented in a database. This chapter describes entity-relationship models. What other database models are commonly used, and how might you choose amongst them?

5. Explain the role of hashtags in a Twitter message or of metadata on a Web page.

6. Find the names of some widely used terminologies and ontologies in healthcare or biology.

7. The human genome is the Rosetta stone needed to decipher the origin of human disease. Discuss.

8. A picture is apparently worth a thousand words. Assume each word is six letters. How big a picture do we get, in bits? Hint: How many bits are needed to encode each letter of the alphabet?

9. If everything we understand is subjective, what does it mean to 'know' something?

Chapter summary

1. Information is derived from data and knowledge.

   a. Data are collections of facts.

   b. Knowledge defines relationships among data.

   c. Information is obtained by applying knowledge to data.

2. Knowledge can be thought of as a set of models describing our understanding of the world.

   a. These models are composed of symbols.

   b. A symbolic model is created using a language that defines the meaning of different symbols and their possible relationships among each other.

3. Inferences are drawn when data are interpreted according to a model.

   a. Data on their own have no intrinsic meaning.

   b. A language identifies concepts within the data.

   c. Next, the knowledge stored in a model can be used to draw an inference from the labelled data.

4. This process of data interpretation actually requires different kinds of information model. Specifically we need a *database, a knowledge base, an ontology* and an inference procedure.

5. Assumptions in the knowledge model affect the quality of the inferences drawn from it.

   a. Assumptions may implicitly define the context within which the model was created.

   b. These design assumptions include the language used if the model is symbolic.

6. Knowledge acquisition and application are examples of the cycle of model abstraction and template-based construction.

7. Once a model and data have been sufficiently formalized, the interpretation can be automated using a computer.

   a. Computers can store data according to data models.

   b. Computers can provide different views onto data according to user models.

   c. Computers can interpret data when they have a knowledge base and an inference procedure.

CHAPTER 3

Information systems

> One doesn't add a computer or buy or design one where there is no system. The success of a project does not stem from the computer but from the existence of a system. The computer makes it possible to integrate the system and thus assure its success.
>
> *C. Caceres in Dickson and Brown, 1969, p 207*
>
> Computers and automation have captured man's imagination. That is to say, like the psychiatrist's ink blot, they serve the imagination as symbols for all that is mysterious, potential, portentous. For when man is faced with ambiguity, with complex shadows he only partly understands, he rejects ambiguity and reads meaning into the shadows. And when he lacks the knowledge and technical means to find real meanings in the shadows, he reads into them the meanings in his own heart and mind … Computers are splendid ink blots.
>
> *Simon, 1965*

A system is commonly understood to be a routine or regular way of working. One can have a system for betting on a horse race or a filing system for storing and retrieving documents. These types of systems are models providing templates for action in the world. Systems can also be models of aspects of the world, such as an ecosystem. In this chapter, we first introduce the general topic of systems and identify a few of their key characteristics. The main focal points of the chapter are what is formally meant by an information system and how information systems are used to control the way decisions are made.

3.1 A system is a set of interacting components

Just as there is ambiguity with the normal meaning of words such as data or information, the notion of a system is equally nuanced. Systems pervade healthcare, and there are countless examples of them. In physiology, one talks of the endocrine system or the respiratory system. In clinical practice, we develop systems for questioning and examining our patients. Indeed, the whole of healthcare itself is often described as a system. The simplest thing connecting these examples is that *each system consists of a collection of component concepts, processes or objects.*

We saw in Chapter 1 that models are the basis for building artefacts and interacting with the world. We can use these ideas to understand that the collection of entities we call a system can be one of three things:

- A model acting as an abstracted description of a set of objects or processes observed in the real world.
- A model consisting of several interlinked elements acting as a template to action.
- An artefact constructed by the process of instantiating the template in the real world.

So when you read the words 'the health system', there are three different possible meanings. The health system could be someone's description of how he or she sees healthcare, based upon observation of the world. It could be a proposal or plan for how healthcare should work, or it could be the physical collection of people, buildings and infrastructure that collectively come together to deliver healthcare.

As abstract descriptions of the world, like all models, systems help compartmentalize some portion of the world in a way that makes it more understandable. For example, a collection of anatomical structures whose function is closely related may constitute a system. Thus, we speak of the nervous system and collect within its definition organs such as the peripheral nerves, the spinal cord and the brain.

The collecting of such elements into a system is a powerful way of enhancing our understanding of the way things work. When Harvey first proposed the notion of a system of circulation for blood through the body in 1628, he essentially constructed a model that, for the first time, connected the arteries, veins and heart into a functioning whole. So powerful was this model that it was adopted despite its inadequacies at that time. It was, for example, not until 1661 that Malpighi finally demonstrated that the capillaries connected the arterial and venous systems (Schafer and Thane, 1891).

As templates or blueprints, systems allow us to develop clear models of how entities will interact. There are separate blueprints for different systems in a building, including the electrical system, the plumbing system and the air-conditioning system. *Complexity* often refers to the number of interconnections that exist among such system components, and complexity increases with the number of interconnections. A *complex system* is thus one in which there are a relatively large number of connections among components. Complex systems are sometimes informally distinguished from a *complicated system,* which may have a large number of components but relatively few interconnections.

The discipline of decomposing a composite structure into sub-elements that carry out different functions simplifies the design process and will more likely result in something that is well designed for its intended purpose. Most machinery, for example, is designed as a set of complicated modules, to limit interconnection and minimise complexity. Modular systems are common features of modern technology. Cars have separate fuel, suspension and brake systems, and this separation into component systems means that each can be maintained and repaired fairly independently of the others.

3.2 A system has an internal structure that transforms inputs into outputs for a specific purpose

Systems have inputs and outputs

Systems usually have a set of *inputs,* which are transformed by the components of the system into a set of *outputs* (Figure 3.1). The inputs to a coffee maker are ground coffee, water and heat. The output is hot liquid coffee. The inputs to a leaf are water and carbon dioxide, and the photosynthetic system produces as output oxygen and carbohydrates. The inputs to a hospital emergency room are the clinical staff, patients and supplies – the outputs are patients who have been in some way transformed by their emergency room visit.

In the process of transforming inputs into outputs, the *state* of a system may change. For example, a car may have as its state a location, and the input of fuel, oil and a driver transforms the state of the vehicle to a different location. An influx of patients may rapidly change an emergency room from the state 'able to receive patients' to 'full'. Further, the state of a system may determine just how it will change inputs into outputs. If a human's state is 'physically fit' then that person transforms food into energy more efficiently than someone in the state 'unfit', who with the same food inputs may tend to deposit more of the food as fat.

Systems have behaviour

For a system to be distinguishable from its environment, it should have a characteristic behaviour. Thus, a weather system may be a set of related pressure bands, whose collective behaviour stands out and demands attention. One of the behaviours of the vascular system is that it can be observed to contain flowing blood. This behaviour distinguishes the vascular system from, say, the nervous system. It is this identification with a particular behaviour that helps conceptually separate a system from other parts of its environment.

Critically, a system's behaviour cannot usually be predicted by an examination of its individual components, but it emerges from the way the components interact with each other. Thus, the behaviours of social groups, communication networks, roads and neural processes are all emergent properties of the interactions among their components (Box 3.1). The emergence of system behaviour means that the effects of anything we build are not directly predictable from an examination of individual components, but rather from an understanding of how the components interrelate.

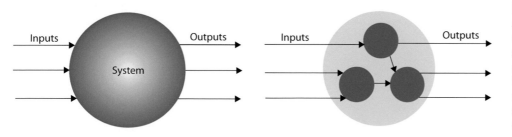

Figure 3.1 A system is characterized by a set of inputs and outputs and can be internally decomposed into a set of interacting components or sub-systems.

Physical systems are embedded in an environment

To be distinguishable from everything else, there must be a *boundary* between a system and the rest of the environment. However, that boundary may be difficult to define precisely. Depending upon the integrity of the boundary, three different kinds of systems are possible:

- *Closed systems* have no external inputs and outputs, and they behave like a black box that is unaffected by the external world.
- *Relatively closed systems* have precisely defined inputs and outputs with their environment.
- *Open systems* interact freely with their surrounding environment.

Except for the rare closed system, which does not interact with its environment, a system can never be completely separated from its external world. It is for this reason that emergent

Box 3.1
Braess' paradox

Simple cause and effect analysis predicts that putting more resource toward achieving a goal should improve performance, but this is not always the case. The creation of new roads can lead to greater traffic congestion. The installation of new telephone or computer network elements can lead to degraded system performance. Introducing new workers to a team may actually result in a decrease in the team's performance.

To understand these apparently paradoxical results, one needs to examine events from a system view. Studying the effects of new roads upon traffic, Dietrich Braess discovered that if a new road is built in a congested system, everyone's journey unexpectedly lengthens (Bean, 1996). He explained this result by examining the behaviour of drivers, who made individual decisions about their journey, and the emergent effects of all these individual decisions upon the whole system. Consider a journey from A to D that can follow several routes, such as ABD or ACD.

The delay on any link is a function of f, which is the number of cars on that link. As shown in Figure 3.2 (a), there are 2 equidistant path choices. With 6 cars in the system, they will tend to distribute equally, with 3 cars on each path ABD and ACD. If they did not distribute equally, the congestion on one link would over time cause drivers to choose the less congested path. The expected delay is thus 83 on both routes. As shown in Figure 3.2 (b), a new link BC is added, thus creating a new path ABCD. Assuming previous path costs, drivers think that ABCD is now the quickest route. Users take the new path to try to minimize their journey (Glance and Huberman, 1994), but the choice hurts the whole system. Equilibrium eventually occurs when 2 cars choose each of the paths ABD, ACD and ABCD. This puts 4 cars on the link AB. Now, the new road has increased the expected delay for everyone to 92.

Figure 3.2
(a) and (b) The effect
on travel time of
building a new road
in an already
congested system.

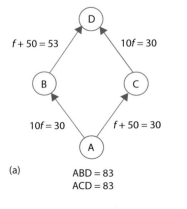

(a)
$f + 50 = 53$ $10f = 30$
$10f = 30$ $f + 50 = 30$
ABD = 83
ACD = 83

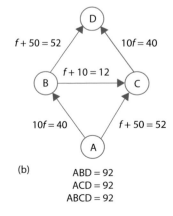

(b)
$f + 50 = 52$ $10f = 40$
$f + 10 = 12$
$10f = 40$ $f + 50 = 52$
ABD = 92
ACD = 92
ABCD = 92

behaviour of a physical system is even more difficult to predict because that behaviour is in part determined by the environment in which the system is embedded, and we usually do not know the exact state of the environment. For practical purposes, we usually restrict the description of a system to include a limited set of elements of the environment that are of immediate interest (Box 3.2). Thus, one cannot divorce a physical system from the environment within which it exists because, by doing so, the very context for the system's existence disappears, and its function will alter.

Systems have internal structure

Systems have component parts that together constitute their internal structure. These components are often decomposed into sub-systems for ease of understanding, manufacture or maintenance. A health system is decomposed into community and hospital services. A hospital is decomposed into different departments or services. The amount of internal detail that can be described within a system is probably limitless. The description of the cardiovascular system could descend to the cellular level, the molecular level and beyond. The amount of detail in a system description is usually determined by the purpose of the description.

For a system to function, each of its sub-systems or components must interact or communicate. This means that they may share inputs and outputs, with the output of one component providing the input to another. Inputs to a factory may be raw materials and energy, and its outputs could be manufactured products such as cars or foodstuffs. These products in turn are inputs into the retail sector, which uses them to generate a financial output.

The introduction of antibiotics in the second half of the twentieth century heralded a period of optimism. Infectious diseases were soon to be a thing of the past, and every year saw the discovery of new drugs that attacked an ever-wider spectrum of bacteria. Then, as time went on, the tide started to turn, as individual organisms such as penicillinase-producing bacteria developed resistance to specific drugs. Through a process of natural selection, the drugs that were created to kill bacteria were actually selecting individual organisms that were immune to their effects, thus allowing these organisms to survive and dominate the gene pool. Some organisms now have such widespread resistance that their detection can shut down large sections of a hospital.

Modern medical science is often challenged by critics who cite examples such as the development of antibiotic resistance as proof that its methods ultimately do more harm than good. This 'fight-back' of natural systems following the introduction of technology is not a phenomenon confined to healthcare, but potentially affects every technological intervention made by humans (Tenner, 1996).

From a systems viewpoint, whenever a technology is introduced, the fight-back effect is not so much a fault of the technology as it is an inevitable consequence of the way that we understand systems. When we model the world, we intentionally simplify or exclude whole sections of reality to create a point of view. When a technology is applied, it is aimed at solving a particular problem within a system, with the assumption that its effects are predictable, 'everything else being equal'. This clearly is never completely possible.

The assumption that everything that can be known is known is called the *closed-world assumption* in logic (Genesereth and Nilsson, 1987). Its function is to allow reasoning to proceed even if our knowledge is incomplete. It serves a similar role when a technology is introduced into a system because without this assumption we would never be sure we understood all the possible consequences of the technology's actions.

So rather than being a specific consequence of technology, unexpected outcomes are a result of the imperfect way in which we understand the world. Our only way around it is to assume, at some stage, that we know enough to try things out. The alternative is to do nothing.

Box 3.2
Penicillinase and the closed-world assumption

Systems can regulate their output by using feedback as input

A special case of connecting output and input between systems occurs when some or all of the output of a system is taken back as its own input. This is called *feedback* (Figure 3.3). In this way a system can influence its future behaviour based upon measurement of its past performance.

Feedback systems can become quite complicated in their design and are used to create what are known as *cybernetic* or *control systems,* which are systems that are able to adapt their output to seek a particular goal. Most feedback control systems are more open and use a measurement sub-system to sample their output and use this feedback to determine what the next input should be (Figure 3.4).

The simplest feedback control system consists of three components:

- A *sensor,* which measures the parameter that is to be controlled.
- A *comparator,* which determines whether the measurement deviates from the desired range.
- An *activator,* which creates an output that then alters the environment in some way to change the value of the parameter being measured.

For example, bank account interest is determined by measuring an account value and adding back the interest to the account. A thermostat is part of a feedback system for controlling temperature. The thermostat samples the temperature of a room, which is being warmed by the heating system. As the temperature rises, the system shuts off when a pre-set temperature is reached, or it turns on when the temperature drops below the *set point.* A patient with insulin-dependent diabetes samples his or her blood sugar level with a glucometer and uses the glucose

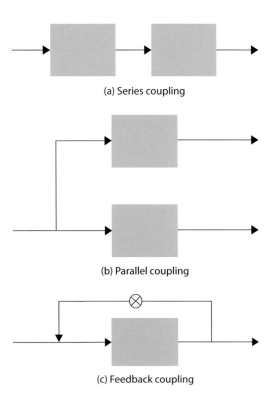

(a) Series coupling

(b) Parallel coupling

(c) Feedback coupling

Figure 3.3 (a), (b) and (c) Sub-systems may be coupled by joining their inputs to their outputs. In the special case of feedback (c), a sub-system takes some of its own output to modify its input.

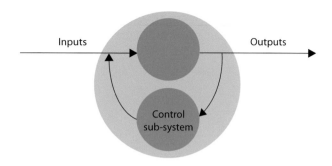

Figure 3.4
The output of a system may be regulated by a control sub-system that measures the system's outputs and uses that measurement to regulate the subsequent system inputs.

value to adjust the next dose of insulin to be administered, based upon a rule or a formula that aims to keep blood sugar within a set range. The input to the diabetic patient's 'system' is a dose of insulin and food, and the output is an effect on blood sugar that is then used to alter the next input of insulin and food. The thermostat and the glucometer are both measurement devices that form an integral part of a feedback controlled system.

There are two basic types of feedback system (Figure 3.5).

- In a *negative feedback arrangement,* the output of a system is subtracted from the next input. This restricts a system to working within a steady operating range. Physiological systems mostly use negative feedback to provide homeostasis – the maintenance of a desired pre-set physical state, despite variations in the external world. Homeostatic mechanisms maintain everything from body temperature to the concentration of ions within cells.
- In a *positive feedback system,* the output of a system is added to its next input; the result is that the system's output increases with time. For example, a savings account increases in value over time as interest is added to it.

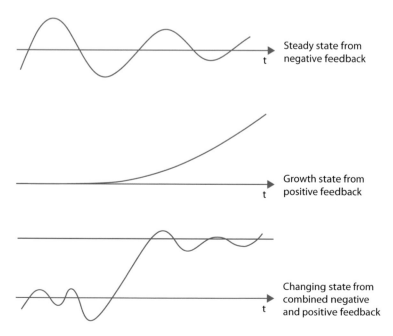

Figure 3.5
System states can be maintained or varied depending upon the type of feedback control being used (After Littlejohn, 1996).

During the French Revolution, a method was devised to create logarithm tables en masse. Individuals called computers each carried out a small calculation, and as a result the team of individuals was able to carry out a large number of intricate calculations. In his seminal treatise On the Economy of Manufacture *(Babbage, 1833), Babbage reasoned that because such lengthy calculations could all in principle be broken down into simple steps of addition or subtraction, these calculations could be carried out by machine. This thought inspired Babbage to devise his difference engine, which was the first proposal for a general purpose calculating machine.*

- Positive and negative feedback systems can be combined to allow a system to change from one to another of a number of predefined states. The positive feedback component permits the system to move from one state to another, and the negative feedback comes into play when the new state has been reached and keeps the system there.

Systems are arbitrary

We create descriptions of systems to help us understand the observable world. So by their very nature, system descriptions are arbitrary human creations. There can never be something called 'the correct' definition of a system, whether it is a description of something in the world or a design to accomplish some function.

There are many possible ways that one could choose to describe a system, and it is often only a matter of convention and practicality that one description is chosen over another. It should come as no surprise that two competing system descriptions may overlap and have common elements. Are the pulmonary arteries more properly part of the cardiovascular system, or are they part of the respiratory system? It depends entirely upon one's point of view.

Systems are purposive

This brings us to a key point. Descriptions of a system are constructed with a function or purpose in mind (Box 3.3). The intent behind modern descriptions of different physiological systems is to treat illness. The reason that one particular system begins to gain common acceptance over another is that it is inherently more useful for that purpose. Thus, phrenology, the study of bumps on the skull, was replaced by a system of thought we now call neurology because this newer viewpoint proved itself a more useful approach to treating illness. So, over time, whole systems of thought gradually fall into disuse as newer and more useful ones appear.

Box 3.3
Network systems

There are many ways to conceive of systems and to represent their individual elements and the ways in which they interact. Networks are a particularly important and universal systems construct. We can, for example, describe networks of biological and social processes (see Figure 3.6). As templates to action, and as real world artefacts, we invent transportation, communication and energy networks, to name a few.

The basic elements of any network are its *nodes,* which represent the atomic entities that inhabit the network, and the *edges* between those nodes, which record their possible interactions. In a *social network,* nodes are people and edges are their relationships (see Chapter 20). In a *metabolic network,* the nodes are molecules and the edges are their reactions. With a *computer network* such as the Internet, nodes are individual computer machines, and edges are the communication links between them.

Network theory is the study of network behaviour at a general level, and it tells us that despite the wide variety of networks we see in the world, they all share commonalities. Network behaviour is directly related to network structure. The number, distribution and type of links among the nodes in a network strongly influence the network's properties.

For example, the *average path length* in a network measures the average number of steps it takes to travel from one node to another. Typically, the shorter the average path length, the easier it is for a network to function, whether transporting packets of information across a computer network or minimizing power loss as energy is transported across a power grid. Many networks share a *small world* property because of commonalities in their structure, meaning that they have a small average path length. The small world effect famously explains why it is usually easy to connect two strangers to each other through shared acquaintances.

Other important network properties that help explain their behaviour include *node centrality* (a measure of how influential a node is in a network, based on how many connections it has to other nodes) and *connectedness* (which describes the degree to which nodes are directly or indirectly connected). The presence of highly connected and central *hubs*, for example, appears to confer stability on networks.

Defining the borders of a network is analogous to finding the boundaries of any system. Some networks are highly isolated. Some are coupled to other networks, upon which they depend, through shared nodes. Dependencies are both a source of system richness and a potential weakness. For example, cascading failures can propagate among networks, as sometimes occurs when blackouts move across connected power grids.

Further reading
Newman M., A-L. Barabásii and D. Watts (2006). *The Structure and Dynamics of Networks*. Princeton, NJ, Princeton University Press.

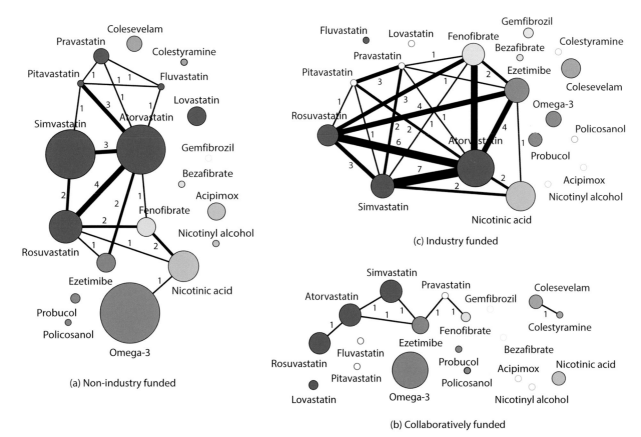

Figure 3.6 (a), (b), (c) Networks showing the number of clinical trials comparing different cholesterol-lowering drugs, depending on whether the comparative effectiveness studies were funded by industry or not. Node size corresponds to the number of trials of a drug. Network structure differences show the different priorities of industry and academic scientists (Dunn *et al.*, 2012).

3.3 Information systems contain data and models

People develop systematic routines because they find themselves doing the same task again and again. We abstract the elements of our actions that recur and give them some objective existence by describing the routine. When the recurring routine is a decision, it should require access to the same kind of data and use the same knowledge. In these circumstances, one can develop a regular process or *information system* to accomplish the decision task. An information system could thus be anything from the routine way in which a clinician records patients' details in a pocket notebook or the way a triage nurse assesses patients on arrival in an emergency department through to a complicated computer system that regulates payments for healthcare services.

An information system is distinguished from other systems by its components, which include data and models. Recall from Chapter 2 that there are different kinds of information models, including databases and knowledge bases. These different information components can be assembled to create an information system. For example, consider a calculator that can store data and equations in its memory. The data store is the calculator's database, and the equation store is its knowledge base. The input to the calculator becomes the equation to be solved, as well as the values of data to plug into the equation. The database communicates with the knowledge base by using a simple *communication channel* within the device, and the output of the system is the value for the solved equation (Figure 3.7).

Many potential internal components could be included within an information system including a database, a knowledge base, an ontology and decision procedures or rules of inference. The different components of an information system are connected by input-output channels, which allow data to be shifted among the components as needed.

A patients' record system is a more complicated example of an information system. Its purpose is to record data about particular patients in some formalized fashion to assist in patients' management. The record system is composed of a database, organized according to data models that are based upon the way clinicians use the data in their decision-making process. A patients' record system also requires an ontology that stipulates the medical language or terminology to be used in the records. The record system may also include access control rules that govern the way that records are to be accessed and possibly the individuals who are permitted to see the records. The record system itself is a component of a larger system, which may be the particular institution within which it exists or the health system as a whole.

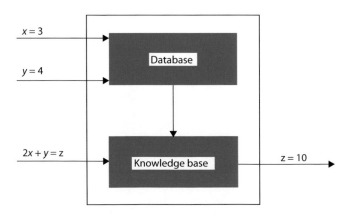

Figure 3.7
A calculator with a stored equation is an information system. The inputs are the equation to be solved and the data values, and the answer output by the system depends on the input values.

We saw at the beginning of this chapter that there are actually three different meanings of the word 'system' – a system can be an abstracted description of the real world, a template to action or an artefact constructed in the real world. Consequently, an 'information system' may be one of three things:

- A simplified description of an existing set of information processes. For example, one could produce a document or diagram cataloguing the different input and output flows of information that connect a number of different organizations.
- A plan for implementing a new set of information processes.
- An actual physical system. Medline is an information system organized to allow access to the biomedical literature. The Internet is an even larger information system consisting of computer hardware, software, data such as text and graphics stored as Web pages, network connections and the people using these technologies.

Information systems can be created for a number of reasons. In the main, a system is devised because an information process is very common, very complicated or in some way critical. In the first case, the goal of introducing an information system is to reduce the effort of decision making by streamlining the process. In the case of complex or critical decisions, the role of the information system is either to reduce complexity or to minimize the likelihood of error.

Information systems share all the characteristics of systems described in earlier chapters. We collect together decisions, data and models that are of interest for some purpose, and then we look upon them as a system. An information system exists within an environment and is built to interact with an environment. Information systems can never fully capture the richness of the real world, and as with all model-based constructs, they become increasingly less accurate over time as the world changes around them. Information systems built for one set of environmental assumptions may not work as well when transplanted to another environment.

Conclusions

We have now reached a point where we can look at an information system in a fairly rich way, based upon an understanding of the basic principles of models, information structures and systems. Through a variety of examples, we have seen how information systems are often designed to be part of a feedback control system used to manage clinical activities. Whenever a decision is important enough, or is made often enough, an information system is built to manage the process. With this background, it is now possible to move on and look at how information is used to support clinical activities. In Chapters 4 through 8, we will learn how to search for, structure and use information in the support of clinical processes, and in Chapters 9 through 14, we see how healthcare is structured from an informational viewpoint and how information systems reflect and contribute to that structure.

Discussion points

1. Why may a patient object to being considered an input to a 'health system'?

2. What are the inputs and outputs of a patients' record system?

3. How many states can you identify for the cardiovascular system, and how does each state change the way the system handles its inputs and outputs?

4. What is the purpose of the health system? What are the components of the health system? What is the purpose of each component?

5. Compare the structure of the health system in the United States and the United Kingdom. If the purpose of both systems is the same, how do you explain the differences in their components?

6. How many people separate you and Kevin Bacon? Why is it such a short list?

7. When is a model not a system? When is a system not a model?*

8. Identify one positive and one negative feedback system in the health system. What are the inputs and outputs? Which components act as sensors, comparators and activators? What is the purpose of the system in terms of control?

9. Identify the different information models used to create the Medline biomedical literature system.

10. Why is it often necessary to upgrade the software in a computer?

Chapter summary

1. A system is a collection of component concepts, processes or objects.

2. Systems transform inputs into outputs and may change their state in doing so.

3. A system has behaviour that cannot usually be predicted by an examination of its individual components but that emerges from the way the components interact with each other.

4. Physical systems are embedded in an environment; closed systems have no external inputs and outputs; open systems interact freely with their surrounding environment.

5. Systems have internal structure.

6. Networks are used to describe the internal structure of many systems. The properties of a network arise out of the way in which the network connects its nodes and edges.

7. Systems can regulate their output by using feedback as input; in a negative feedback arrangement, the output of a system is subtracted from the next input; in a positive feedback system, the output of a system is added to its next input.

8. A feedback control system consists of the following: a sensor, which measures the parameter that is to be controlled; a comparator, which determines whether the measurement deviates from the desired range; and an activator, which creates an output to change the value of the parameter being measured.

9. Systems are arbitrary and purposive.

10. Information systems contain data and models, which include databases and knowledge bases that interact via a communication channel.

---

* If a model has no decomposable parts, no inputs and outputs, then it is not a system. If a system is an artefact or a process in the real world, then it is not a model. However, if that system has been constructed, then it is probably an instantiation of a model.

PART 2

Informatics skills

CHAPTER 4

Communicating

> "The chart is not the patient."
>
> *Gall, 1986*

Every clinical action – every treatment choice and investigation made – is shaped by the available information. We can think of this information as the clinical evidence that informs a judgement about the right course of action. Clinicians gather evidence through communication with others, either through what is said now or what has been documented from before.

There are many different sources of clinical evidence used in the routine care of a patient, and these include:

- The patients themselves, who give information about their symptoms and their problems, as well as demonstrate clinical signs through physical examination.
- Clinical colleagues, who exchange messages containing information about the state of patients, their opinions, own workload and needs, or background clinical knowledge.
- The scientific clinical literature, which captures past knowledge about disease and treatment.
- The patient's record, which is a history of the patient's past state, including clinical observations and laboratory and imaging reports, as well any treatments given and their impact on the disease.
- Measurement and imaging devices, from simple instruments such as a blood pressure cuff or glucometer, through to cardiograms, polymerase chain reaction gene tests, ultrasound probes, multisensor patient monitors in intensive care and positron emission tomography scanners.

The information contained in these clinical 'messages' is stored in a variety of media and formats and can be delivered in a variety of ways, including face-to-face conversations, letters, e-mail, voicemail and electronic or paper medical records.

When this exchange of information works well, clinical care is solidly based upon the best evidence. When information exchange is poor, the quality of clinical care can suffer enormously. Poor presentation of clinical data can lead to poorly informed clinical practice, inappropriate repeat investigation, unnecessary referrals and waste clinical time and resources (Wyatt and Wright, 1988). For example, the single most common cause of adverse clinical events is medication error, which accounts for about 19 per cent of all adverse events; the most common prescription errors can be redressed by the provision of better information about medications or the patients receiving them (Bates *et al.*, 2001).

In this chapter we examine this communication process and explore how variations in the structure of clinical messages affect the way in which they are interpreted and can influence the quality of care. If the motto for Chapter 1 was 'a map is not the territory', then the motto for this chapter is 'the chart is not the patient'.

4.1 The structure of a message can influence how it will be understood

What a message is meant to say when it is created and what the receiver of a message understands may not be the same. What humans understand is profoundly shaped by the way data are presented and by the way we individually interpret what is presented. It is thus as

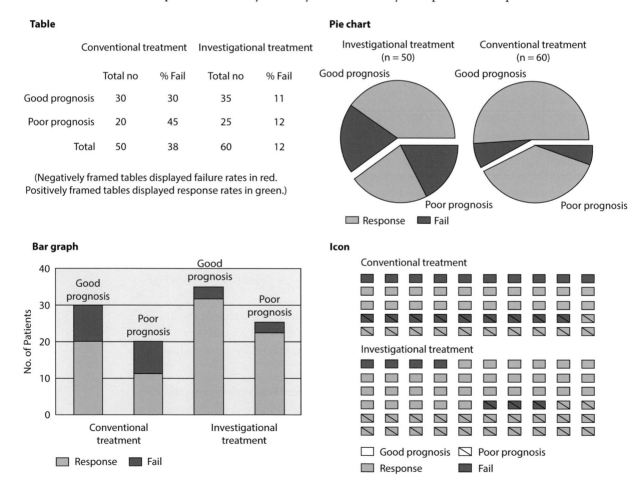

Figure 4.1   Table, pie chart, icon and bar graph displays of the same data from a hypothetical clinical trial each resulted in a different percentage of correct decisions being made. The icon display (bottom right) was most effective for the decision to stop the clinical trial. (From Elting *et al.*, 1999.)

important to structure data in a way that maximizes the chance that it will be understood as it is to ensure that the data are correct.

What a clinician actually understands after seeing the data in a patient's record and what the data actually show can be very different. In Figure 4.1, identical patient data are presented in four different ways (Elting *et al.*,1999). The data show preliminary results from two hypothetical clinical trials of a generic 'conventional treatment' compared with a generic 'investigational treatment', both for the same condition. In an experiment to see whether clinicians would decide to stop the trial because the data show that one treatment is obviously better than the other, the decision to stop varied depending on how the data were displayed. Correct decisions were significantly more common with icon displays (82 per cent) and tables (68 per cent) than with pie charts or bar graphs (both 56 per cent).

If this example was reflected in actual clinical practice, up to 25 per cent of the patients treated according to data displayed as bar or pie charts would have received inappropriate treatment. This finding underlines just how important the choice of data presentation method is. The way data are structured has a profound effect on the conclusions a clinician will draw from the data. There is an enormous difference between simply communicating a message to a colleague and communicating it effectively.

4.2 The message that is sent may not be the message that is received

Messages can be misunderstood both because of the limitations of the agents interpreting them and because the very process of communication is itself limited. To explore the nature of communication, we will develop a simple general model that describes the process of sending a message between two agents. The agents may be human beings or a human and a computer. A communication act occurs between the two agents A_1 and A_2 when agent A_1 (the sender) constructs a message m_1 for some specific purpose and sends it to agent A_2 (the receiver) across a *communication channel* (Figure 4.2).

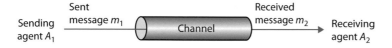

The second agent A_2 receives a message m_2, which can be different from the intended message m_1. The effectiveness of the communication between the agents (how closely m_1 and m_2 match) depends upon several things – the nature of the communication channel, the state of the individual agents, the knowledge possessed by the agents and the context within which the agents find themselves.

Figure 4.2

When a message is sent between two agents, it is transported over a communication channel. The sent and received messages may not be identical.

Communication channels distort messages

Many different communication channels are available, from face-to-face conversation, digital channels such as the telephone, e-mail and videoconferencing through to non-interactive channels such as the medical record or letters.

The signal to noise ratio measures how much a particular message has been corrupted by noise that has been added to it during transmission across a channel.

A message is sent as a signal across a selected channel (e.g. as sound waves or electronic impulses). Channels vary in their *capacity* to transport such signals. The more limited a channel's capacity, the less of the original message can be transmitted per unit time. Simply put, the thinner the channel 'pipe', the fewer data can flow through at any given moment.

Channels also have different abilities to keep a message exactly as it was sent, and a signal can be distorted during transmission. This distortion is usually called *noise*. Noise can be thought of as any unwanted signal that is added to a transmitted message and that distorts the message for the receiver. It can be anything from the static on a radio to another conversation next to you that makes it difficult to hear your own. Thus, 'one person's signal is another person's noise'. Standard *information theory* describes how the outcome of a communication is determined in part by the capacity and noise characteristics of a channel (Box 4.1).

Therefore, in general, when an agent sends a message, that message may be modified by the chosen communication channel and, through delay or distortion, arrive as a slightly different message for the receiving agent.

Box 4.1
Information theory

Claude Shannon developed the mathematical basis for information theory while working at Bell Laboratories in New Jersey during the 1940s. Motivated by problems in communication engineering, Shannon developed a method to measure the amount of 'information' that could be passed along a communication channel between a source and a destination.

Shannon was concerned with the process of communicating using radio, and for him the transmitter, ionosphere and receiver were all examples of communication *channels*. Such channels had a limited capacity and were noisy. Shannon developed definitions of channel capacity, noise and signal in terms of a precise measure of what he called 'information'.

He began by recognizing that before a message could enter a channel it had to be *encoded* in some way by a transmitter. For example, a piece of music needs to be transformed through a microphone into electronic signals before it can be transmitted. Equally, a signal would then need to be decoded at the destination by a receiver before it could be reconstructed into the original signal. A high-fidelity speaker thus needs to decode an electronic signal before it can be converted back into sound.

Shannon was principally interested in studying the problems of maximizing the reliability of transmission of a signal and minimizing the cost of that transmission. Encoding a signal was the mechanism for reducing the cost of transmission through *signal compression,* as well as combating corruption of the signal through *channel noise*.

The rules governing the operation of an encoder and a decoder constitute a *code*. The code described by Shannon corresponds to a model and its language. A code achieves reliable transmission if the source message is reproduced at the destination within prescribed limits. After Shannon, the problem for a communication engineer was to find an encoding scheme that made the best use of a channel while minimizing transmission noise.

With human verbal communication, the information source is the sender's brain and the transmitter is the vocal cords. Air provides the communication channel, and it may distort any message sent because of extraneous noise or because the message is dampened or *attenuated* the further the distance grows between the communicating parties. The receiver in this model is the listener's ear, and the destination that decodes what has been received is the listener's brain.

Although Shannon saw his theory helping us understand human communication, it remains an essentially statistical analysis over populations of messages and says little about individual acts of communication. Specifically, information theory is silent on the notion on the meaning of a message because it does not explicitly deal with the way a knowledge base is used to interpret the data in a message (Figure 4.3).

Further reading
van der Lubbe, J. C. A. (1997). *Information Theory.* Cambridge: Cambridge University Press.

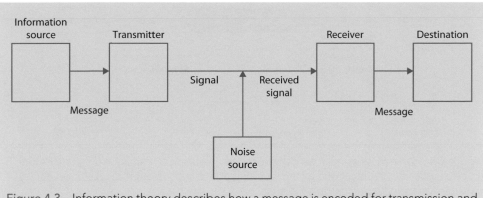

Figure 4.3   Information theory describes how a message is encoded for transmission and then decoded by the receiver.

Individuals do not know the same things

In Chapter 2 we saw that the inferences drawn from data depend on the knowledge base used to make that inference. Because each individual 'knows' slightly different things, he or she may draw different inferences from the same data. Variations in diagnosis and treatment decisions, based upon the same data, may simply reflect differences in clinical knowledge among individual clinicians.

When sending a message, we have to make assumptions about what the receiver already knows and shape the message accordingly. There is no point in explaining what the receiver already knows, but it is equally important not to miss important new details. Thus, notionally identical messages sent to a clinical colleague or to a patient end up being very different because we often assume that the colleague requires less explanation than the patient.

The knowledge shared among individuals is sometimes called their *common ground* (Coiera, 2000). This explains why we communicate more easily with others who have similar experiences, beliefs and knowledge. It takes greater effort to explain something in a conversation to those with whom we share less common ground. Conversely, individuals who are particularly close can communicate complicated ideas in terse shorthand. One of the reasons agents create common ground is to optimize their interactions. By developing common ground, less needs to be said in any given message, thus making the interaction less costly and more effective (see Box 21.3).

Returning to our simple communication model, each agent now possesses knowledge about the world in the form of a set of internal models K. Critically, the private world models of the two communicating agents in our model, K_1 and K_2, are not identical. Thus, agent A_1 creates a message m_1, based upon its knowledge of the world K_1 (Figure 4.4). A_2 receives a slightly different message m_2 because of channel effects and then generates its own private interpretation of the message's meaning based upon its knowledge K_2. Further, agent A_1 makes a guess about the content of K_2 and shapes its message to include data or knowledge it believes agent A_2 will need to make sense of the message being sent. The effectiveness of the message depends upon the quality of the guess agents make about what the receiving agent

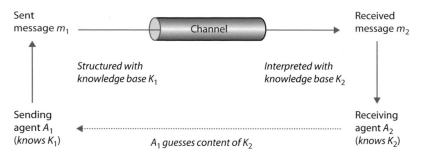

Figure 4.4 When a message is sent between two agents, it is built according to a model that we think will be understood by the receiving agent and is potentially distorted during transmission by the communication channel.

knows. Usually, agents send more than is needed because some redundancy in a message improves the chance that what the receiver needs is actually sent.

The receiver's knowledge alters the effectiveness of a message

Agents vary in the terminology they are familiar with, and communication is often difficult because one agent uses technical terms or jargon with which the other is unfamiliar. When communicating to patients, the decision to avoid jargon is essential. In one UK study that looked at educational leaflets about asthma that were written for patients, the investigators found that most leaflets assumed a 'reading age' close to secondary school entry level. However, to ensure that most of the population can understand such leaflets, the leaflets should have a much lower reading age, around mid-primary school level (Smith *et al.,* 1998). Because 22 per cent of the UK population at the time of the study were judged to have low literacy, they would have had great difficulty in understanding the content of the health messages contained in those leaflets.

More profoundly, it is not just that clinicians and patients do not share the same training and language; they may not even share the same goals during the conversation. A clinician may be sending messages based upon the medical model of the purpose of a conversation, but the patient may have very different needs (Mathews, 1983).

Message complexity and jargon also have an impact on effectiveness of messages aimed at health professionals. For example, clinicians are less likely to comply with clinical guidelines if the guideline is written in a complex way (Grilli and Lomas, 1994). Using a measure of document complexity, guidelines with high complexity had a significantly lower compliance rate (41.9 per cent) compared with those judged to be low in complexity (55.9 per cent).

A channel is selected based upon its suitability to the task

Given that different communication channels have varying characteristics such as bandwidth and noise, we may prefer to choose one channel to another for a given task. However, the choice to use one communication channel over another is often not considered explicitly.

For example, some channels, such as the telephone or pager, immediately interrupt the receiver of the message. Others, such as voicemail or e-mail, can be accessed at a time of the receiver's choice. Interruptive channels are called *synchronous* channels because they demand real-time interaction. Non-interruptive channels are called *asynchronous* channels because the interaction between agents can occur at separate moments over an extended period. Many clinicians use synchronous channels or even face-to-face interruption 'in the corridor' as their preferred way of communicating, without any conscious attention to the cost of that choice on the receiver.

Some channels allow point-to-point communication, meaning that they connect only pre-designated individuals. Others are broadcast channels, where anyone can listen in on the conversation. Social media are interesting as communication channels in that they often allow both types of communication, by allowing point-to-point conversations to be visible to the public. The decision to use such channels for clinical conversations thus needs to be carefully weighed, given that privacy is not often guaranteed.

Research has also shown that different types of messages are more effective when transmitted with some channels than with others (see Chapter 18). For example, are public health messages better transmitted using mass media, such as television, or as more personal messages, such as a letter? The answer is complex, but it seems to relate both to the cost of using a channel by the receiver and to the benefit the receiver expects to receive from the message (Trumbo, 1998).

Messages are constructed and received according to imperfect models of the world

Sending and receiving messages are model-based processes. Consequently, the process of communication is fundamentally limited not just by the physical limitations of transmission channels, but also by the inherent limitations of modelling, as described in Chapter 1.

Model theory tells us that the sender of a message is operating with models of the world that will always be inaccurate in one way or another, and that equally, the receiver must attempt to interpret messages according to models also somehow flawed. Consequently, communication can never be perfect, and misinterpretation at some level is unavoidable.

Human communication also suffers from limitations in the way humans use models to interpret physical symbols received by our senses:

- *Perceptual limitations*: Humans may misperceive the symbols that they see or hear. This misperception may simply occur when symbols are poorly constructed and therefore ambiguous. Drug names can be confused because of illegible handwriting. Equally, perception can be distorted because each human sense is a communication channel with its own unique capacity and noise characteristics. At a more fundamental level, the human perceptual system distorts sense data by exaggerating some characteristics and minimizing others. For example, the visual system emphasizes edges, and the auditory system responds better to some sound frequencies than to others. They do this presumably because the brain has evolved to recognize some signals or signal patterns over others because of their survival benefit. Consequently, what we perceive and what actually *is* are not the same thing (Figures 4.5 and 4.6).
- *Cognitive biases*: The distortions introduced by our cognitive architecture do not stop at sense data, but they extend to the interpretation we draw from them. Perception is an active process in which we try to map what arrives as sense data to our internal models

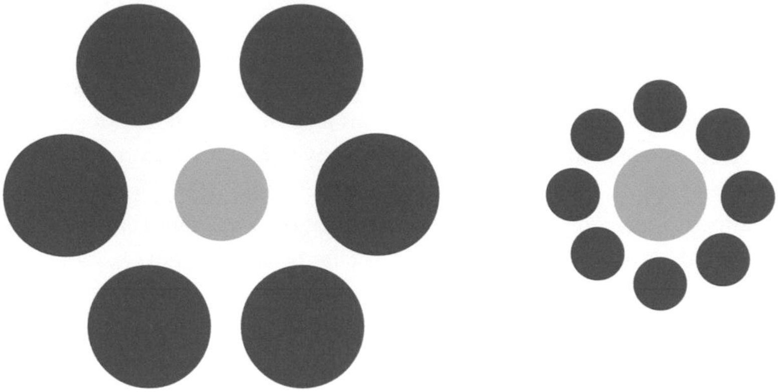

Figure 4.5
The Ebbinghaus illusion demonstrates how human perception distorts sense data. The two central circles are the same size, but the left one seems smaller (Rose and Bressan, 2002).

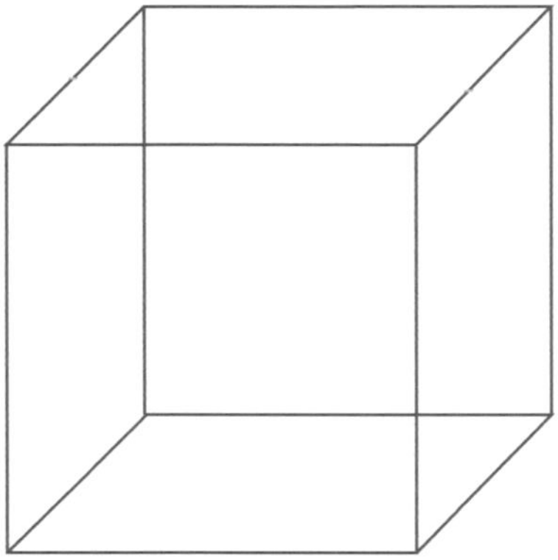

Figure 4.6
There are two possible interpretations of this cube, depending on whether you think the rightmost square surface is at the back or the front of the three-dimensional cube.

of the world (Van Leeuwin, 1998). Humans try to match what we sense through sight, sound, touch and smell to our pre-existing models of what we think *should* be there (see Figure 4.5). If you think there is an intruder in your house, then you will interpret any sounds you hear from that perspective. Put simply, we hear what we want to hear or think we should hear. Further, an inherent set of cognitive biases leads us to draw conclusions not supported by the immediate evidence (see Chapter 8). For example, recent events can bias us to recognize similar events, even when they are not present. A recent encounter with a thyrotoxic patient can bias a clinician to overdiagnose the same disease in future patients (Medin *et al.*, 1982). Humans also react to positive information differently from negative information. The way in which treatment results were framed in the experiments shown in Figure 4.1 made a significant difference. Negatively framed tables (reporting treatment failure rates) resulted in significantly more decisions to stop treatment than did positively framed displays reporting success rates (Elting *et al.*, 1999).

- *Human attentional limitations*: Human attention is a cognitive resource with a very limited capacity to process items (see Box 8.2). Therefore, when individuals are distracted by other tasks, they are less likely to have the capacity to attend to a new message fully. When one is receiving a message, the amount of cognitive resource available to an individual determines the quality of the inferences that person can draw. When a message is constructed, we should therefore consider the cognitive state of the individual receiving the message. For example, in a stressful situation, a clinical flow chart that makes all the steps in treating a patient explicit and requires less attention than the same information presented as paragraphs of unstructured text may be beneficial.

4.3 Grice's conversational maxims provide a set of rules for conducting message exchanges

How is it that agents, whether they are human or computer, manage to communicate effectively given the many limitations of message exchange? More importantly, given that poor communication can have a profound negative impact on healthcare delivery, what makes a good message?

One of the most influential answers to these questions comes from the work of H. Paul Grice, who took a pragmatic approach to the mechanics of conversation. Grice suggested that well-behaved agents should all try to communicate according to a basic set of rules to ensure that conversations are effective and that each agent understands what is going on in the conversation (Grice, 1975).

Grice's *co-operative principle* asks that each agent participating in a conversation should do their best to make it succeed. Agents should only make appropriate contributions to a conversation, saying just what is required, at the appropriate stage in the conversation, and only to satisfy the accepted purpose of the conversation. Grice proposed a set of *four maxims,* which explicitly defined what he meant by this principle of co-operation:

1. *Maxim of quantity*: Say only what is needed.
   1.1. Be sufficiently informative for the current purposes of the exchange.
   1.2. Do not be more informative than is required.
2. *Maxim of quality*: Make your contribution one that is true.
   2.1. Do not say what you believe to be false.
   2.2. Do not say that for which you lack adequate evidence.
3. *Maxim of relevance*: Say only what is pertinent to the context of the conversation at the moment.
4. *Maxim of manner:*
   4.1. Avoid obscurity of expression.
   4.2. Avoid ambiguity.
   4.3. Be brief.
   4.4. Be orderly.

There are some overlaps in the maxims, but they do lay out a set of rules to guide how conversations should proceed. Clearly, people do not always follow these maxims. Sometimes it is simply because agents are not well behaved. At other times, the maxims are broken because agents share insufficient common ground. A message that an expert thinks contains too much unnecessary information may be just right for a novice.

Agents can also break these rules on purpose to communicate subtle messages. For example, if someone asked you 'How much do you earn?' a wry answer could be 'Not enough!' or something as vague. Such an indirect answer clearly is unco-operative and violates the maxims of quantity, relevance and manner. However, the clear message behind the answer might be 'This is none of your business'. The intentional violation of maxims allows us to signal things without actually having to say them, either because it may be socially unacceptable or because there are other constraints on what can be said (Littlejohn, 1996).

4.4 Interruptions disrupt cognitive task processing and can lead to mistakes and harm to patients

Grice's maxim of manner recommends that a conversation should be orderly, meaning that each agent takes its turn and does not disrupt conversational flow. In reality, people often interrupt each other. Interruptions are very common in many clinical settings, especially hospital wards and emergency departments, but they are also a feature of life in apparently quiet settings such as surgery or the induction phase of anaesthesia. The frequency of interruption varies with clinical setting and patient load. Senior clinical staff often have higher interruption rates because others seek their opinion. Hospital doctors and nurses can be interrupted anywhere from once every 2 hours to more than 20 times every hour in the emergency department (Li *et al.*, 2012). The interrupting agent is not always human. The ring of a telephone and an alert when a message or e-mail arrives are demands to stop the current task and to attend to a new task.

An interruption can be defined as any disruption to a primary task caused by the arrival of an unexpected message. Interruptions happen because the interrupting agent assumes that its goals are more important than those of the receiving agent or that the receiver can return to the primary task with minimal penalty. The correctness of this assumption determines the impact of the interruption. A life critical situation may demand that clinicians be interrupted to attend to the emerging situation. In contrast, interrupting someone who is preparing an intravenous medication or calculating a drug dose can lead to a medication administration error and harm to a patient. Interrupting the administration of medications in hospital, for example, is associated with a 12 per cent increase in both procedural and clinical errors, and it exhibits a dose-response relationship in which more interruptions significantly increase the risk of error (Westbrook *et al.*, 2010). For this reason, managing interruptions has become a significant patient safety issue.

Not all interruptions are harmful, and there are settings in which interruptions appear well tolerated (Magrabi *et al.*, 2010). Indeed, interruptions are often effective tools for getting work done, for managing urgency and for opportunistic completion of tasks when appropriate individuals appear (Rivera-Rodriguez and Karsh, 2010).

Interruptions pose a risk when an interrupted primary task occupies significant attentional and memory resources. Humans are thought to have a small amount of working memory in which we can keep about five items. This mental 'to-do' list can become full when busy, and interruptions can push items from the list, leading to forgetting that a task needs to be done (Box 8.1). Where primary tasks are very similar and often repeated, memory errors can also lead to recalling that a task has been done when it has yet to be done or forgetting that a task was done and repeating it. When the task is medication administration, these types of error can be particularly dangerous.

If an interruption occurs during a sequence of sub-tasks, then its position in sequence is important. Interruptions earlier in sequence are less risky than those toward the end because recovery is more difficult. Interruptions also create time penalties. It takes time to suspend a primary task and switch to the interruption, and there is also a resumption lag before

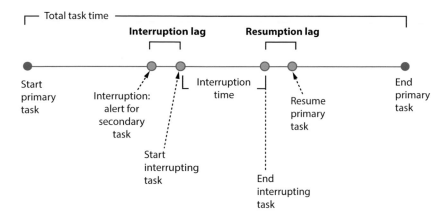

Figure 4.7
Temporal structure
of events as an
interruption intrudes
on a primary task
shows time lags at
task switching
boundaries.
(Adapted from
Trafton and Monk,
2007.)

returning to the primary task (Figure 4.7). Depending on the nature of the primary task and the interruption, one will need to suspend the primary task entirely and return to it later, or alternatively *multitask,* carrying out both tasks at the same time. When a primary task is suspended, a small period called the interruption lag occurs to allow task switching, and this is a time when mental cues about the suspended task can be stored in memory. After dealing with an interruption, a resumption lag period occurs when switching back to the primary task, at which point memory cues are retrieved to allow reorientation with the state of the primary task (Trafton and Monk, 2007).

Individuals can develop strategies to reduce the number of times they interrupt colleagues, as well as manage their work when they are interrupted. For organizations, interruption management requires policies and procedures that keep interruptions at a safe and appropriate level (Box 4.2). For safety critical tasks, some organizations use no interruption zones

Box 4.2
Informatics skill
set – interruption
management

Personal interruption management strategies

1. Interruption reduction.

Principles: Minimize the number of times you interrupt others, and use interruptions only for tasks that are both urgent and important. If worried and in doubt, interrupt.

Avoid creating risk: Check that the individual you intend to interrupt is not involved in a task that involves clinical risk. Avoid interrupting during preparation or administration of medications, injectables and chemotherapy, procedures (e.g. inserting central lines, anaesthetic induction) or concentrated quiet work (e.g. writing up medication orders or notes).

Substitute sources: Instead of interrupting, are easily available alternate information sources available? For routine information needs, consider online resources, help manuals or dedicated individuals (e.g. telephone help lines).

Substitute channels: If there is no urgency, replace synchronous interruptions with asynchronous messages (e.g. e-mail, voicemail, text notes).

Delay: Come back when the individual is less busy or no longer engaged in high-risk clinical tasks.

Status asymmetry: Do not avoid necessary interruptions because an individual is more senior than you.

Escalate your concern: If you are ignored, escalate your concern through repetition, indication of concern for the matter or seeking an alternate individual.

(Contd.)

Box 4.2
(Contd.)

2. Interruption handling.

Principles: Reduce interruptions either by signalling uninterruptibility or removing sources of interruption. Actively manage unavoidable interruption to minimize impact on memory and task execution.

> *Be in control:* Actively manage the way you respond to interruptions because this is less disruptive to task performance. In anticipation of interruptions:
> - *Signal unavailability:* When commencing a risky procedure or quiet time is needed, physically indicate unavailability (e.g. wear a 'no interruption' vest, avoid common area workspaces, use signs or say 'no' to interruption requests).
> - *Reduce availability:* Turn off interruptive devices (e.g. message alerts, telephone) when they would be disruptive to task.
> - *Record resumption cues proactively:* Keep a task list, write down intermediate calculations or place in task sequence, to assist with task resumption after the interruption.

At the time of interruption, have a repertoire of different pre-planned interruption handling strategies to deal with varying circumstances (Colligan and Bass, 2012). Options include:
> - *Immediately suspend and engage:* If the interruption brings a high-priority secondary task, then suspend the primary task and resume it after completion of the secondary task.
> - *Multitask:* Where the nature of primary task and interruption permit it, and both have similar priority, divide attention between them to allow parallel execution. Usually, tasks need to use different visual and auditory cognitive processing elements to permit this (e.g. talking while visually scanning a monitor is possible, but writing a medication chart and discussing a patient will require one task to be suspended).
> - *Delay engagement and cue:* To support effective resumption of the primary task, create memory cues that record the current state of the primary task or complete a subtask of the primary task before switching to the interruption. Cue strategies include mentally rehearsing your current or next task before dealing with an interruption (e.g. name of the next medication or patient) or creating a note if details are more complex.
> - *Delegate the interruption:* Quickly reallocating the interrupting task to another worker means that it does not need to be attended to, and it minimizes its impact on attention and memory.
> - *Block:* Just say 'No'. If the primary task is high priority, then it takes precedence over any interruption, and new secondary tasks are blocked.

Organizational interruption management strategies

1. Interruption reduction.
   Support information needs: Provide alternate information sources for routine requests such as telephone numbers, equipment location or how to use information systems. Research can identify the most common local requests.
   Create 'sterile' workspaces: Provide physical cues to staff that they are entering a zone where interruptions pose a safety risk. Wearing 'no interruption' vests or clear signs may be sufficient.

2. Interruption handling.
   Educate: Train clinical staff in the impact of interruption on patients' safety and how to avoid unnecessary interruption. Focus on status asymmetry rules, interruption handling strategies and training in multitasking.
   Provide memory cues: Recovery from interruption is aided when the state of the interrupted task is recorded. Clinical software should indicate progress in task and record intermediate calculations. Provide personal tools for task management.
   No blame: Allow for decisions requiring human judgement. Worried staff should be free to interrupt in a non-judgemental atmosphere.

(NIZs), taken from the idea of a sterile cockpit in aviation (Hohenhaus and Powell, 2008). NIZs can reduce interruption numbers and lead to improvements in outcome measures (Anthony *et al.*, 2010; Scott *et al.*, 2010).

Clinical environments and computer technologies can also be designed to deal with interruption. For example, an individual's capacity to recover from interruption is aided by environmental memory cues (Altmann and Trafton, 2004). When calculating a drug dose on paper, after an interruption the paper acts as a cue to re-engage with the task, thus minimizing error. Clinical systems such as electronic prescribing technologies can be designed to be tolerant of interruption (Magrabi *et al.*, 2010). User interfaces can make it clear what the current task is, where the user is in the process and display intermediate calculations, decisions or data used in the task.

Conclusions

In this chapter, we have used the idea of models and templates to develop a rich picture of the process of structuring and communicating information. Grice's maxims provide a foundation for understanding how such structuring should be carried out to maximize the effectiveness of communication. In common events such as dealing with interruptions or handing over care, these basic principles can help develop the skill sets needed to ensure that care is both safe and effective. In Chapter 5, we take this communication model and related ideas to explain the ways we can structure one of most common clinical 'messages' – the patient's record.

Discussion points

1. 'The chart is not the patient'. Explain why people may confuse the two, perhaps thinking back to Chapter 1, and explain why they should keep the two separate, perhaps thinking of the principles in this chapter.

2. Marshall McLuhan famously said 'the medium is the message'. What did he mean? Do you agree?

3. The way we interpret a message is shaped by the way a message is constructed. Give examples of the way public figures such as politicians shape their messages to have a specific impact on public opinion.

4. Politicians shape their messages differently depending upon which medium they are using at the time. Compare the way the same message will look on television news, in the newspaper, in a magazine article or when delivered over the phone or face to face.

5. In the game Chinese whispers, a message is passed along a chain from one individual to the next. By the time the message reaches the end of the chain, it is highly distorted compared with the original. Explain the possible causes of this message distortion.

6. Within healthcare, a message can be passed down long chains of individuals. What mechanisms do we have to prevent the 'Chinese whispers' effect distorting critical clinical data?

7. You need to send a copy of a 200-page paper medical record to a colleague in another institution. What is the best channel to use? Consider the impact that urgency, distance or cost could make on your answer.

8. You have a question about your patient's treatment. What is the best channel to use to obtain an opinion from a colleague?

9. What is the bandwidth of Twitter, and how does that shape the type of message sent?

10. Are all clinical interruptions bad?

11. If e-mail is asynchronous, then why is it often so interruptive?

Chapter summary

1. What a message is meant to say when it is created and what the receiver of a message understands may not be the same.

2. The structure of a message determines how it will be understood. The way clinical data are presented can alter the conclusions a clinician will draw from the data.

3. The message that is sent may not be the message that is received. The effectiveness of communication between two agents depends upon:

   a. The communication channel, which will vary in capacity to carry data and noise, which distorts the message.

   b. The knowledge possessed by the agents and the common ground between them.

   c. The resource limitations of agents, including cognitive limits on memory and attention.

   d. The context within which the agents find themselves that dictates which resources are available and the competing tasks at hand.

4. Grice's conversational maxims provide a set of rules for conducting message exchanges:

   a. *Maxim of quantity:* Say only what is needed.

   b. *Maxim of quality:* Make your contribution one that is true.

   c. *Maxim of relevance:* Say only what is pertinent to the context of the conversation at the moment.

   d. *Maxim of manner:* Avoid obscurity of expression, ambiguity; be brief and orderly.

5. The channel is selected based upon its suitability to the task:

   a. Interruptive channels are often called *synchronous* channels because they demand real-time interaction between agents.

   b. Non-interruptive channels are called *asynchronous* channels because the interaction between agents can occur at separate moments over an extended period.

6. An interruption is a disruption to a primary task caused by the arrival of an unexpected message, and it can lead to errors because memory of events is affected.

7. Different strategies can reduce the rate of interruption or mitigate the impact of interruption, including creation of no interruption zones, communication rules, provision of alternate channels and memory supports.

CHAPTER 5

Structuring

> Everyone writing in the medical record is an information designer, and is responsible for making the data recorded there easy to find and interpret.
>
> *Wyatt and Wright, 1988*

Grice's maxims give us a set of rules for conversational economy. The co-operative principle is a bargain between agents to not waste each other's time and genuinely try to say what is needed. In healthcare, the stakes are higher because time-wasting or misleading behaviour can have a negative impact on the efficiency of clinical work and patient care.

Consequently in health communication Grice's maxims are not a social nicety, but a professional necessity. When constructing a message, it is therefore insufficient simply to pass on information. It is critical that the intended individual actually receives the information, that he or she correctly interprets it and that the effort expended in understanding the message fits within the work constraints of the receiver.

How does one decide what should be put into a clinical conversation, message or document? What is 'sufficiently informative' and not obscure or ambiguous? Using the model of communication developed in Chapter 4, we now set out a process for determining the structure and content of such messages. Two clinical communication tasks – the handover of patient care and the creation of medical records – are explored using these basic principles because they both depend vitally on the approach taken to information structuring and presentation.

5.1 Messages are structured for a specific task to suit the needs of the sender and receiver

A message carries a package of data and some of the models needed to interpret the data. A message is therefore typically created to accomplish a specific purpose. For example, a request for a radiological investigation should contain both the historical patient data needed to assist a radiologist interpret the images as well as the details of the clinical conditions to be investigated. The more specific the request is about the clinician's goals in ordering the test, the more precise will be the answer.

The degree to which the purpose for which information is used can be anticipated dictates how much of that task can be embedded into the message. Compare, for example, a simple telephone directory in which companies are arranged according to their business with a directory in which companies are organized according to user tasks. In the former, which we will call a *data-oriented* directory, telephone numbers appear under headings such as 'travel agents'. In contrast, in a *task-oriented* directory, under a heading of 'planning a holiday' you could find entries to book a flight, arrange accommodation or organize health checks and vaccinations.

The data-oriented directory assumes that users have a model of their task. Although it is space efficient (most entries will appear once), an informed user will need to make multiple accesses to the directory for a complex task. The data-oriented directory is suited to handle a wide variety of tasks, many that its creators have not anticipated, because it assumes that the user knows what he or she is doing. In contrast, the task-oriented directory provides both a task model and its associated data, but the directory is only useful for a narrow range of tasks. Further, the task-oriented directory is space inefficient. One business could reappear under many different task headings. Finally, if a user's task is not supported, then the directory is of little value.

A third *template-based* approach avoids the pitfalls of both these approaches by creating a data-oriented directory along with a separate knowledge base containing the task models. Each task model describes the different steps involved in completing the task and contains cross-references into the database indicating where the data needed to instantiate this template are stored. This *template-directed* directory is optimal in terms of space usage because data duplication is minimized, and it can be used whether or not a user's task appears in the knowledge base. However, a *template-oriented* directory is a more complex information structure because the database and knowledge base need to be defined as separate entities and then cross-linked.

The Gricean 'bargain' between agents thus does not say that the message is always created to maximize the benefit of only the receiver of the message. Conversational economy means that agents agree to create messages that, on average, satisfy the needs of both sender and receiver. The cost of creating a message is as important a consideration as the cost of receiving it. The point of maximal cost may be borne by the sender, or the receiver, or shared equally, depending upon the nature of the message and the nature of the relationship between sender and receiver.

Hence we can never make the case that a specific message class is 'best' for all messages (Table 5.1). For example, when the sender and receiver share much common ground, then much of their communication will be data oriented. When ease of use rather than efficiency is the primary concern, then a task-oriented approach may be best. For example, procedures meant to be read during an emergency are probably best to be task oriented.

Messages should be structured to emphasize key elements to enable rapid and accurate understanding

When messages are crafted to support a specified task, message structure can emphasize some elements above others to minimize effort and misunderstanding. For example, the

Table 5.1 Costs and benefits of different message classes

Message class	Predominant content	Space utilization	Cost to build	Receiving agent	Cost to use	Scope of utility
Data-oriented	Data	Best	Least	Knows task	Most	Broad range of tasks
Task-oriented	Data intermingled with task knowledge	Worst	Moderate	Does not need to know all steps in task	Least	Narrow, limited to defined tasks
Template-oriented	Data and task knowledge separate but cross-linked	Worst	Most	May or may not know task	Variable, depending upon task	Broad range of tasks

classic map of London's underground train system is designed to support route planning and thus emphasizes connection and route, rather than distance and geography.

In Figure 5.1, an example of a poor clinical message is shown along with a better version. In the original radiotherapy summary, the data are organized exactly as they were dictated by the clinician. Date formats are used inconsistently, and important data lie buried within the text. The radiation dose given in the therapy is written as the abbreviation *42.9 Gy*, but *43 Gray* would probably be clearer. If the reader had never encountered the Gray as a scientific unit for the measurement of radiation, then an explanatory note defining the units in non-specialist terms would make the report even easier to understand. Using the principles in Table 5.2, the revised format is more structured and allows clinicians to find data such as the dose or duration of radiotherapy more rapidly and to interpret these data more reliably. Non-specialists can also understand more of this message.

A standard template is used to structure a message when many different people will receive it

In the game of 'Chinese whispers' a message is passed from one individual to the next along a chain. By the time the message has passed through many different agents, it typically is distorted both in structure and content. In healthcare, messages pass among many different individuals. Patient data, for example, may travel from laboratory to hospital medical record to primary care physician to patient. Indeed, the number of possible pathways a message may travel is enormous, and the combination of agents it may pass through is equally complex.

A common strategy to minimize message distortion is to adopt a public standard against which messages are constructed and against which agents can interpret a message if they receive it. If a message starts to deviate from the standard, it is a warning to agents that the message's quality may not be acceptable. For example, there are standard ways to record data obtained from a patient's history and examination, such as the use of a 'system review' that methodically categorizes data into different organ systems. Journal articles adopt a common framework of structured abstract, methods and results to ensure that studies are reported in a uniform way, thereby maximizing the chance that the articles will contain the necessary

Re **Anne Patient d.o.b 10.10.46**
    29 Some Road, Sometown, Somecounty SC9 9SC
    Node positive carcinoma of the left breast treated by
    mastectomy, chemotherapy, and radiotherapy

Radiotherapy treatment summary: the left chest wall and draining nodal areas received a dose of 42.9 Gy in 13 fractions treating three times a week with 6 MV photons. Treatment started on 15 September and was completed on 14 October 1995.

The patient will be followed up for one visit at Dr X's clinic and thereafter follow-up will be with Mr Y and Dr Z.

RADIOTHERAPY TREATMENT SUMMARY

Name: Anne Patient
Born: 10 October 1946, age 49
Address: 29 Some Road, Sometown, Somecounty SC9 9SC

Status before radiotherapy

Diagnosis	**Carcinoma left breast**
Spread	**Left axillary nodes**
Previous treatment	**Mastectomy, chemotherapy**

Radiotherapy given

Treatment type	**6 MV photons**
Site	**Left chest wall and draining nodes**
Total dose given	**43 Gray**
Schedule	**3 fractions/week from 15 September 1995 to 14 October 1995 (13 over 4 weeks)**

Follow-up plan

Radiotherapy department	**One visit – Dr X**
Other departments	**Mr Y (surgery), Dr Z (ICRF clinic)**

Summary date: 20 October 1995

Figure 5.1 Extract from an actual radiotherapy summary and below it a version revised to improve communication. (Gy = Gray, a unit of radiation measurement). (Adapted from Wright *et al.*, 1998.)

information to understand the study, as well as permitting some form of comparison among different studies. As we shall see in Chapter 22, the use of standard terms and their associated codes means that messages written by humans can be understood by computers and that computer messages can be constructed into terms likely to be understood by healthcare workers.

Standards work because all agents know they exist and are therefore motivated to learn the necessary standard structures and terminologies. These standards are a sort of publicly agreed common ground. Standards support Grice's maxims because agents know that if they use them, other agents are likely to understand them. Agents also know that if they receive a message, they have a good chance of understanding what it means. Box 5.1 summarizes the steps involved in shaping the content of a message, based on the task at hand and our understanding of the capabilities of those who will receive the message.

The remainder of this chapter turns to two specific clinical communication tasks – the handover of patient care and the crafting of medical records – in which the approach taken to message structuring is central to success.

Table 5.2   Six principles of information design that can aid interpretation of medical record data

Set the context.
For example, give the date and main purpose of the consultation.

Write informative headings.
Rather than a generic heading 'Symptoms', use a more specific heading, 'Eating problems', to aid interpretation and future retrieval.

Limit the information given under each heading.
Records with more subheadings, and fewer data under each, will be more easily used than the reverse.

Include signposts and landmarks within the records.
These can be specific locations for certain kinds of information or marking of abnormal values or adverse reactions with highlighter or marginal symbol.

Organize information to meet the needs of more than one profession.
Visual separators, such as lines or boxes, can distinguish instructions to other professionals, such as clinic nurses, from data.

Make the organization of the material visually explicit.
Vertical space between sections and horizontal indents help to signal the relationships among different parts of a medical record.

Adapted from Wright *et al.*, 1998.

1. Determine the specific purposes for which the information will be used.

2. Break down the information elements needed to achieve the task. What is needed in the database and in the knowledge base?

3. Determine who will be using the information. Is it a named individual, someone in a defined role with specific training or a general group of individuals?

4. Determine the capabilities of the receiver to interpret the message. What are you assuming is in their database and their knowledge base?

5. Determine the context in which the message is likely to be received. How much time will be available to the receiver, and how many competing tasks will they have?

6. Decide whether the message should be data oriented, task oriented or template oriented based upon the characteristics of the task(s), the agents and the available resources.

7. Arrange the information elements in a way to maximize the ease of use, and minimize misinterpretation, by the receiver.

8. Select a communication channel from those available based upon impact of the channel on the receiver, cost of channel use and bandwidth based upon message length and risk of noise corruption.

Box 5.1
Summary of the steps involved in shaping the content of a message

5.2 Clinical handover requires messages that successfully transfer responsibility for care

A *handover* or a *handoff* is a transfer of responsibility and accountability for the care of a patient from one clinician to another on a temporary or a permanent basis. Handoffs are a routine and essential feature of healthcare, and they occur at different *transitions of care,* including:

1. Inter-institution – When a patient is transported from one facility to another, including the transition of care between hospitals, and outpatient and inpatient settings.
2. Inter-departmental – When a patient moves between two departments within the same facility (e.g. from an intensive care unit [ICU] to a ward).
3. Inter-shift – The transfer of care across shifts, including night and weekend care.
4. Inter-professional – The transfer of care between individuals or teams (e.g. between specialties such as medicine and surgery).
5. Intra-team – The transfer of care between members of the same team.

At handoff, clinicians exchange information and sometimes jointly plan the next stages in care. Effective handoff is clearly critical to ensuring care continuity and patient safety. Unfortunately, there is much evidence to show that handoff practices are often deficient, and some handoffs are informal and unstructured events with highly variable content and process. Failure to communicate critical information during handoff can lead to necessary tasks not being done or repeated or to unnecessary or incorrect decisions being made in the absence of crucial information.

The consequences of handoff failure often harm the patient (Ong and Coiera, 2011). In a review of 122 malpractice claims in which patients had alleged a missed or delayed diagnosis in the emergency department, inadequate handoffs contributed to 24 per cent of the cases (Kachalia *et al.*, 2007). Another study of 889 malpractice claims found that communication failures during handoff were implicated as the cause in 19 per cent of cases involving medical trainees and in 13 per cent of other cases (Singh *et al.*, 2007).

The root cause of much handoff failure is a failure to follow the edicts behind Grice's maxims, which ask that individuals consider the needs and capabilities of those with whom they are communicating. The reasons for such failure are often found in the complex and stressed nature of clinical work:

- *Diversity of teams* – Handoff can involve multiple teams, which have differing expertise, work processes and culture. Even within the same team, the level of knowledge and experience among team members can vary greatly. Diversity is necessary to deal with complex care, but it means that individuals may not share sufficient common ground, thus leading to misunderstanding or assumptions of shared knowledge that are incorrect.
- *Ambiguity of roles and processes* – Clinicians often report not knowing when a transfer of care takes place or to whom handoff should be given (McFetridge *et al.*, 2007; Smith *et al.*, 2008). Indeed, poorly defined boundaries of responsibility are not uncommon even within teams (Williams *et al.*, 2007). Tasks that are not explicitly assigned to an individual can easily be overlooked. Conversely, more than one clinician may assume responsibility for a task, thereby leading to task duplication or conflicting actions.
- *Time and resource constraints* – When workloads are high, communication can be rushed and less interactive than normal (Horwitz *et al.*, 2009). Handoff from the emergency department to wards, for example, may often be inadequate when there is urgency in treating emergency patients. Fatigue is also a cause of reduced communication efficiency and increased error.

Safe and effective handover occurs when all parties understand their roles and responsibilities, and appropriate information is communicated. Making that happen in a setting of clinical pressures and constraints, between individuals with often different backgrounds, requires a systematic approach to handover.

As we have now seen, a common mechanism for minimizing breakdowns in communication is to develop standard communication protocols. These protocols lay down the structure and content of handover messages. Message standardization leads to consistency in message structure, reduces the opportunity for misunderstanding and assists in the detection of errors of omission.

Such protocols typically cover both verbal and written communication. Verbal handoff allows interaction between sender and receiver; points of confusion can be clarified, and the ability of the receiver to manage the patient can be assessed. Written handoff creates a persistent copy of critical information that can be accessed long after the sender has become unavailable (e.g. at night shift). Standard templates have been shown to be effective ways of ensuring that critical information is communicated at care transitions, by providing both a script for the verbal component of communication and a robust persistent record of what was said (Clark *et al.*, 2011; Wayne *et al.*, 2008).

Structuring can extend beyond the act of handover and extend into shared information that is always accessible to clinicians. For example, creating structured daily goals for patients in the ICU produced a significant improvement in the percentage of residents and nurses who understood the goals of care for the day and reduced ICU length of stay (Pronovost *et al.*, 2003). Standardizing the handoff process can diminish hierarchical barriers between senior and junior clinicians. Several methods for standardization of handover are summarized in Box 5.2.

5.3 The patient record can have many different structures

Of all the messages the clinicians receive, none receives more attention than the patient record. To ensure that the patient record supports effective communication between different healthcare practitioners, it is almost always created according to a standard structure, as would be expected from the previous discussion. There are four common record structures (Figure 5.2):

- *Integrated-record* – Data are presented in a strictly chronological way, identifying each episode of care by time and date. Data arriving from an investigation such as radiology may be followed by progress notes written by a clinician, followed by a change in medication orders. A variation of this is the *time-oriented medical record*, developed for chronically ill patients, in which data are arranged in two dimensions, according to axes of time and data type (Tange, 1996).
- *Source-oriented medical record (SOMR)* – The SOMR is organized according to the source that generated the data, typically different hospital departments. There are separate sections for medical notes, nursing notes, laboratory data, radiological results and so forth. Within each source section, data are sometimes further subdivided, for example, according to the different types of test, and then arranged chronologically.

Box 5.2
Informatics skill
set – clinical
handover

The quality and effectives of the handover of patient information can be enhanced by the adoption of several strategies, including:

Read-backs: To help ensure critical information is not missed or misunderstood, repeat back the information you have understood from the sender.

Structured goals: Create a set of daily goals for a patient's care, and place these goals in an accessible part of the medical record, to ensure that any clinicians who take over care can quickly inform themselves of the current situation, independent of the handover process.

Standardized templates: Use a pre-defined handoff structure to gather information, and then use it to structure a verbal presentation. The template should include critical fields that need to be communicated (e.g. allergy status, medication history and preference for treatment).

One such message structure is *SBAR (situation, background, assessment, recommendation)*. SBAR asks for a brief description of the clinical situation, followed by relevant background, your assessment of the situation, followed by a complete recommendation (Haig *et al.*, 2006). When a message is communicated using a well-understood standard, cognitive load is reduced. This is especially beneficial when communicating urgent messages with time or resource constraints. The SBAR template has the following elements:

Situation
What is the problem? Describe the situation, including:

● Patient's name, physician and unit.
● Brief statement of your concerns.

Background
What are the circumstances leading to this situation? Provide a brief history of the patient or situation, including:

● Admission diagnosis and admission date.
● Pertinent medical history.
● Treatment to date.

Assessment
What do you think the problem is? Assessment of the patient or situation may include:

● Vital signs.
● Changes since last assessment.

Recommendation
What needs to be done to correct the situation?

● *Protocol-driven patient record* – When a patient is being given a standard treatment for a well-understood condition such as asthma or diabetes, a standard template can be used to guide the construction of the medical record. The template or protocol is captured in a pre-structured form that dictates what specific data are to be obtained and recorded by the clinician and what the treatment plan for the patient will be.
● *Problem-oriented medical record (POMR)* – The POMR has four components – a problem list, an initial plan, a database containing all patient data and progress notes (Weed, 1968). The POMR organizes data according to the list of the patient's problems, which may be anything from symptoms through to well-defined diagnoses. The

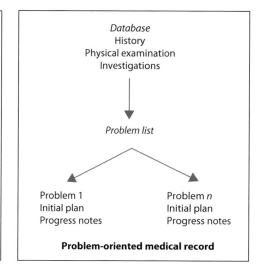

Care episode 1
Care episode 2
.
.
.
Care episode *n*

Integrated patient record

Data collection protocol

History
Physical examination
Investigations

Pre-defined treatment plan
Follow-up notes

Protocol-oriented patient record

Admission sheet
  History
  Physical examination
Doctor's progress notes
Nurse's progress notes
Medication orders
Reports e.g.
  Chemical pathology
  Microbiology
  Imaging
  Surgical
  Anaesthesia
  Intensive care
Consent forms
Correspondence

Source-oriented patient record

Database
History
Physical examination
Investigations

Problem list

Problem 1
Initial plan
Progress notes

Problem *n*
Initial plan
Progress notes

Problem-oriented medical record

Figure 5.2
Typical arrangement of different patient record structures from a hospital admission.

problem list is dynamic and is used to name, number and date each problem, and it acts as an index to the whole record. The plan describes what will be done for each problem. All progress notes, laboratory tests, treatment notes and medications are numbered according to the problem to which they relate. Progress notes are often written according to the SOAP (subjective, objective, assessment, plan) template (Table 5.3).

Looking at the different message types discussed in this chapter, it should be easy to see that:

● The *integrated record* is a data-oriented message. It provides little to no structure to data beyond a time stamp, and consequently guidance is not offered on navigation through the record or for what elements may be more important than others for a given task.

Table 5.3   Components of the progress notes in a problem-oriented medical record

S = Subjective.	What the patient states the problem is.
O = Objective.	What is identified by the practitioner via history, physical examination and tests.
A = Assessment.	Conclusion based on subjective and objective data.
P = Plan.	The method to be used to resolve the problem.

- The *SOMR* is a variation of a data-oriented record, still strongly focussed on presenting data in a simple indexed form, much like a telephone directory. There is no concept of clinical task in the SOMR, and it is up to clinicians to extract data that they need for different tasks.
- The *protocol-oriented record* is clearly a task-oriented message. It is designed to guide both the message creator and anyone who will receive it through all the necessary steps in a task.
- The *POMR* is a template-driven message because there is clear separation between some of the data, which are stored in a separate database, and the problem-specific information. However, this structure is not applied uniformly across the whole record. Some data are stored in the progress notes directly associated with individual problems, rather than in the database. Further, although there is a link from a problem to different items in the database, it points only one way. There is no link from the individual items in the database back to the different problems to which they relate. Therefore, at least in its paper-based format, the POMR is a hybrid incorporating features of both task-oriented and template-oriented messages.

No single patient record structure will suit every purpose

It is often claimed that the POMR is the 'best' patient record structure, but as we saw with different message types, this is not so for all circumstances. In some settings the POMR may be best, but in others, one of the other structures may be superior.

The integrated record seems particularly weak as a message because data are not categorized other than by time, and it is therefore difficult to integrate data according to the source of the data or the patient's problem. Yet it may be the best way to present data for patients with complex or long-standing diseases. Patient charts in intensive care are often time-oriented records so that clinicians can look across the time progress of different data sources.

The SOMR also makes it is difficult to assemble a clear picture of a patient's condition, given that data are scattered among different sources. Yet it probably remains the most popular method of structuring patient data, probably because it is a very flexible record structure and because clinicians know where they can look up specific data very rapidly.

The protocol-oriented record clearly is a very prescriptive document format, but it finds favour in highly repetitive situations, such as patient clinics, or the formal trial of new treatments. It not only guarantees that the standard of the record is uniform across different authors, but also tends to be more complete because the pre-defined structure acts as a prompt to remind clinicians to ask specific questions or carry out specific investigations. Even the most skilled clinicians can be overloaded and forget elements of a patient's work-up. Clearly, a disadvantage of the protocol-based approach is that it is best suited to single-problem patients who have well-defined diseases and treatment pathways. It is not possible to pre-define protocols for every problem a patient has, so sometimes we need a more flexible approach.

Although the POMR solves this to an extent, allowing flexibility in defining patient problems, it demands a large amount of time and commitment to write. The POMR is clearly attempting to create task-oriented messages *for the reader* of the document, by grouping data according to patients' problems, but there are no task-specific guides for the author. Consequently, it is up to the author of the POMR to decide what a distinct problem is, and different authors may label the same patient's problems in different ways. In contrast, the protocol-driven patient record pre-defines the task template for common conditions *for the writer* of the document.

The use of distinct problems as a record structure encourages integration of data within the scope of individual problems. However, the POMR also creates barriers to integration of data by clinicians. Compartmentalizing data into separate problems may inhibit a clinician from considering how one problem could relate to another, and it encourages the thinking that each problem is separate. The end result may be that a patient receives multiple medications, each addressing different problems, but no attention is paid to the total number of medications given or to a unified dosing schedule optimized to the patient's needs rather than the problems' demands (Feinstein, 1973).

The POMR may have repetition of data entries across different problems because specific data may be relevant to more than one problem. This has the impact of making the paper version of the POMR large, and this effect itself may obscure trends in data. Thus, the POMR is organized to optimize making inferences for particular problems, rather than recording and storing patient data. As a consequence, the paper POMR shows unchanged speed and accuracy of data retrieval compared with SOMRs, and as a result it has been argued that it does not improve clinical practice substantially (Fernow *et al.*, 1978; Fletcher, 1974).

Many of these problems disappear when the patient record migrates from paper form to a computer version. Computer record systems usually store a specific patient datum only once and then call up a subset of the data into different 'views' as needed. Thus, data are stored only once in the electronic POMR and are then called up when we view the patient database from the perspective of a given patient's problem. Indeed, there is no reason why in a computer-based patient record we cannot merge the different record types further. When a patient's problem is well understood, then a pre-defined protocol could be used, and when it is not, a clinician-defined problem would appear. If a time-oriented or source-oriented 'view' of data is considered more helpful, then the same data can be reassembled into these different displays. Thus, computer-based patient records have the inherent flexibility to vary their message structure to suit the needs of different clinical tasks.

Conclusions

In this chapter, we use the idea of models as templates to develop a rich picture of the process of structuring and communicating information. Communication is a complex phenomenon that is usually not explicitly thought about in routine clinical practice, yet getting it right has profound implications for the quality of patient care. We have also seen that an understanding of the communication process also helps explain the process of clinical handover and also structure of the most common of clinical 'messages' – the patient record.

Discussion points

1. Should a textbook be source oriented, task oriented or protocol directed?

2. Look at the two versions of the radiology report in Figure 5.1. Explain how the principles in Table 5.2 were used to transform the first report into the second.

3. Look again at the radiology report in Figure 5.1. Identify two different users of this report and two different ways in which the information in the report is used. Now design two new versions, each one optimized to suit the specific needs of the two different users and their tasks.

4. How much information should be conveyed during a handover of patient care?

5. What do you think about the notion in SOAP progress notes that patient-presented data are subjective and clinician-presented data are objective? What does model theory from Chapter 1 tell us about the notion of 'physician objectivity'?

6. Try and repeat Question 2, this time using Grice's maxims to explain the changes.

7. Can you justify any of the six principles of message design in Box 5.1 by using Grice's maxims?

8. Which sets of principles, Grice's or those in Table 5.2, are more useful? Explain why this may be so, by discussing the different roles in which we use a specific set of principles such as those in Table 5.2 and the more general set of Grice's maxims. Hint: Think of each set of principles as a message. Are they more like source-oriented, task-oriented, or protocol-directed messages?

Chapter summary

1. Messages are structured to achieve a specific task by using available resources to suit the needs of the receiver:

   a. Data-oriented messages contain only data.

   b. Task-oriented messages contain data structured according to specific task models.

   c. Template-oriented messages contain both data as well as separate task models cross-linked to the data.

2. Messages should be structured to emphasize key elements to enable rapid and accurate understanding. A message template is a standardized method used to structure a message when many different people will receive it.

3. Clinical handover requires messages that successfully transfer responsibility for care.

4. The patient record can have many different structures:

   a. The integrated record presents data chronologically and is data oriented.

   b. The source-oriented record is organized according to the source that generated the data and thus is also data oriented.

   c. The protocol-driven patient record is pre-structured and dictates what data are to be recorded, as well as the treatment plan, and it is task oriented.

   d. The problem-oriented record organizes data accord to a patient's problems and has four components – a problem list, an initial plan, a database containing all the patient's data and progress notes. It aims to be template oriented.

5. No single patient record structure will suit every purpose, and computer-based patient records have the inherent flexibility to vary their message structure to suit the needs of different clinical tasks.

CHAPTER 6

Questioning

Knowledge improves patient care. The more we know about our patients, their diseases and treatments, the better is the chance that patients will receive the best care possible. As a result, patients will require fewer health resources, recover more quickly and have fewer complications.

In one major study, it was shown that hospitals could save up to 70 per cent of the cost of managing patients with complex illness if clinicians conducted literature searches as part of routine care, by looking for new research data on the most appropriate treatment for diseases (Klein *et al.*, 1994). If conducting a literature search is so cost effective then it should be a standard element of clinical care, alongside laboratory tests, and perhaps even be reimbursable by insurance companies.

If searching for knowledge improves patient care, then by implication those not searching are missing key information about patient management. Indeed, individual clinicians vary widely in how well they manage different patients, depending upon their knowledge. This has led to the realization that 'knowledge of content is more critical than mastery of a generic-problem solving process' (Elstein *et al.*, 1978). In other words, having excellent clinical reasoning skills alone does not compensate for lack of clinical knowledge.

In the previous century, there was a model that clinicians, and doctors in particular, 'knew best', meaning that their opinions could not be challenged. Today, we understand that no single individual can know all the evidence to support one course of action over another and that good clinical practice is not so much 'knowing about' diseases and their treatments, but 'knowing where to find out' that knowledge.

Consequently, one of the generic skills needed by all clinicians is the ability to formulate questions that will find the answers to the gaps in their knowledge. In this chapter we explore the reasons why asking questions is an essential component of the process of patient management and examine the sources of knowledge that can be used to answer questions. We also focus on how questions can be structured to deliver answers that matter.

6.1 Clinicians have many gaps and inconsistencies in their clinical knowledge

Although an individual clinician may be very experienced it is unlikely that they will be completely up-to-date in every aspect of clinical knowledge or even know which parts of their knowledge base needs updating.

Clinicians' knowledge decays over time

The accuracy of a clinician's knowledge is statistically correlated with the number of years since graduation, and younger clinicians are more likely to have up-to-date knowledge of clinical practice compared with older colleagues (Evans *et al.*, 1984). This difference has nothing to do with ability, but is simply due to exposure to the latest knowledge. When older clinicians are exposed to up-to-date knowledge, they quickly match the knowledge of younger clinicians. This problem of knowledge decay is created by the relentless *growth* in the volume of scientific knowledge and the resulting *obsolescence* of past knowledge.

Depending upon the discipline, the number of scientific articles in existence doubles at 1- to 15-year intervals, and a new article is added to the medical literature every 26 seconds or less. As a consequence, the growth in the research literature is exponential. In a study of the knowledge associated with a single clinical disease over 110 years, 3 per cent of the literature had been generated in the first 50 years, while 40 per cent had been generated in the last 10 years (Arndt, 1992).

As knowledge grows, it also changes, and what was once believed to be true becomes obsolete. This has given rise to estimates of the 'half-life' of knowledge (the period over which half of what is believed to be true is replaced). Although the survival time of knowledge in some domains can be short (less than 5 years in physics), in some clinical domains it can stretch out to 45 years. More than half of systematic reviews, which summarize the best evidence for treatment of different conditions, need to be updated on average every 5 years, and many need to be updated within 2 years (Hersh, 2009).

It is thus no longer physically possible simply to keep 'up-to-date' by reading the latest literature. The volume of published material exceeds any human capacity to read it, let alone synthesize its meaning (Coiera and Dowton, 2000).

Clinicians' beliefs about appropriate treatment often do not accord with the facts

Clinicians' beliefs strongly influence the choices they make about patient management. Even if a clinician is exposed to the knowledge about the best course of action for a disease, the 'message' he or she hears may be distorted, for any of the reasons discussed in Chapter 4. The result is overuse of ineffective or dangerous practices or underuse of effective practices.

In one study of the beliefs of general practitioners about the effectiveness of various cancer screening procedures, there was a wide variation between the best available evidence at the time of the study and the beliefs of clinicians (Young *et al.*, 1998). Clinicians believed that many cancer screening approaches that were unsupported by evidence were effective, including skin or breast examination, digital rectal examination and flexible sigmoidoscopy. Equally concerning, although the evidence strongly supported the effectiveness of faecal occult blood testing, the practitioners believed it to be relatively ineffective.

Clinicians have many more questions about patients than they look for answers

Several studies have tried to measure the base requirement for knowledge support during routine patient care. In a ground-breaking study, 47 internal medicine physicians in an office-based practice in Los Angeles County in California were interviewed (Covell *et al.*, 1985). Although the doctors interviewed believed that they needed information once per week, the researchers estimated that actually two unanswered questions were raised for every three patients seen (about 0.67 questions per patient) – a very large gap between what is believed and what actually is. Of these questions, 40 per cent were questions about medical facts (e.g. 'What are the side effects of bromocryptine?'), 45 per cent were questions about medical opinion (e.g. 'How do you manage a patient with labile hypertension?') and 16 per cent were about non-clinical knowledge (e.g. 'How do you arrange home care for a patient?'). About one third of the questions were about treatment, one fourth about diagnosis and 14 per cent about drugs. Most importantly, only one third of questions were answered. The doctors in the study claimed that when they did search for answers, they used sources such as textbooks and journals, but in fact they were actually most likely to consult another doctor.

Many other studies have looked at these questions since that study and have mainly focussed on doctors (Smith, 1996). The studies show that:

- Knowledge gaps are routinely identified when clinicians see patients. Doctors can have anything between 0.07 and 5.77 questions per patient encounter, depending upon the study method, how a 'clinical question' is defined and the clinical setting.
- Although doctors are usually aware that they have gaps in their knowledge, they significantly underestimate their needs or overestimate the quality of their own knowledge.
- In medical practice, many of the questions relate to treatment and are most often about drug therapy.
- Further, doctors actually pursue answers to questions in only about one third of cases (Ely *et al.*, 1999). Doctors are most likely to pursue questions about drug prescription (see Table 6.2). Two factors have been shown statistically to predict whether a doctor would pursue a question – whether the doctor believed that an answer actually existed to the question and the urgency of the patient's problem (Gorman, 1995). If evidence is immediately available, then a clinician is more likely to access it, but when evidence is not readily available, clinicians rarely search for it (Sackett and Straus, 1998).
- Answers are found for between 25 per cent (Gorman, 1995) and 90 per cent of those questions that are pursued (Sackett and Straus, 1998). Doctors spent about 2 minutes searching for an answer (Ely *et al.*, 1999).
- Of the methods used to access knowledge, most studies also agree that clinicians prefer to ask another human if possible, ahead of accessing formal sources such as textbooks and drug manuals. Searches of the primary literature are rarely performed.

● When questions are answered, it does appear that the evidence found changes the approach of clinicians. When evidence was sought in one study, at least one member of a hospital team changed the approach 48 per cent of the time (Sackett and Straus, 1998). Accessing evidence seems to change clinical decisions about 13 per cent of the time, initiate it 18 per cent of the time and confirm existing plans 70 per cent of the time (Haynes *et al.*, 1990).

If keeping your knowledge up-to-date is no longer feasible because the growth in knowledge exceeds your capacity to read it, then searching for changes in clinical knowledge is a basic component of patient care. The difficulty in even keeping textbooks up-to-date has caused some investigators to argue that we should burn all our textbooks and instead use online information technology to find the answer to clinical questions (Sackett *et al.*, 2000). Thus, the whole notion of ongoing clinical education changes from one of periodic updates to a clinician's knowledge to a 'just in time' model in which a clinician checks the medical knowledge base, potentially at every clinical encounter (Coiera and Dowton, 2000).

6.2 Well-formed questions seek answers that will have a direct impact on clinical care

Answers to questions should make a difference. They should return knowledge that has a direct impact on the task that initiated the question. Given that most clinicians work in time-pressured environments and that the range of potential questions that could be asked is enormous, it is essential that the question posed be focussed on accessing the knowledge that is most likely to influence decision-making.

In any field of expertise, there are general principles and theories that underpin the discipline. Such knowledge has sometimes been called *background knowledge,* to reflect that the knowledge sits in the background and is brought forward to solve different problems from time to time. In contrast, individual situations may require very specific knowledge that has little application beyond that context. Such knowledge is called *foreground knowledge* (Sackett *et al.*, 2000). A background question could be 'What are the causes of asthma?' and a foreground question could be 'What is the treatment for an episode of severe bronchoconstriction in a child?'

As a general rule, the number of background questions that arise in a clinical situation diminishes as an individual becomes more experienced and builds up a knowledge base. With experience, the questions asked are more likely to be foreground ones about the specifics of managing a particular situation.

Because background questions are about general principles, they are likely to have a smaller impact on the immediate situation and can be asked at another point in time. Foreground questions that have a high impact on care ask for *patient-oriented evidence that matters* (POEM) and should therefore be asked and answered as an integral part of clinical work (Slawson *et al.*, 1994). In contrast, background questions usually ask for *disease-oriented evidence* (DOE) (Table 6.1).

Typically, the medical literature contains much more DOE than POEM. One way to distinguish POEM from DOE is to determine how many assumptions the knowledge requires us to make before it can be applied. For example, DOE may help identify cancer earlier. However, until a clinical trial actually shows that identifying the cancer earlier causes a

Table 6.1 Examples of disease-oriented evidence and patient-oriented evidence that matters*

DOE		POEM
Many assumptions needed to ascribe benefit.	Some assumptions needed.	Few assumptions needed to ascribe benefit.
Drug A lowers cholesterol.	Drug A decreases cardiovascular disease mortality and morbidity.	Drug A decreases overall mortality.
Antiarrhythmic A decreases PVCs.	Antiarrhythmic A decreases arrhythmia symptom.	Antiarrhythmic A decreases mortality.
Antibiotic A is effective against common pathogens of otitis media.	Antibiotic A sterilizes middle ear effusions in patients with otitis media.	Antibiotic A decreases symptoms and complications of otitis media.

DOE, disease-oriented evidence; POEM, patient-oriented evidence that matters; PVCs, premature ventricular contractions.

*The number of assumptions needed to apply the evidence to a specific patient decreases from left to right as the evidence becomes more case specific.

After Slawson et al., 1994.

reduction in morbidity or mortality, or in resource use, then its value is unclear. When one studies the type of question that clinicians are most likely to ask, the most frequent questions are all POEMs (Table 6.2).

Because clinical knowledge is incomplete, it will not always be the case that specific patient-oriented evidence can be located. In such circumstances, it makes sense to turn to the next best available evidence, which in this case may be disease-oriented knowledge. Using DOE does require the making of assumptions, and sometimes the process of thinking this way is called *reasoning from first principles*. For example, knowing that insulin has the effect of reducing blood levels of glucose, one could conclude that giving insulin to a patient with chronically high blood sugar levels would help reduce the sugar levels. One typically reverts to reasoning from first principles when exposed to a new set of circumstance, for which no prior first-hand knowledge is available to help.

Table 6.2 The 10 most common question structures asked by family doctors and the likelihood that once asked, it would be pursued

Generic question	Frequency asked (%)	Frequency pursued (%)
What is the cause of symptom X?	9	9
What is the dose of drug X?	8	85
How should I manage disease or finding X?	7	29
How should I treat finding or disease X?	7	33
What is the cause of physical finding X?	7	18
What is the cause of test finding X?	4	40
Could this patient have disease or condition X?	4	14
Is test X indicated in condition Y?	4	29
What is the drug of choice for condition X?	3	47
Is drug X indicated in situation Y?	3	25

After Ely et al., 1999.

2008). *Decision velocity* measures the time it takes to make a clinical decision when aided by information retrieval, and it is useful when we need to understand the impact of system use in time-pressured settings (Coiera *et al.*, 2008). Ultimately, one needs to measure the downstream impact of using a search system on clinical decisions and patient outcomes (see Chapter 11). For example, we may want to compare the number of correct and incorrect decisions clinicians make when aided by information retrieval and when unaided (Westbrook *et al.*, 2005).

Conclusions

Clinicians need to ask questions if they are to deliver safe and effective healthcare. With so many gaps in their knowledge clinicians need to consider seeking knowledge to support their practice as a routine part of clinical work, no different from ordering a laboratory test or conducting a physical examination. In this chapter we focussed on how such questions should be structured to maximize the quality of information received. In Chapter 7, we take a step back from the specific content of clinical questions and look at the overall process of searching for information. It is not enough to know what to ask. One also has to understand the process of knowing whom to ask and how to proceed if you are not immediately successful.

Discussion points

1. Will it always be the case that DOE is less useful than POEM?

2. Using Venn diagrams, follow the logic used to demonstrate DeMorgan's theorem for the union of two sets in Box 6.1, to prove the truth of the equivalent law that *not (A and B) = (not A) or (not B)*.

3. Using a similar approach, demonstrate the truth of the law of absorption for: the union-intersection case: *A and (A or B) = A*; for the intersection-union case *A or (A and B) = A*.

4. Is exact-match or partial-match searching more appropriate when searching for evidence to inform clinical decision-making?

5. What are the advantages and limitations of conducting a Medline search using the pre-defined clinical queries contained in Table 6.3?

Chapter summary

1. Clinicians have many gaps and inconsistencies in their clinical knowledge because:

    a. Clinicians' knowledge of treatment decays over time.

    b. Clinicians' beliefs about appropriate treatment often do not accord with the facts.

    c. Clinicians have many more questions about patients than they look for answers.

2. Well-formed questions seek answers that will have a direct impact on clinical care.

    a. Foreground questions that have a high impact ask for patient-oriented evidence that matters (POEM).

    b. Background questions usually ask for disease-oriented evidence (DOE).

(Contd.)

3. *Partial-match search engines* take a set of terms and return documents with the highest weight, calculated by parameters including term frequency, term scarcity and document importance (e.g. as measured by the number of links to the document or number of times it has been accessed).

4. *Exact-match search engines* use Boolean logic and a query language to construct well-formed search expressions.

5. Well-formed questions are both accurate and specific. Performance can be measured by:

   a. The number of *false-positive* documents retrieved.

   b. The number of *false-negative* documents missed.

   c. The *precision*, which is the proportion of relevant documents returned by the search.

within any agent is also a search space that can be drilled down into to find the specific piece of knowledge we are after.

For example, in seeking the answer to a clinical question raised in the care of a patient, the initial search space could consist of several colleagues, a bibliographic database such as Medline and some textbooks. Choices need to be made about which agent to ask first, and the way the agent is to be interrogated, as we explore the knowledge that an agent possesses. The 'search' through the knowledge base of a fellow human requires a different process from the way we ask questions of Medline.

Consider, for example, the way questions are structured and pursued in a legal cross-examination of a witness in a courtroom. Although the lawyer is not constructing well-formed Boolean statements to a database, the process of question formation and sequencing is just as deliberate. Whereas a database is deterministic, by returning the same result for a given question time and again, humans vary in their responses to a question. Cognitive biases may be in operation, and cognitive loads or lack of common ground may limit their capacity to answer.

7.4 Search strategies are designed to find the answer in the fewest possible steps

For search to occur, there needs to be a structure or map through the search space to act as a reference point. Otherwise, the search is essentially a random process in which we hope eventually to bump into the thing we are seeking by chance. For example, a book has a structure of chapters and subheadings, as well as an index, that can be used to guide the search process. We have already met such directory structures in Chapter 4, where they were introduced to explain the different types of message. Each of the patient record structures discussed in Chapter 4 is also an attempt at creating a structured search space to assist data and knowledge retrieval.

Search spaces are often thought of as a branching tree-like structure, with a hierarchy of nodes corresponding to particular elements in a search space. The links between the nodes represent the path the searcher must follow from one to the other. The table of contents of a book is a good example of a search space, structured according to a hierarchy of chapters, sections and subsections (Figure 7.2).

The topmost node of the tree to which everything else connects is called the *root* node. Sometimes the final nodes at the end of the tree are called *leaf* nodes, the node above another

Figure 7.2
Search spaces can be represented as a tree, with the entry point to the space at the topmost or 'root' node, which is connected via links to other nodes, eventually terminating in 'leaf' nodes.

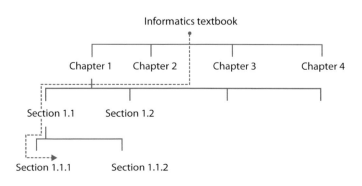

node is called its *parent,* and the node below a parent is its *sibling,* beautifully mixing botanic and genealogic metaphors. The different collections of nodes and links are called *branches,* and the route we take as we 'walk' through the tree is the traversal *path,* adding a recreational flavour to the metaphors. In Figure 7.2, 'Textbook' is the root node, and 'Subsection 1.1.1' is a leaf node. The dotted line connecting these two nodes follows a path that descends the branches of the tree, and 'Chapter 1' is a parent of 'Section 1.1'.

A *search strategy* is the plan that directs the way an agent searches in a space. If the search space is constructed like a tree, then the strategy directs the choices made in walking along the branches of the tree, by looking for a node that has the information we want.

Any strategy for navigating through a search tree is constructed from various combinations of three basic actions:

1. Move down a link from a parent node to a sibling node.
2. Evaluate a node to see whether it matches the search criteria.
3. Backtrack up a link, moving from sibling back to parent.

So, for example, a simple strategy could be to:

1. Start at the root node.
2. *Repeat* the following steps:
   a. *If* the node satisfies the criteria, then we can stop the search.
   b. *If* the node does not match search criteria, then we continue down the tree moving from parent to the next leftmost sibling that has not been searched.
   c. *If* we have reached a leaf node, then we backtrack up one link and continue the process from there.

There are several different classic search strategies that can be followed when navigating a search space (Figure 7.3). We can search the space *systematically,* where we start at the beginning and then keep looking at every item until we find what we want:

- The search strategy described earlier is a systematic process called a *depth-first search* because we keep diving more deeply into the search space until we can go no further and only then come back somewhat reluctantly, to resume the dive. Looking for information in a textbook, the depth-first strategy starts at the first chapter, opens it up and then reads each section before returning to open up a new chapter.
- A *breadth-first search,* in contrast, will examine a node, backtrack immediately if it does not find an answer and continue to explore all the nodes at the same level. Only then, if it is unsuccessful, will the strategy move to a deeper level. So, in looking for a section in a textbook, a breadth-first search would first browse all the chapter headings, to look for a match, and only then do go down one level and open up a chapter.

Systematic searches are bound to find an answer if one exists in the search space, but it may take a long time to get there. When time is short, it makes sense to try to use an *analytic search* strategy, in which the searcher uses prior knowledge to focus on areas of the space that are most likely to contain the information being sought:

- A *heuristic search* uses approximate rules of thumb based upon past experience to point the search in the right direction. For example, a rule of thumb could be 'if you are

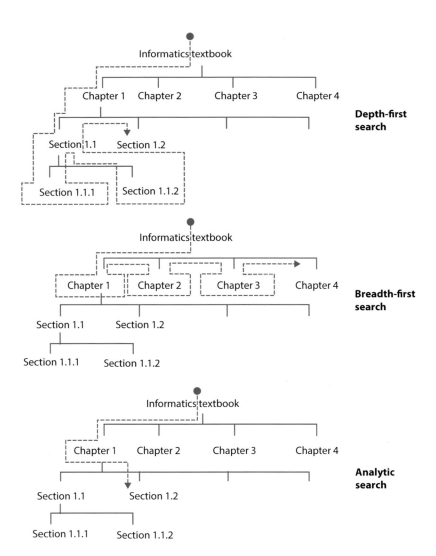

Figure 7.3
A search space can be explored systematically by using a depth-first or breadth-first strategy, eventually terminating when the required item is found. When specific knowledge about the location of an item exists, the search can be analytic and ignore parts of the search space, by targeting the most likely spots where the item can be found, using heuristics or more complex models.

looking for the final diagnosis of a patient in the medical record, first look for it in the most recent medical discharge summary'. Table 7.1 lists some commonly used heuristics to track down papers in the biomedical literature.

- A *model-based search* uses a precise model to guide the search. For example, a search party hunting for a lost hiker may use satellite maps, the known direction in which the hikers were heading and a mathematical estimate of how far they are likely to have walked since they set out, to identify the most likely area to start the search. When looking for evidence, a clinician may use Medical Subject Headings (MeSH) keywords that model the content of journal articles, along with a limit on publication date to identify the part of the search space that is most likely to contain the documents being sought.

Heuristic search has the advantage that it usually is simple and, more often than not, will come up with the right answer if the heuristics are based upon real experience. Experts often

Table 7.1   Example heuristics that can guide a search through the biomedical literature

Heuristic	Description of search strategy
Journal run	Having identified a journal that is central to one's topic of interest, one reads or browses through issues or volumes of the journal.
Citation search	Using a citation index or database, one starts with a citation and determines what other works have cited it.
Area scan	After locating a subject area of interest in a classification scheme, one browses materials in the same general area.
Footnote chase	One follows up footnotes or references, thus moving backward in time to other related materials.
Index or catalogue subject search	One looks up subject indexing terms or free text terms in a catalogue or abstracting and indexing service (online or offline) and locates all references on one's topic of interest.
Author subject search	Having found an author writing on a topic of interest, one looks up that author in catalogues, bibliographies or indexes to see whether he or she has written any other materials on the same subject.

Adapted from Bates, 1990.

have the best heuristics because they have refined them over many years of use. Model-based strategies require more calculation and reasoning to identify the target area, and if time is short, they may not be optimal. Neither the heuristic nor the model-based strategies can guarantee success, unlike the systematic search strategies, because analytic methods exclude parts of the search space. Unless we can guarantee that the thing being looked for is within the area defined by the analytic method (and we usually cannot do that with clinical evidence), then there is a chance we are looking in the wrong place.

The process of search is often an iterative one, as shown in Figure 7.1. Depending on how well the search process is advancing, it may make sense to keep the current strategy, or if it looks like the right answer is not going to be forthcoming within an acceptable time, the strategy may be changed.

For complex search tasks, it may make sense to combine different search strategies, to maximize the likely outcomes. For example, when looking for a specific section in a textbook, it may be reasonable to start with a breadth-first search of the table of contents in the knowledge that the textbook is hierarchically structured. Once a likely chapter is identified, perhaps using some heuristic knowledge about where the answer is likely to reside, then the reader could switch to a depth-first search of the chapter, combing it systematically until the relevant sections are found. If this does not succeed, then the reader could switch to a different representation of the search space and use the book's index to identify likely pages.

Database search terms are used to create a working document search space

Sometimes a search space is given to us explicitly, such as a table of contents listing. In other cases, we use tools to create a search space for a specific task. For example, when searching a document database for specific articles, such as Medline, the potential search space is many millions of documents. In such a situation, it does not make sense to search all the documents individually. Instead, we extract a subset of documents that are most likely to contain the specific documents in which we are interested. For example, we may ask only for documents published in the last 6 months or documents that match specific keywords.

To start a search with a database, one should try to ask the most specific question possible. For example, rather than using the keyword 'diabetes', the more specific term 'insulin-dependent diabetes' would be used. Once the database query has been made, the database returns a set of documents, which constitute the working search space the searcher will actually look through. When a search space of tractable size is generated, then the items can be inspected directly to see whether they contain the target items.

As the search progresses, it may be necessary to refine the strategy. For a given question, there are two search space refinement strategies possible:

- *Specific to general enlargement* – If it seems that the target of the search is not present in the search space retrieved, for example, because it contains only a very few documents, then the question may have been too specific. We then need to generalize it, which has the effect of enlarging the working search space.
- *General to specific narrowing* – Alternatively, if the space is too large, with too many documents, then the question may have been too general. We may wish to restrict it by becoming more specific in our question.

There are two different ways of changing how specific or general a question is. One way of performing such *query reformulation* is essentially mechanical, in which we play with the syntax or structure of the query, and the second is semantic, in which we play with the meaning of the query (Figure 7.4).

Syntactic query reformulation – Most queries consist of several words, usually implicitly joined together with the logical operator 'and'. As a rule, the more keywords given as search terms, the more specific is the search, and the fewer items will match the search specification. The fewer the number of terms in a query, the more general it is. Consequently, we can make a query more or less specific by simply adding or subtracting terms from the query. For

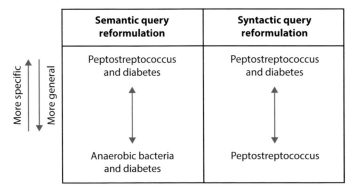

Figure 7.4   When an initial query to a database does not yield results, it may be because the question is either too specific or too general. To improve its performance, the query can be reformulated by altering either its syntactic structure or the semantics of the concepts being explored.

Table 7.2 A record of the sequence of actions taken as a clinician searches for an answer to a clinical question by choosing which knowledge sources to interrogate and by refining the question posed to each knowledge source, based upon the success of the query in retrieving appropriate documents

What anaerobic microorganism is most commonly found in osteomyelitis associated with diabetic foot?			
Knowledge source	Query	No. documents retrieved	Query action
PubMed	Anaerobic bacteria AND osteomyelitis	90	First guess
PubMed	Anaerobic bacteria AND osteomyelitis AND diabetes	8	Syntactic specification
Medline Plus	Anaerobic bacteria AND osteomyelitis AND diabetes	0	Change knowledge source
Medline Plus	Anaerobic bacteria AND diabetes	0	Syntactic generalization
Medline Plus	*Peptostreptococcus* AND diabetes	0	Semantic generalization
Textbook	*Peptostreptococcus* AND diabetes	6	Change knowledge source
Textbook	*Peptostreptococcus*	9	Syntactic generalization

example, in Table 7.2, the query 'anaerobic bacteria and osteomyelitis' can be made more specific by adding on the term 'diabetes'. Conversely, it can be made more general by dropping a term such as 'osteomyelitis'.

Instead of altering the terms, we can also manipulate the logical operators joining them. For example 'diabetes and osteomyelitis' is a more specific query than 'diabetes or osteomyelitis' (see Box 6.1). Some databases allow queries to contain exact phrases such as 'diabetic osteomyelitis', and phrase searches are very specific because they look for the exact appearance of the phrase. In contrast, breaking the phrase down into its component words to produce 'diabetes and osteomyelitis' requires only that both words appear in the same document or perhaps near each other and therefore should yield more matches.

Semantic query reformulation – It is also possible to make a question more or less specific by changing the words used. For example, 'chair' is a more specific term than 'furniture' and more general than 'dining chair'. Similarly, *'Peptostreptococcus'* is a more specific concept than 'anaerobic bacteria'. Making this type of change to a query requires knowledge of the meaning of the question and the terms in the query. We can imagine that words come from a hierarchy that organizes them conceptually, much like a taxonomy, and move up or down the hierarchy to make the term more or less general (see Figure 22.3).

● A semantic reformulation can also simply restate the query by using synonyms or alternate wording. For example, 'kidney stones' and 'renal calculi' are semantically equivalent expressions. However, if a database is unable to check for such semantic equivalents automatically (e.g. by using MeSH), then the two searches will potentially retrieve very different document sets. If completely different semantic concepts are chosen in the reformulation, the effect is not to narrow or expand the existing search space, but rather to define a new and entirely different space (Figure 7.5).

Figure 7.5
When search spaces (S) are large, a subset is usually selected to produce a working search space, W. Using knowledge about the likely location of the search target, there is a good chance that the item being looked for will be found in W. W can be modified if the initial working search space is too small, too large or looks like it does not contain the target of the search.

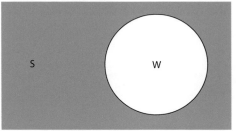

When searching in a database, we usually retrieve a working subset **W** of the total search space **S** to search through.

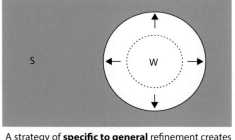

A strategy of **specific to general** refinement creates the smallest, most specific, working search space and then expands it until the search is successful.

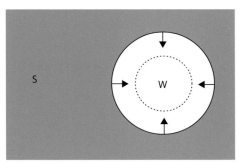

A strategy of **general to specific** refinement creates the largest, most general, working search space and then contracts it until the search is successful.

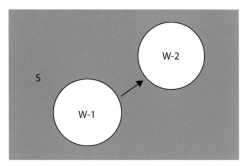

If the initial working search space is fruitless, a new working search space can be generated using different criteria to select candidate items.

If, after using such strategies, the item is not found, it may be necessary to reconsider the overall search strategy. It may be that the wrong terms are being used to locate the search items, in which case a complete re-thinking is needed to describe the search target in other ways. Alternatively, the item may not be in the sources being searched, and it may be necessary to alter the knowledge sources in which the search is conducted. This may mean looking at different databases or consulting an expert for advice on where to look next.

Patient history taking and examination combine analytic and systematic search methods

When a map exists, we use it, and when none exists we build our own map, much like leaving breadcrumbs through a forest. Consequently, when no search structure exists, it is up to the individual asking the question to impose a structure on the search space, which will then act as a reference point to guide the knowledge seeking process.

The process of patient history taking can be seen as a search for information (Figure 7.6). No map comes purpose built with a patient's history, so it is necessary to impose a map to guide the search. Taking a patient's history is actually a controlled traversal of a search space, structured according to an externally imposed model of organ systems. There are many different ways to take a patient's history, but one of the most common approaches is to:

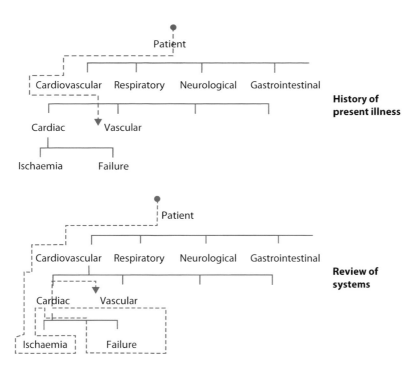

History of
present illness

Review of
systems

Figure 7.6
Taking a patient's
history is a process of
search with an
imposed template to
guide the search.
The standard review
of systems is a
systematic process,
examining each
physiological system
in turn, in an
approximately
depth-first manner. In
contrast, taking the
history of present
illness is much more
analytic, requiring
the use of knowledge
to guide the search
to identify specific
issues identified by
the patient.

1. Take a history of present illness (HPI).
2. Conduct a review of systems (ROS).
3. Take a past, family and social history.

Each step approaches search in a different way. The ROS is systematic in that it forces an exploration of different physiological systems and ensures that the whole search space is covered. It is thus a kind of depth-first search. The ROS is a series of questions that systematically explores body systems in an effort to identify relevant signs or symptoms from a patient. An ROS asks a few key questions for each system that is covered and will probably examine in turn the cardiovascular, respiratory, gastrointestinal, genitourinary, musculoskeletal, neurological, endocrine and other systems (Mikolanis, 1997).

In contrast, taking the HPI is an analytic search, and it is here that a clinician's experience, accumulated knowledge and rules of thumb helps home in on the key issues presented by the patient. Starting with a chronological description of the present complaint, the clinician then tries to determine what the core problem may be with a targeted set of questions.

By combining the systematic aspects of the ROS with the analytic of the HPI, the process of history taking attempts to be both efficient, homing in rapidly on the most likely issues, and comprehensive, ensuring that key issues that may be hidden to the patient may also surface. The systematic nature of the ROS also ensures that less experienced clinicians have templates to guide their search, and this increases the likelihood that relevant patient data are discovered.

In most circumstances there is a trade-off between a comprehensive history-taking process, which is time consuming, and the focussed analytic process, which may miss some details, but usually targets the key problem. In clinical situations in which time is of the

8. Search query reformulation may be semantic or syntactic.

9. Patient history taking and examination combine analytic and systematic search methods. A review of systems is like a depth-first search, whereas a history of present illness is an analytic search.

10. An answer is evaluated to see whether it is well formed, specific, accurate and reliable by examining:

    a. Syntax, its terminology, its complexity and structure.

    b. Semantics, by looking at its meaning and the quality of that answer.

11. The quality of an answer can be ascertained by the level of evidence used to create it or, if nothing else is available, the existence of a quality label that attempts to guarantee the pedigree of the information provided.

CHAPTER 8

Making decisions

> Evidence does not make decisions, people do.
>
> *Haynes* et al., *2002*
>
> You only see what you look for. You only look for what you know.
>
> *Anon*

Nothing gets done without someone making a decision. Patients are treated, or not treated, because someone has looked at the facts of the case, the available scientific evidence, thought through the consequences of the different options and made a choice. Often these clinical choices arise out of mutual agreement between patient and clinician or among different members of a clinical team.

In previous chapters we saw how a question should be structured and communicated and how the search for an answer should proceed. Now, we take a step back and look at where questions come from in the first place and what we do once we have our answers.

Decision-making is rarely a clear-cut affair, and most decisions are inevitably compromises. Decisions reflect not just 'the evidence', logic and probability, but also our goals, our values and the available resources. Decisions are almost always compromised by uncertainty and, when humans are the decision makers, by our in-built cognitive biases.

8.1 Problem solving is reasoning from the facts to create alternatives and then choosing one alternative

Clinical care can be thought of as a set of problems presented to patients and clinicians. Clinical problems can come in many forms. They may, for example, be diagnostic – 'What is the cause of my chest pain?', therapeutic – 'How do I treat rheumatoid arthritis?', prognostic – 'How long do I have to live?' or about resource management – 'What is the most cost-effective way to run a hospital emergency department?'

Figure 8.1   The problem-solving process is an iterative cycle of discovering data, reasoning from it to form hypotheses and, when no further data would improve the likely outcome, selection of the most plausible hypothesis. The process of search is captured in the 'question and answer' box and can be expanded into the smaller steps shown in Figure 7.1.

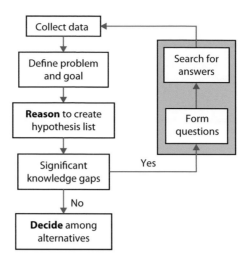

The process of problem solving is essentially the same for most tasks (Figure 8.1), and it begins when new data suggest there is a problem. For example, the presentation of new clinical symptoms or a cash-flow shortfall in a departmental budget could indicate the presence of a new problem that requires attention.

Once a problem is identified, we next decide what it is to be done about it. For example, if a department will always be given operating funds, whether or not it goes into deficit, then overspending may not really be a problem. If, conversely, failure to keep to budget threatens the operation of the organization, then action is needed. Consequently, it is important first to define the exact problem and to ascertain whether it needs to be solved, and its relative importance, because this information determines what happens next. Time is short and resources scarce, and it is probably just as harmful to solve unimportant problems as it is to set out to solve the wrong problem.

The next step in the problem-solving process is to think through what the alternative solutions may be. This is often described as the process of *hypothesis generation* and creates a list of alternatives from which the best choice is selected. If the problem is diagnostic, then the hypothesis list contains potential diagnoses. If the problem is therapeutic, then the list contains potential treatments.

At this stage there may not be enough evidence at hand to generate a satisfactory list of candidate hypotheses. This is the 'knowledge gap' that we encountered in Chapter 6. As we now know, in such situations, appropriate questions are formed and a process of search commences, to look for answers to those questions. In clinical practice, the evidence surrounding a given case may be obtained from the patient's history, physical examination or laboratory investigations. The wider evidence may be contained in knowledge about similar situations that comes from the scientific literature.

A successful search results in the arrival of new evidence that will then be integrated into the problem-solving cycle. The impact of the new evidence could simply be to reduce the number of active hypotheses by eliminating some candidates. New evidence may be sufficiently informative that it allows a choice to be made among different hypotheses, or it may cause the whole problem to be re-evaluated and new hypotheses generated.

Potentially, many iterations of this cycle of data gathering and hypothesis generation can occur, until the decision maker believes that there is enough clarity to move on to choosing among hypotheses. The key to this stage of the problem-solving process is to keep the initial goal in mind. For example, if the goal is to quickly stabilize a critically ill patient who has presented to an emergency department, then the problem-solving goal is not to come up with a detailed diagnosis and therapy plan, which may take many days, but to stabilize the patient. In such circumstances, the problem-solving goal determines a rapid resolution to the process. In contrast, a clinician managing a patient who has presented with a complicated and slow-onset auto-immune disorder may need many problem-solving cycles, with the potential diagnoses refined as different test results are returned.

The final step in the problem-solving process is to make a decision. This involves examining the list of competing hypotheses, supported by the assembled evidence, and choosing the one that is most appropriate. The criteria for making that choice need to reflect the initial goal. For example, a patient may have an incurable disease, and some treatment options may prolong life but make the patient's life unbearable because of pain and stress. Other treatment options may lead to an earlier death, but through the use of palliative treatments will ensure that the patient is relatively comfortable for that time. Clearly, in such cases, the choice of treatment is not simply derived from the scientific evidence, which could favour the treatment that most prolongs life. The choice is as much one of the patient's values and preferences, and in situations such as this, there is no right answer, but a spectrum of preferences that causes different individuals to draw different conclusions from the same evidence.

8.2 Hypotheses are generated by making inferences from the given data

Problem solving begins with data and the need to draw some conclusions from the data. In Chapter 2, we saw that this process requires a *database,* a *knowledge base* and *rules of inference.* Rules such as 'if the pH is greater than 7 then it is abnormally high' may be part of a clinician's knowledge base. The *rules of inference* specify how we apply the knowledge base to data. There are many different possible rules of inference, but the two most important from a clinical viewpoint are the rules of logic and the rules of probability.

The rules of logic infer what is known to be true, given the facts

If asked, most clinicians would say that the logical process of diagnosis is most like the process of *deduction,* often associated with the fictional detective Sherlock Holmes. In fact, a diagnosis is obtained by using a logical rule called *abduction.* Along with *induction,* these three together form the basic rules of logical inference (Figure 8.2).

The differences among these logical rules are straightforward. We start by assuming there is a *cause and effect* statement about the world that we know to be true. For example, assume that 'pneumonia causes fever' is always true. Pneumonia in this case is the cause, and fever is the effect. Another statement could be that 'septicaemia causes fever'.

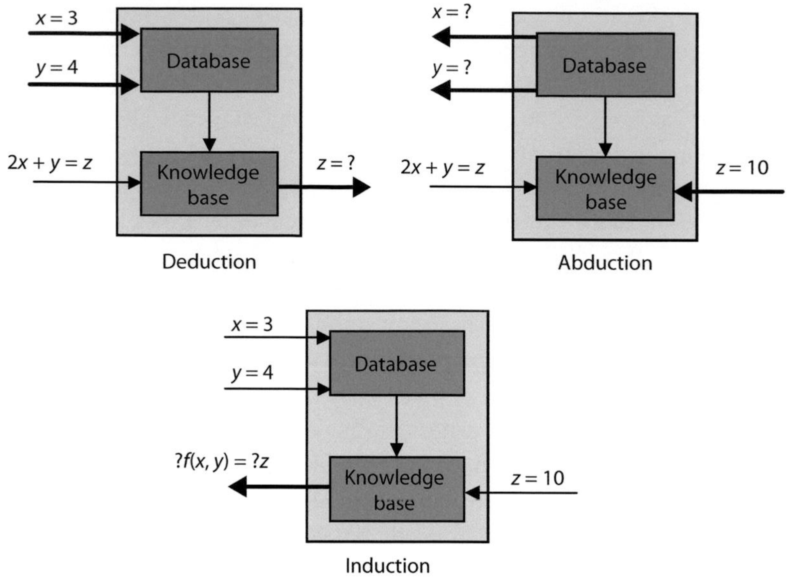

Figure 8.2
The three basic types of logical reasoning are deduction, abduction and induction. Each method proceeds from a different set of inputs to infer their logical consequences.

We can write these 'rules' in the following way:

If pneumonia *then* fever.
If septicaemia *then* fever.

For the process of deduction, we are told that a cause is true and then infer all the effects that arise naturally as a consequence. Having been told that a patient has pneumonia, deduction will tell us that the patient will therefore develop a fever.

In contrast, abduction takes the cause and effect statements we know and, given an observed effect, generates all known causes. In this case, we may be told that a patient has fever. Abduction would say that both pneumonia and septicaemia are possible causes.

Abduction allows us to produce a list of alternate hypotheses to explain the given data. Note that whereas deduction produces statements of certainty, abduction produces statements of possibility. To choose amongst the options generated by abduction, one may need to seek further information that clearly differentiates among the hypotheses. In some cases, the data are so clear that a single hypothesis is confirmed. When the pattern is so distinctive of a disease that it can be nothing else, the pattern is labelled pathognomonic (literally, 'naming the disease').

The basic rules of logic use simple operators such as *if, then, and, not* and *or,* which we already encountered in Chapter 6, in which quite complex rules of inference such as DeMorgan's theorem were introduced.

In contrast to abduction and deduction, which use cause and effect statements, the role of induction is to discover these statements from observations. For example, a doctor may have observed many patients who have had fevers. Some of these patients die, and post-mortem examination shows they all have an infection of the lung, which the doctor labels 'pneumonia'. The doctor then may hypothesize the (incorrect) rule that 'fever causes pneumonia'.

Unlike the other rules of logic, induction is unsound. In other words, it may lead to false conclusions. Thus, when our doctor finds a feverish patient who does not have pneumonia on autopsy, the original conclusion becomes invalid. Perhaps then, the doctor re-uses induction to hypothesize the reverse statement 'pneumonia causes fever'. Induction then is the process of generalization which creates our models of the world.

The rules of probability infer what is most likely to be true, given the facts

In classical logic, things are either true or they are not. There is no space for imprecision. However, such clarity is often lacking in the real world, and it is more useful to talk about how likely an event could be. A middle-aged smoker with known heart disease and chest pain may have any number of conditions that could plausibly cause pain, but given our past experience with similar patients, the likelihood is that the pain is caused by myocardial ischaemia. As we saw in the previous section, the rules of logic allow us to generate a candidate list, but in clinical medicine, the full list of possible diagnoses may be very long. Consequently, it makes sense to consider only those hypotheses that are most likely. Statistical rules of inference allow the likelihood that a hypothesis is true to be calculated and therefore permit the list of candidate hypotheses to be reduced to a manageable size.

Typically, a probability is an expression of the frequency of an event in the past. Assigning the event myocardial ischaemia a probability of $p = 0.8$ says that in 8 out of 10 similar past cases the outcome was myocardial ischaemia. In 2 out of those past 10 cases it was not, so the probability of not having myocardial ischaemia is $(1 - p) = 0.2$ because the probability of all events together always sums up to 1.

One of the most famous probability theorems used to estimate the likelihood of clinical events is Bayes' theorem, which estimates the likelihood that a patient has a disease, given a certain symptom. For example, the theorem would help answer the question 'What is the probability of a patient having myocardial ischaemia, given that the patient has chest pain?' This expression is known as a *conditional probability* and is written p(ischaemia | chest pain).

Bayes' theorem (Box 8.1) states that the probability of a disease given a clinical finding p(D|S) depends on the following:

- The *prior probability* that anyone in the population has the disease p(D), before any information is known about the current patient.
- The probability that the patient will have a clinical finding p(S | D) given that the patient has the disease. This is simply the likelihood that anyone with the disease has the symptom.
- The probability that the patient has a clinical finding p(S | not D) given that the patient does not have the disease. This is simply the likelihood that anyone has the symptom but not the disease.

Bayes' theorem states that:

$$p(D|S) = \frac{p(S|D) \times p(D)}{p(S|D) \times p(D) + p(S|not\ D) \times p(not\ D)}$$

We sometimes call the result of the theorem p(D | S), the *posterior probability*, because it reflects how our belief in the likelihood of an event has changed from the prior probability, given our new information about the state of the symptom in the patient.

Box 8.1
Bayes' theorem

Bayes' theorem can be derived in the following way. First, from Figure 8.3, we note that the conditional probability of a disease D occurring, given a sign S, is:

$$p(D\,|\,S) = \frac{p(D+S)}{p(S)}$$ [1]

Next, from Figure 8.3, we also note that p(S) is simply the sum of the probabilities of those patients who have S and D, p(D and S), as well as those patients who do not have D but do have S, p(not D and S). So, we simply replace p(S) in the denominator of equation [1] with this new expression to give:

$$p(D\,|\,S) = \frac{p(D+S)}{p(D+S) + p(not\ D+S)}$$ [2]

Next, we need to rewrite the right-hand side probabilities into a form that is more clinically useful. We first note that any p(X and Y) is identical to p(Y and X). So we can gently modify the right-hand side of [2] to give us:

$$p(D\,|\,S) = \frac{p(S+D)}{p(S+D) + p(\ S+not\ D)}$$ [3]

We next use our first conditional probability equation [1] as a model to rewrite each of the terms on the right-hand side of [3] into the following forms:

$$p(S+D) = p(S\,|\,D) \times p(D)$$

$$p(\ S+not\ D) = p(\ S\,|\,not\ D) \times p(not\ D)$$

These expanded forms are then substituted back into equation [3] to give us the full version of Bayes' theorem:

$$p(D\,|\,S) = \frac{p(S\,|\,D) \times p(D)}{p(S\,|\,D) \times p(D) + p(\ S\,|\,not\ D) \times p(not\ D)}$$ [4]

Further reading

Hunink, M. G. M., M. Weinstein (2014). *Decision Making in Health and Medicine: Integrating Evidence With Values*, **2nd edition**. Cambridge, Cambridge University Press.

Sox, H., M. Blatt, M. Higgins and K. Marton (1988). *Medical Decision Making*. Stoneham, MA, Butterworth-Heinemann.

Bayes' theorem as presented here requires some very strict assumptions to be true for it to be used. This requirement can restrict the clinical applicability of the theorem in some circumstances. Specifically:

● Each hypothesis must be mutually exclusive. One hypothesis cannot depend on any other candidate hypothesis.
● The symptoms, signs and test results that form the patient's data must be independent of each other. No data type should influence the likelihood that another data type will take on a certain value.

The theorem is also often restricted in its practical use because not all the probabilities may be known.

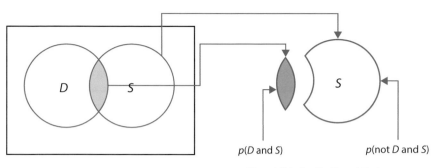

p(D and S)   p(not D and S)

p(S) is the likelihood that a patient has a clinical sign and **p(D)** is the likelihood the patient has the disease.

p(D and S) is the likelihood that a patient has both a clinical sign and the disease. **p(not D and S)** is the likelihood the patient does not have the disease but has the sign.

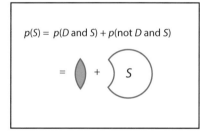

$$p(S) = p(D \text{ and } S) + p(\text{not } D \text{ and } S)$$

$p(D \mid S)$ is the likelihood that a patient has a disease given on the condition that they have a sign S.

p(S) is the sum of those with **D and S** and those **without D but with S**.

Figure 8.3
For a clinical sign S and a disease D that are not independent, we can derive expressions to calculate the conditional probability of D being present, given S. The probability expressions shown here are the foundations of Bayes' theorem (see Box 8.1).

Bayes' theorem assists in the interpretation of new diagnostic data

Bayes' theorem shows how new evidence changes our belief in the existence of an event. Specifically, our belief in the likelihood of an event depends on what our belief was before the arrival of the new evidence arriving and is modified by the likelihood that the new evidence is true. Bayes' theorem can be used to update the belief in the likelihood of a disease, given a new test result. When dealing with test results, the prior probability is called the *pre-test probability* and the posterior probability the *post-test probability*.

For example, a patient with chest pain may be asked to take a stress test, to see whether exercise causes ischaemic changes in the electrocardiogram. A positive test result increases the likelihood that disease is present. However, if the pre-test probability of cardiac disease was low in the first place, then the presence of a positive test result, while increasing our belief in cardiac disease, is still much lower than for a patient in whom we had a high suspicion of cardiac disease before the positive test result (Figure 8.4).

In Chapter 6 we examined the notion of the accuracy of asking a question and introduced explicit measures such as the true-positive rate (TPR) for information searches. A test can be thought of in exactly the same way, by asking whether or not a condition is present. The sensitivity and specificity of test results are routinely calculated to give an estimate of how well they perform in identifying a condition.

Figure 8.5 A decision tree represents the different alternatives from a chance event, then branches using a chance node show the possible consequences of each alternative. The leaf nodes of the decision tree are associated with a specific outcome of the event. HIV, human immunodeficiency virus. (After Hunink et al., 2001.)

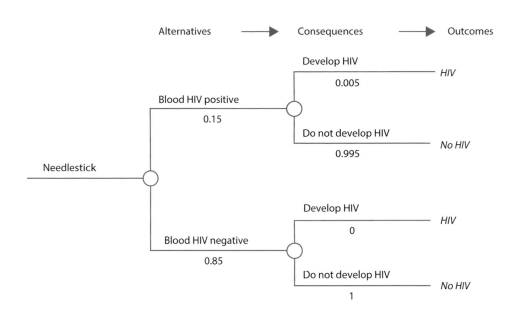

conditional probability of developing HIV infection, given exposure either to HIV-positive blood or HIV-negative blood. Let us assume that about 5 per 1000 cases of needlestick with HIV-positive blood lead to HIV infection.

The decision tree also allows us to combine the probabilities to determine the overall probability associated with each outcome. The likelihood of a given path is simply the product of the probabilities along all the branches it takes to reach the outcome. To determine the likelihood of HIV infection, we now sum up all the paths that end in this outcome: $(0.15 \times 0.005) + (0.85 \times 0) = 0.001$. Similarly, the probability of not contracting an HIV infection is $(0.15 \times 0.995) + (0.85 \times 1) = 0.999$. Note that, by definition, the sum of probabilities of all possible outcomes must always add up to 1.

8.4 An individual's preferences for one outcome over another can be represented mathematically as a utility

Most decisions have an element of choice in them. Individuals may have to choose among alternatives, and the measures of the likelihood of one event over another are not sufficient to help in making the choice. For example, should an individual who has suffered a needlestick injury with potentially HIV-positive blood choose to be treated prophylactically? As we saw in the previous example the odds of becoming HIV positive are low. However, an individual in such a situation may nevertheless choose to undergo prophylactic treatment, just in case. This is because whilst the treatment may carry some negative consequences, the individual believes that the risk or cost of being treated still outweighs the cost of doing nothing, which carries a higher risk of infection. The individual has expressed a preference for one outcome over another.

The preference for one uncertain outcome over others can be represented with a quantitative value called a *utility*. A utility is a number between zero and one, and the outcome with the highest utility is the preferred outcome.

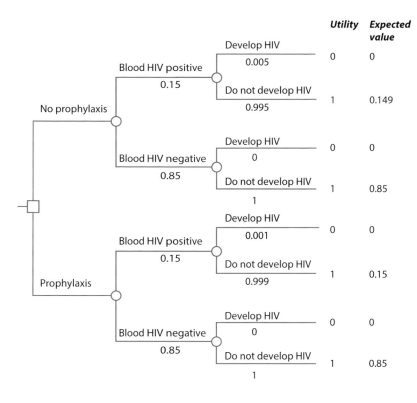

Figure 8.6
The expected utility
of two alternative
choices can be
determined by
summing the
individual path
probabilities for all
possible outcomes
of that choice, with
each probability
individually
weighted by the
utility of the
associated outcome.
The expected utility
of prophylaxis after
needlestick injury is
greater than
choosing no
treatment. HIV,
human
immunodeficiency
virus. (After Hunink
et al., 2001.)

In Figure 8.6, the decision tree for the HIV needlestick example has been redrawn to show it as a choice of having or not having prophylactic treatment following the injury. These different treatment choices can be represented in a decision tree with a *decision node*, which is traditionally drawn as a box. Two separate branches of the tree are now created. The tree from Figure 8.5 forms the 'no treatment' arm, and we now need to calculate the probabilities for the outcomes if prophylactic treatment is chosen.

If we assume that prophylactic treatment following a needlestick injury with HIV-positive blood has an 80 per cent chance of protection, then from Figure 8.5 we know that the chance of developing HIV infection is reduced from 0.005 to $(1 - 0.8) \times 0.05 = 0.001$ (i.e. only 20 per cent of those treated now go on to be HIV positive). Similarly, the probability of not seroconverting to HIV positive now increases from 0.995 to $(0.8 \times 0.995) = 0.999$. Finally, our needlestick victim assigns being infected with HIV a utility of zero and of being free of HIV with a utility of one.

The *expected utility* of making one choice over another is simply the product of its probability and utility:

$$e(x) = p(x) \times u(x)$$

Expected utility is a measure of the actual benefit that can be expected from an event over multiple trials, given uncertainty about the occurrence of the event.

To calculate the expected utility of treatment versus non-treatment, each utility value is multiplied by the different path probabilities to give the final expected utility of each option. Thus, the expected utility of prophylaxis is the sum of the expected utilities of each of the

7. Decision trees are used to determine the most likely outcome among several alternatives. The likelihood of a given path is the product of all branches it takes to reach it. The likelihood of an outcome is the sum of all paths that lead to it.

8. An individual's preferences for an outcome can be represented mathematically as a utility. The expected value of an outcome is the product of different path probabilities and their utility.

9. Utilities can be determined in many different ways, including subjective rating scales, the standard gamble and the time trade-off method.

10. Humans overweigh the impact of a loss compared with a gain when assigning utilities.

11. Human assignment of event probabilities is also biased. In decisions based upon experience, people underestimate the importance of rare events. When making decisions from description, rare events are assigned a higher likelihood than they deserve.

12. The way that personal experience samples the true distribution of an event underpins a number of common biases and heuristics that are often associated with clinical decision-making including the availability, representativeness and anchoring and adjustment heuristics.

13. The process of hypothesis formation by clinicians sees a few hypotheses generated early using pattern matching, new hypotheses added reluctantly and improvements with direct experience of the disease in question.

PART 3

Information systems in healthcare

CHAPTER 9

Information management systems

> He will manage the cure best who has foreseen what is to happen from the present state of matters.
>
> *Hippocrates, The Book of Prognostics*
>
> If you can't measure it, you can't manage it.
>
> *Bill Hewlett, paraphrasing an older aphorism of Lord Kelvin*
>
> Not everything that can be counted counts, and not everything that counts can be counted.
>
> *Bruce Cameron, 1963*

Information is care. Every clinical decision is predicated on information about the patient and about the patient's treatment choices. We saw in Part 1 that whenever a decision is important enough, or is made often enough, an information system can be built to support it. In this chapter we examine both how and when healthcare processes and decisions need to be structured from an informational viewpoint. Two key concepts are examined. Firstly, the central notion of an information management cycle is introduced. Second, we explore why it is not always necessary or indeed appropriate to formalize this cycle completely. To do so can be counterproductive, by introducing excessive bureaucracy, especially when flexibility in decision-making is needed. Consequently, we see that many information processes are left in an unstructured or informal state and are more likely to be supported by communication processes.

9.1 Information systems are designed to manage activities

The main reason that a clinical information system is built is to manage healthcare activities such as the delivery of therapy or administrative tasks such as deciding staffing levels for a hospital unit. An information model is created to describe the process, including the data elements needed to measure its possible states, and the way that decisions are to then be made based upon those data.

For example, consider the case in which a patient is being treated for an acid–base disorder. The *goal* of management is to maintain the patient's acid–base status in a range consistent with good health. Measurements such as pH and serum bicarbonate provide the data about acid–base state. The model used in this case is physiological. It could include rules that describe the relationships between the measured acid–base parameters in health and in disease. Based upon this model of acid–base disease, one can then interpret the measurement data of a given patient (see Figure 2.3). Associated with each interpretation, there usually exists a set of *management actions* that can be taken. In this example, the actions are a set of therapeutic interventions.

The process of activity management generally consists of the following steps:

- Define a set of management goals.
- Construct a model of the system that incorporates these goals, as well as which measurements are needed to track performance in achieving goals.
- Measure the system state by gathering those data specified in the model.
- Assess the state of the process being managed by interpreting the measurements using the model.
- If needed, manage the process by taking action to alter its state, and move the process to the target state described in the management goals.

This process is usually iterative. Once an action is taken, a new check usually needs to be made to see whether the process has responded in the right way. When a treatment is given to a patient, measurements are usually taken to see whether that treatment has been effective. If the outcome is not as hoped for, further action may be needed. In this way the result of the first decision feeds a further decision-making round, thereby creating a feedback control loop. Depending on the task, the loop can cycle through many times.

This control loop is the *model-measure-manage cycle,* and it is at the heart of nearly every information system (Figure 9.1). It is the way in which computer-based information systems are used from the delivery of clinical care to the administration of services and organizations to clinical research. The cycle can be mapped directly onto the model abstraction and application cycle described Chapter 1 (see Figure 1.2), and it is a simpler way of thinking about how models are used to manage activities.

Figure 9.1
The model-measure-manage cycle. When the outcome of a management decision is fed back into another cycle, a feedback control loop is formed.

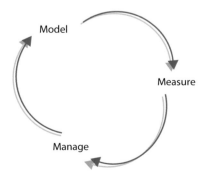

There are many alternate ways of describing this process. The *plan-do-study-act* methodology of system control and organizational management (also known as the Shewhart cycle) has been popularized by Deming and is perhaps the most widely known (Deming, 1968; Shewhart, 1931).

9.2 There are three distinct information management loops

It is useful to distinguish three distinct model-measure-manage cycles. These are responsible for the *application, selection* and *refinement* of knowledge. Together, they come together to form the *three-loop model* (Phaal, 1994), which describes the main ways that information is used within an organization, or indeed any system requiring informed control (Figure 9.2).

We start with a set of models of the system we want to manage. In the case of clinical medicine, these models correspond to medical knowledge. If we are administering an organization such as a hospital, then the models could capture our understanding of economics, historical demands on the service, organizational dynamics and so on. Such models may exist in books and journals, in the software of an information system or in people's heads.

In the first loop, data are used to manage directly a specific activity, such as the selection of a diagnostic test for a patient. The second loop manages the models used in the first loop. For example, a treatment model may need to be replaced or customized more closely to the circumstances of a patient, if sufficient progress has not been made. In the third loop, the performance of all these models is assessed. For example, the clinical effectiveness of a procedure may be measured after its use over a large number of patients, thereby resulting in its modification once problems are identified. Each loop thus has a different role. Each involves different data sources and different operations on the data. As a result, each cycle has different requirements for the kind of information or communication system needed to support it.

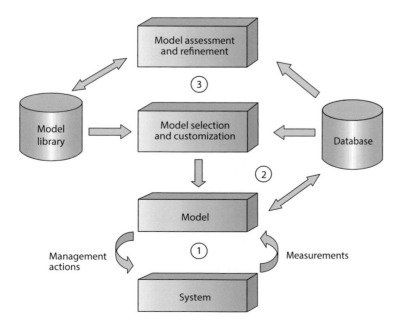

Figure 9.2
The three-loop model. Three separate information cycles interact within the health system. The first and second cycles select and apply models to the management of specific systems. The third information cycle tries to assess the effectiveness of these decisions and improve the models accordingly.

Loop 1 defines the direct application of a model to a task

The first loop is simply the model-measure-manage cycle. Using knowledge contained in a model, measurements are made and actions are taken. For example, a clinician may choose an insulin dosing regimen for a diabetic patient. Having chosen that regimen, the clinician uses it to manage the care of the patient. Measurements of blood sugar levels are taken, and the dose of insulin is varied according to the rules specified in the regimen. Similarly, a hospital has a formula for determining the number of nurses needed to staff a ward adequately. This formula may take into account the number of patients in a ward and their level of dependency. On any given day, based upon measurements of patients' numbers and dependency, a nurse manager will use the formula to decide upon staffing levels for different wards.

Loop 2 defines the way models are selected and customized

Usually, there are a number of different ways in which a task can be completed – there are many ways that the world can be modelled and many ways in which that model can be translated into a prescription for action. Loop 2 describes the process of deciding which of these models are most appropriate for a specific task.

Returning to the example of the diabetic patient, a clinician must decide which insulin regimen or set of rules is the most appropriate for a given patient. The choice could be based upon an assessment of the severity of disease or on the patient's ability to test his or her own blood sugar and self-administer insulin. The regimen may be varied many times during the period in which the clinician manages the patient. When the patient is ill, the clinician may prescribe 'sick-day' rules that alter the doses of insulin that can be given. If a patient has an implanted insulin delivery device, then the rules for frequency, timing and dose of insulin are different from those for self-administered subcutaneous doses.

In a hospital ward, a nurse manager may need to apply a different formula for staffing levels based upon on the type of ward. A different set of rules may be applied to an intensive care unit, which has different requirements for staff skills and different levels of patient dependency from those of a general surgical ward.

Sometimes local variations need to be considered. Patients have specific circumstances that may require a treatment to be tailored to their specific needs. A patient with particularly 'brittle' diabetes may need to be closely monitored and the treatment varied because of the unpredictability of the disease. Nursing staff on a ward in a teaching hospital may need to vary the balance of their daily activities if they are expected to train students as well as carry out clinical duties. Sometimes these variations in approach reflect very particular circumstances and are not frequent enough to be turned into general policy.

Loop 3 is responsible for model creation and refinement based upon the results of application over time

All knowledge is constantly re-examined, and our understanding of the world evolves with time. In loop 3, the knowledge used to complete a task is examined against the outcome of application. The results of repeated application of a model are pooled, and assessments about its effectiveness are made. When several different approaches to execute a task exist, historical data may help identify the most successful approach. If the models selected in loop 2 are regarded as hypotheses about the best way to approach a task, then loop 1 is where each hypothesis is tested. Loop 3 is where inductive reasoning is applied in the scientific examination of these theories and drives the modification or creation of new theories.

Thus, the many different treatment regimens used in the management of diabetes have all hopefully been tested in trials across large numbers of patients. As the outcomes of the treatments are examined, decisions are made about which regimens should be retained and which should be modified and under which conditions particular regimens should be best applied.

Equally, over time, the way in which hospital units are staffed is modified when measurements such as patient outcomes, staff retention and satisfaction levels are examined. Those hospitals that perform best on these measurements can be used as role models by other hospitals that want to improve in a similar fashion.

9.3 Formal and informal information systems

Just because it is possible to define an information system, it does not follow that it is always reasonable to go and build it. If that were the case, our lives would be regulated in minute detail. What happens in reality is that most organizations, small or large, try to find a balance between creating formal processes and allowing individuals to behave freely and informally. Large organizations gain stability through formal processes, but they are often criticized for being overly bureaucratic. Although smaller organizations may be flexible and able to respond rapidly to change, they may be chaotic to work in as a result. The difference between such extremes lies in an organization's view of the need to formalize its internal systems.

So, although structuring processes have clear advantages, including improved reliability, efficiency and consistency, this approach comes with a cost. There are several such costs that need to be considered before a system is formalized:

- First, the creation of a process, by definition and intent, limits flexibility of response. A particular view of how things should be done is captured within the rules, regulations and procedures that describe any formal process. Alternative views exist, and in some circumstances they would produce better results. Choosing to adhere to a single formal process is a trade-off. The number of times it produces a good result is balanced against the cost of those times when an alternate approach would have been better. If the situations being dealt with are highly variable, then it is probably better to come up with a way of handling them from 'first principles', rather than looking to a formal cookbook solution.
- Second, formalizing the information elements that describe a process usually requires considerable effort. An explicit model of the process needs to be created, and this includes definitions of the data that need to be collected. In some situations it is just too costly to engage in this formalization process, given the likely return.

What should now be apparent is that, before a formal information system is created to manage a process, there needs to be an explicit cost benefit analysis. In many circumstances, the result of that analysis may be that it is preferable not to build the system.

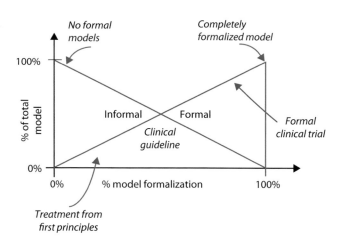

In Chapter 2 we saw that there is a continuum that describes how much of a model is incorporated into a computer and how much is left in the heads of humans (see Figure 2.5). A similar continuum describes those situations in which everything needs to be formalized and those in which a process can be left informal. In between these two extremes, depending upon specific needs, one can formally define some parts of a system and leave the remaining interactions undefined (Figure 9.3). The proportion that is formalized depends on the cost benefits of formalization of a given situation.

Thus, although a hospital has many formally defined procedures for managing different activities, most activities are left informal. Similarly, the way that patients are managed falls along this continuum of formality. Patients enrolled in a clinical trial have their management completely regimented, to maximize the scientific significance of any results. Patients with common conditions may be treated according to well-defined guidelines, but some aspects of their treatment are modified to match individual needs. At the other end of the spectrum, a patient's problems may be approached in a non-standard way, perhaps because of the uniqueness of circumstances. Although there may be a few general guidelines on how to approach such patients, most of what occurs has to be created 'from scratch'. This does not mean that such a treatment, if repeated over time, will not slowly become part of the formal treatment of similar patients.

Not all data need to be made available for computer interpretation

Given that not all processes need to be formalized, it follows that just because data are stored in a computer system, the data will not always be analyzed. Consider, for example, a recorded voice message left by a member of a healthcare team for a colleague that contains an update on a patient's progress. The message is likely to be loosely structured and cover a number of topics that would not normally be predictable in advance. It is also likely that the message will be of interest to the few individuals associated with the patient's care. There may be no formal agreement in advance on the content of the message or the ways in which it will be used. Such agreements are at the heart of traditional computer-based information systems, in which data formats are specified in advance of the system's construction. Nevertheless, the recorded message constitutes data that are stored, perhaps even on a computer system, and clinical decisions may be altered based upon the content of the message.

As a consequence, the message data are treated in a very different way from those data that are formally recorded in a patient's record. The model and the interpretation of the data are owned by the recorder and listener of the message. The machine that stores and transmits the data takes on a passive role. It is used as a data repository or as a channel between the communicating parties, rather than for any active interpretation it may make.

This does not mean that no one would ever want to develop a model that allowed a computer to analyze such a message. Text and speech processing algorithms can be used to do exactly that. When there is a clear cost benefit to doing so, messages may be screened for the appearance of key words or phrases. This may be done for quality control processes or as part of a root cause analysis to understand the circumstances that led to a patient's being harmed.

In general, we can make a distinction between information systems in which data are explicitly modelled and those in which data are intentionally left unmodelled:

1. A *formal Information system* contains an agreed model for the interpretation of data, and data within the system are structured in accordance with that model.
2. An *informal information system* is neutral to the interpretation of data, containing no model and imposing minimal structure on any data to allow it to be stored, retrieved and shared.

Thus, an informal system does not imply the absence of a model or the inability to interpret data in the light a model. It is just that the model and the act of interpreting the data within an informal system are held somewhere external to that system. In practice, these models are often kept in the heads of those who create or access the informally stored data or in other information systems designed to retrieve and interpret that data using different methods (e.g. text or speech recognition).

In general, informal information systems are used when data are of temporary value, of interest to a very few people, are complex or when the content of the data is not predictable in advance (Coiera, 2000). There is thus no sense in which the data in an informal system are less valuable than formally structured data. Data can be used in fundamentally different ways and in different situations.

Communication systems frequently support informal exchanges

Some tasks, such as storing and retrieving telephone numbers, lend themselves to being formally organized. Other tasks, such as writing quick notes, can be impaired by such structure. People often use simple tools such as pen and paper to manage a variety of unstructured tasks. The key requirements for any tool used to support informal tasks are that it provides a means of creating and then managing information that is flexible and can be used across a variety of tasks.

One of the most common ways of supporting informal processes is to use a communication system to channel data between people because such systems have only minimal models of the content of the data they transfer. Thus, a telephone is an informal information system. The models for interpreting the data transmitted across the telephone are not in the machinery responsible for mediating a conversation, but rather are external to it. When examining the flows of information through an organization, it would thus be a mistake to look only at formal processes because this would give a very skewed picture of what really is going on. There is a complementary, and probably significantly larger, body of information coursing through the informal channels of the organization's communication infrastructure.

Many processes are a blend of formal information and informal communication elements. Clinical handover is an example of a communication process that benefits from some structure (see Chapter 5). Structured approaches such as SBAR (situation, background, assessment recommendation; see Box 5.1) describe both the expected content of the handover conversation, as well as the order in which items are to be presented. This structure stays at a very general level, and it is up to the individuals making the presentation to decide upon the level of detail or issues that need to be highlighted.

The following example should make the contrasting roles of communication and information systems in managing information clearer. Consider a primary care physician who wants to share a patient's electrocardiogram (ECG) with a cardiologist during a teleconsultation. There are two ways in which this could happen:

- Informal: *Scanning the ECG* – An ECG can be captured by a scanner either from a printed version or by sending the ECG document electronically to the scanner. The scanner is not configured in any special way to recognize that it is transmitting an ECG. It just as well could be sending text or a photograph. Thus, the scanner is informal with respect to the content of the data. The cardiologist who reads the scanned image possesses the model for the interpretation of the ECG. The advantage of using a scanner is that it is cheap, easy to use and widely available. Because no interpretive model is associated with the data scanned, the scanner can be used on a wide variety of tasks. The disadvantage of using this system is that it requires someone with expertise on the receiving end of the scanned document to provide the model and interpretation.
- Formal: *Transmitting the ECG data file* – If an ECG is captured directly from an electrocardiograph as a data file specifically structured to store ECGs, then any computer that understands that file structure can take the data and recreate the original waveform. The advantages here are the inverse of scanning an image. Having data that are structured according to a model permits flexible manipulation of the data. One could choose to display only some portions of the signal at different resolutions. The computer could automatically interpret the signal if its models included the different patterns that ECGs may take in disease. The disadvantages of this system are that one requires a dedicated system at both the sending and receiving ends to encode and decode the signal.

The decision to adopt one or other approach is a cost benefit trade-off. A primary care practitioner who rarely has the need to transmit an ECG might find the cost of purchasing a dedicated system unjustifiable. A cardiologist, for whom this is a common occurrence, would find the case easier to make.

In summary, an informal information system can be used on many different tasks, but it performs each of them less effectively than a system formally designed for the task. When tasks are infrequent, it is often more cost-effective to use an informal solution. In contrast, as a task starts to become more frequent or important, then more expensive and specific formal tools can be created to support it.

Discussion points

1. Are there any significant differences between the model-measure-manage cycle and the plan-do-study-act cycle?

2. Pick a specific health service or clinical task that you are familiar with, and describe its function in terms of the three-loop model.

3. Is the model, measure and manage cycle a positive or a negative feedback system?

4. When is it not appropriate to introduce a computerized information system into an organization?

5. Describe the ways in which you could design a diabetes information service for consumers, first by using a formal information system approach and then by using only communication technologies.

6. Some clinicians seem to prefer using communication devices such as mobile phones, or speech-driven devices such as dictation recording apparatus, rather than computers. Why may that be?

7. What is the appropriate mix of formal and informal processes at patient handover?

Chapter summary

1. An information system is developed to manage a set of activities, and its function can be characterized as repeated cycles of modelling, measurement and management.

2. There are three separate information loops. Loop 1 defines the direct application of a model to a task. Loop 2 defines the way models are selected and are customized. Loop 3 is responsible for model creation and refinement based upon the results of application over time.

3. There are considerable advantages to structuring information processes, including improved reliability, efficiency and consistency. There are also costs associated with formalization, including lack of flexibility to accomodate varying circumstances and the effort involved in defining the system.

4. Not all data need to be available for computer interpretation. A trade-off exists between creating explicit models that permit formal information systems to be created and leaving the system in an informal state, with minimally defined models and data.

5. A formal information system contains an agreed model for the interpretation of data, and data within the system are structured in accordance with that model.

6. An informal information system is neutral to the interpretation of data, contains no model and thus imposes minimal structure on any data that are contained within the system. The model and interpretation for data contained within an informal system are external to that system.

7. Communication systems are frequently used to support informal exchanges. Information flow through an organization occurs both by formal processes and through the informal channels of the organization's communication infrastructure.

8. Informal information systems are used when data are of temporary value, of interest to very few people or are complex or when the content is not predictable in advance. When tasks are infrequent, it is more cost-effective to use an informal solution. However, if a task requires formalization because of its frequency or importance, more expensive and specific tools can be brought in to support it.

CHAPTER 10

The electronic health record

> The problems of medical practice and hospital functioning are rapidly approaching crisis proportions, in terms of cost, limited personnel resources, and growing demands. The application of computer technology offers hope, but the realization of this hope in the near future will require a much greater commitment than is presently true of ... the medical academic community, and the health services community.
>
> *Barnett and Sukenik, 1969*

In Chapter 9, we saw that three distinct information cycles govern the healthcare system. The information coursing within these cycles ranges from operational details such as staff salaries through to complex data captured during patient care. Although some information is captured formally, a large part is left informal and is communicated without necessarily being recorded.

The health record is the single point of deposition and access for nearly all formal elements of clinical data. The health record is so pivotal a topic in informatics that it makes sense to begin our detailed discussion of healthcare information systems here. This chapter first looks at the benefits and limitations of existing paper-based systems and the major functions that could in principle be replaced or enhanced by the electronic health record (EHR). Because the EHR feeds so many different clinical systems, these topics, including decision support, protocol-based care, population surveillance and clinical audit, are all also introduced here.

10.1 The electronic health record is not a simple replacement of the paper record

The health record has traditionally had a number of distinct functions, both formal and informal:

- It provides a means of communicating among staff members actively managing a patient. Notes left in the record by clinicians assist others who will also share care of the patient at different times.

- During the active management of a patient's illness, the record strives to be the single data access point for workers managing a patient. All test results, observations and plans should be accessible through it. The record thus provides a 'view' into the collected data of a patient's episode of illness.
- The record is an informal 'workspace' to capture ideas and impressions that can build upto a consensus view of what is going on with a patient. The evolution of such a consensus is a form of storytelling or development of a narrative about the patient (Kay and Purves, 1996). In this narrative, clinicians select and assemble different data to tell a story. This imposition of an interpretation upon the patient data explains why the patient record as created by clinicians is never the patient's own story, but rather the story as told by those who care for the patient.
- Once an episode of care is completed, the record moves to becoming a historical archive. It may be used to assist in later episodes in the same patient or be pooled with data from other patients to assist in research.

The amount of patient data stored around the world in patient records is bewilderingly large, complex and often disconnected. Every primary care practitioner's office contains patient records. Every hospital has dedicated professional staff whose main focus is to act as custodians and guides for its precious record store.

Paper health records continue to exist in a multitude of forms. They are sometimes intelligible only to those who created them and often are not accessible to anyone except those who work in the institution in which they are stored. Sometimes, records are not even available within institutions – paper records can be misplaced, lost or used by someone else, and archived records may be stored offsite. One of the roles of patient data is to help the growth of knowledge. With many records in such a scattered and inaccessible state, these records can be only poor participants in this wider process.

With drawbacks both at the point of care and population health, many have turned from paper records to computer-based ones. These computer records are known variously as the EHR, the computer-based patient record (CPR) or the electronic patient record (EPR). Different clinical disciplines sometimes distinguish their own contribution to the record. When describing doctor-generated notes, the term electronic medical record (EMR) is sometimes used. Nursing notes are captured in the electronic nursing record (ENR), and the personal health record (PHR) captures the details recorded by patients themselves.

Electronic health records require significant changes to organizational processes

Without doubt, there has been an enormous amount of controversy, confusion, distress and sometimes disappointment associated with the development of EHRs. At the core of much of this difficulty lie very different views of the role of the electronic record and differences in the motivations for computerizing the record.

For some, the EHR is simply a digital replacement for existing paper medical record systems. The computer is a passive mechanism for capturing information during the clinical encounter, storing it securely and permitting retrieval as needed. The potential advantages for moving to such a computer record system include a reduction in record storage space, the possibility of simultaneous access to records by many individuals and the possibility of using data for a variety of clinical and operational research activities. Individual clinicians, for example, could do rapid searches through their practice records for quality control audits. Data pooled from many patients can be used to study the epidemiology of a disease.

The EHR is, however, often more broadly defined as 'a system specifically designed to support users by providing accessibility to complete and accurate data, alerts, reminders, clinical decision support systems, links to medical knowledge, and other aids' (Dick and Steen, 1991). Even this broader definition is limited because the data captured within an EHR need not just support clinicians, but could also feed almost every clinical and organizational process within a healthcare organization (Figure 10.1).

Such an EHR brings with it an opportunity to refashion the process of care, by changing workflows, altering service-delivery models and introducing many other information and communication systems to support clinical activities. Indeed, workflow change is inevitable even if only the core record elements of an institution's EHR are replaced. Computerization brings with it changes in the type and volume of data that are captured, the time and effort devoted to record creation and the layout of data presentations. Even the places where records are created or viewed may change, depending on what hardware choices are made to access the software. The term 'record' in the 'electronic health record' thus becomes increasingly inaccurate as organizational transformation is undertaken.

With such a wide variation in the functions that could be expected from an EHR, and the significant consequences following its introduction, it becomes clearer why some individuals and organizations undertaking the journey from paper to electronic records are sometimes surprised by the complexity, cost and challenge of the process. The justification for adopting

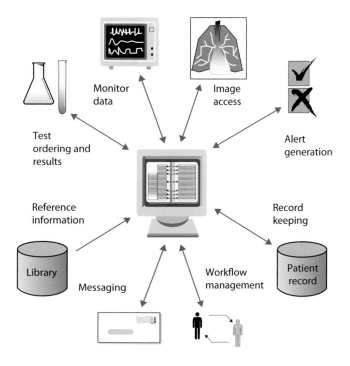

Figure 10.1
The electronic health record supports a variety of clinical functions requiring different degrees of investment and technological sophistication.

an EHR thus rests as much on people's aspirations for transforming clinical practice as it does on the limitations of paper-based methods of recording clinical information. The extent of the transformation undertaken in any one organization depends in part on the resources, needs and expertise of those concerned. It also depends on organizational priorities because, as shown in Chapter 9, it is not always even appropriate to introduce a formal computer system when an informal solution would do.

10.2 The paper-based health record has distinct physical and informational properties

In one form or another, the method of recording patient data on paper has served clinical practice successfully for centuries. Although the physical nature of the paper record has remained relatively unchanged, its formal information structure has undergone much change in the last century. The record has changed from an unstructured chronological record of events to the problem-oriented or task-oriented structures discussed in Chapter 5 (Tange, 1995).

The assertion that a 'computer' record system is always better than a 'paper' one is weak. If we think of a record as a message, then we know from Chapter 4 that the channel of message delivery (in this case a computer) is only one of many factors that shape the ultimate utility of the message for the individual who receives it. Issues such as the informational structure adopted for the record clearly have a large impact on its utility, independent of the medium of delivery.

There are thus two separate aspects of the paper record to consider. The first consists of the physical characteristics of paper as a recording medium. The second comprises the structure and content of the information recorded in it. This distinction is important because it is easy to confuse criticisms of the record structure adopted in a paper system with criticisms of paper as a recording medium. In many cases, the reason a paper record system is poor has much to do with information structure, the effort people make when creating a record and the support processes for record access and storage.

The physical aspects of the paper record bring flexibility in data capture and restrictions in data storage and access

The way paper lends itself to being handled, marked and stored is often taken for granted, but it has some remarkably rich implications. As a physical system, the paper record has many *affordances* or opportunities for human action (McGrenere and Ho, 2000):

- Paper is portable. Apart from needing a light source, there is nothing preventing notes being worked on in most places. A computer system requires a source of electricity and usually a connection to a computer network.
- Paper can be easily annotated, making it readily adaptable to many tasks and users.
- Paper has a high-resolution display surface, which can be produced in small and large sizes.

- Paper and pen require no special training. In contrast, use of a computer system typically requires specific and ongoing training.
- Access to data written on paper is direct. Browsing through a large bound volume of patient notes permits a form of rapid scanning over a large content space.

There are also drawbacks to the physical characteristics of paper, some of which become apparent only when record systems are large:

- Duplication of paper documents is relatively expensive compared with digital duplication.
- Paper records consume space when large amounts of data are recorded. There are methods of reducing this, for example, by scanning paper copies into electronic form or creating copies on microfiche, but these require additional effort and expense, as well as imposing new barriers to easy retrieval.
- A paper record can be used only for one task at a time. Several studies have found that records are unavailable up to 30 per cent of the time in larger institutions (Dick and Steen, 1991). A patient's records may be unavailable during a consultation because other members of the care team are using them. Notes may be physically located in an offsite archive, in a different clinic or in a physician's office or home. Records can also be lost. Even when available, the time and cost required for paper notes to be requested, retrieved and then delivered can be unacceptable.
- Large records for individual patients can be physically cumbersome, heavy and difficult to search through for specific information. Patients whose chronic illness spans a number of years and many episodes of care can generate particularly unwieldy records.
- Paper is fragile and susceptible to damage, and unless it is well cared for, it degrades over time.
- The production of paper has environmental consequences related, for example, to the bleaching processes and forest management.

Informational aspects of the paper record allow a wide variety of structures to be used but hinder population-based analyses

The utility of a paper record can have much to do with the quality of data written in it or the way in which data are structured.

Information entry

One great advantage of paper is how little structuring it demands. The way that data can be recorded on paper is unconstrained in both form and content. A paper record may capture the results of a physical examination with hand-drawn diagrams, or it may be a long and detailed narrative. Paper is thus an informal medium because it imposes no model on the data that are captured. The models to interpret data are contained within the head of the reader. This makes paper a general purpose tool, capturing data on everything from the most personal scribbled note to highly standardized forms. Unfortunately, this freedom of structuring is not without its drawbacks:

- Because the structuring used to create a paper record may be very personal, it may be difficult for others to understand what is recorded. The reader may not possess the model used when the data were captured, thus making interpretation difficult. This may mean that what is recorded is illegible, or its intended meaning is lost.
- In the absence of any formal structure to guide record creation, there is increased opportunity for errors to occur, for example, through the omission of relevant data. The imposition of a formal structure for data capture such as pre-printed forms can improve this situation, at the cost of making the process very directed. In principle however, it is still possible for a well-designed set of paper forms to be far more effective in improving the quality of a health record than a poorly designed computer-based record.

Information retrieval

The way data are structured affects the way they can be searched for and retrieved. There is clear evidence that clinicians routinely fail to find pieces of information that they need during a consultation with a patient from the paper record. One study of 168 outpatient consultations with paper records found that data were searched for but not found in 81 per cent of cases. In 95 per cent of cases, the record was available during the consultation (Tange and Smeets, 1994). Missing information included laboratory tests and procedures (36 per cent), medications and treatments (23 per cent) and patient history (31 per cent). Some consequences of not finding data included the cost of searching alternate data sources, making decisions without data, re-ordering tests unnecessarily or relying on the report of patients or their relatives.

A different type of data retrieval problem arises when population data are extracted from a set of records from many patients. Paper health records are typically accessed using an indexing system that catalogues records by the patient's name or identification number. It would not be possible to use such an index to retrieve the notes of every patient admitted with a particular disease over the last 2 years unless a specific disease-based index (called a *disease registry*) had already been created. The only solution would be to conduct a laborious and expensive record review, by reading each record to check whether it contained the diagnosis in question.

The many positive affordances of paper mean that it persists as a communication medium, even in organizations that are heavily digitized. When paper and digital media co-exist, they can create a communication space or ecosystem in which their different capabilities become clear (Figure 10.2). Although digital systems, as shown later, excel at tasks that require formal information structure, paper's ability to be an informal information tool makes it a highly flexible medium that it is used to fill in the gaps around digital systems. Paper annotations contain *missing information* not captured in digital systems or support the tasks that digital systems ignore or perform poorly (Coiera, 2014).

10.3 The electronic health record

With so many difficulties associated with the paper record, there has been a long-standing drive to replace it with computer-based versions, with varying functionality and variable success. Digital systems bring with them many powerful capabilities and affordances. As with

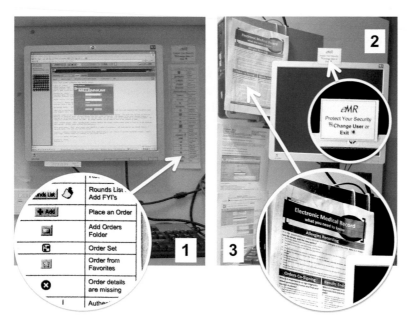

Figure 10.2   Paper and digital documents often co-exist and fulfil different roles. Paper annotations in the space surrounding computer workstations may contain missing information needed to operate a hospital electronic health record, for example: (1) a paper list of software icons and their associated functions; (2) a note on top of a screen reminding users to 'Protect your security', and icons to 'Change user' or 'Exit'; (3) paper sheets behind the workstation with detailed instructions – 'Electronic Medical Record – what you need to know'. (Adapted from Coiera, 2014.)

paper, these affordances arise first from the physical aspects of the digital record and second from the information structures that are imposed upon it.

Physical aspects of the computer-based record

Computer-based systems have a number of powerful physical attributes that make them ideal data capture and storage systems.

- Perhaps first among these is the enormous quantity of electronic data that can be stored in a small physical space. With continued advances in storage technologies, space is rarely an issue. As computer networks become ever more powerful and reliable, even local data storage may not be necessary because data are stored far from the location where they are being used.
- A second physical characteristic of digital data is our ability to create duplicate copies easily and cheaply, for example, as back-ups for security reasons.
- One advantage of paper is its informality. In contrast, computer systems traditionally demand more formal data models and, as a consequence, impose these models on their users during data entry (see Figure 9.3). It is common to hear comments about the rigidity of the way data are entered into a computer and how much simpler it would be to use paper. Data, however, can be entered as a dictated voice recording or as

handwritten notes and diagrams by using a pen-based computer system. Such data can be stored and left uninterpreted, but still permit subsequent retrieval and access in their original form. Further, pattern recognition methods for speech and text recognition can convert voice or handwriting data into text. Ultimately, recognition systems are limited by the way that the meaning of some spoken or written language is based upon an understanding of the context within which a word is used (see Chapter 24).

- It was stated earlier that an advantage of the paper record is its portability, as if to imply that this was not an attribute of a computer-based record. It is now possible to provide networked connections to lightweight portable or handheld computer systems, thus allowing data to be accessed or retrieved in a wide variety of locations.

- The situation in which records are missing, lost or unavailable because they are elsewhere in an organization need not arise with an electronic system. Database technologies permit multiple individuals to read a record simultaneously, and network technologies permit these individuals to be geographically separated. If data exist in electronic files, they should be immediately available to those who have access permission.

Informational aspects of the computer-based record

Many of the advantages of an EHR become apparent when there is a large number of patient records or when information tasks are complex. One of the most immediate benefits of having data available electronically is that the speed of searching for data is significantly improved. While a computer has searched through thousands of records for specific items, a human could still be leafing through one paper record.

Perhaps more importantly, as we saw in Chapter 6, the types of search that can be performed across electronic databases can be complex. A primary care physician can audit the quality of the practice by using Boolean logic to search through practice records and retrieve patient files according to specific attributes, such as age or diagnosis, or perhaps search for patients whose cases are similar to a current case. A researcher can conduct retrospective studies of the epidemiology of specific diseases by accessing records in a region that match specific study criteria. The ability of a computer database to search according to a number of different attributes means that each record is 'indexed' in a large number of different ways – certainly far more than could easily be accomplished by hand-generated indexes. It is possible to move completely away from the notion of creating fixed index structures. In principle, every word in a document can act as an index. Many *search engines* use the frequency of appearance of a word in different documents to retrieve those that are most likely to match the search query.

Given the different and complementary affordances of paper and digital documents, many digital devices are designed to mimic some or all the characteristics of paper, in support of specific tasks. The easy way paper can be annotated can be recreated using digital pen input, and display screens can recreate much of the physical impact of looking at paper, as well as simulate some interactions such as flicking between pages. Tangible user interfaces such as digital paper, which is composed of ultrathin flexible sheets of digital display surface, can be used to create separate pages or book-like devices and may represent a 'best of both worlds' union (Holman *et al.,* 2005; Shaer and Hornecker, 2010).

10.4 The choice of information structure used has a major impact on the utility of electronic records

Information design – decisions about what data to record and how they should be arranged – has a profound impact on the way we see and understand data, as we saw in Chapters 4 and 5. Electronic records (like any information tool) shape human cognition at both data input and output stages. The act of data entry (what we look for in the world) is strongly shaped by the way in which we are asked to input data, and the way data are presented shapes the meanings that are drawn from them (Patel *et al.*, 2000).

The main approaches to clinical record structuring were reviewed in Chapter 5, including the SOAP (subjective, objective, assessment, plan) structure of the problem-oriented medical record. A core message from this chapter is that the information design of a computerized system has a significant impact on its utility – a well-designed paper record could easily out-perform a poorly designed computer record. The choice of information structures is thus central to the success of electronic systems.

Computerized patient records typically have both structured and unstructured elements. *Structured elements* offer clinicians templates (e.g. SOAP) to fill in. Templates ensure that an agreed minimum data set is captured at every encounter, thus maximizing the chances that a patient's care is both safe and effective. Structured records are particularly useful in busy services, in situations where patients' safety is a special concern (e.g. patient handover or surgical checklists), where individuals are non-experts and where services are complex and subsequent steps depend on the data gathered in earlier steps. Structuring is also an important tool in reducing unnecessary variation in the way care is provided (Runciman *et al.*, 2012).

When data are entered into a template, the system knows exactly what the data mean – '120/90' in a blood pressure data field has an obvious meaning, and the data can be easily re-used in other places such as summary views or aggregate graphical charts. Data can also be pooled across multiple patients to allow population-level analyses to be conducted, such as clinical audits, population surveillance and population research. As described later, labelled data can also be used to drive automated processes such as triggering alerts and reminders or orders.

Excessive information structuring, however, can have negative consequences. Asking for more data than is needed at data input wastes time, is distracting and may diminish user trust and willingness to follow the template. Presenting overly complex structures at data output also incurs penalties. Navigating multiple screens of data, or splitting the data needed to make a decision into different structures, may demand more user time and cognitive effort than is appropriate. There is also a trade-off in structure specificity and generalizability. The more detail a structure has (the more formal the information model), the fewer are the circumstances in which it will apply. Thus, SOAP notes, which are intended to be used widely, impose only modest structuring. Overly specific records can be more than a nuisance. For example, forcing a clinician to document a patient's pupilary responses to light before allowing them to proceed to the next section of the record forces a data error when either eye is blind.

Dissonant information structuring can also be a problem. Information structures (whether explicitly intended or not) are models of clinical workflow and clinical knowledge. A template for managing patients who present with a particular condition inherently dictates work process – mandating what questions to ask, what examinations to conduct, what tests to order or which treatments to commence. When the mental models of the user do not match the models in the record, this dissonance among models can be problematic. Use of EHRs in which the information structure does not match those of the user may disrupt the way patient data are gathered, resulting in information loss as well as disruption of a clinician's workflow (Patel *et al.,* 2002). It can generate rework or workarounds, can reduce the trust of users in the integrity of a record and indeed can diminish their willingness to comply with a template or the whole computerized system (Smith and Koppel, 2014).

Information structures thus provide a frame through which clinicians are asked to see patients and the work that they do. By intent, clinicians are inhibited from working outside that frame, and in most cases this is probably desirable with a well-designed system. There are always circumstances, however, when a patient's situation does not match the disease or process model of a template. Patients may present with unexpected co-morbidities, their social circumstances may be challenging or their disease may be rare or unusual. Following instructions, doing the notionally right thing like following a template, but in the wrong circumstance it is known as an *error of commission* (see Chapter 13). When inappropriate instructions come from computer systems, this human behaviour is sometimes called an automation bias (see Chapter 28).

Computerized patient records typically also include unstructured elements such as *progress notes,* which provide an informal space for data capture to complement structured elements. There is a special role for narrative in clinical practice, by telling a patient's story instead of merely documenting their data. The narrative record is where circumstances specific to a patient are recorded and communicated. The rationale for decisions may be recorded where there is a deviation from normal practice. It is also the place where the non-technical human elements of patients' preferences and needs may be expressed.

The act of creating a narrative requires a clinician to look over structured data elements, synthesizing and interpret their meaning, and to highlight the most important developments and problems. This act of synthesis is thus likely to promote an enhanced understanding of the current context. Following structured templates alone may not trigger such a synthesis and may promote a more 'tick the box' approach to data entry and 'out of loop' unfamiliarity with what is really happening.

For a reader of the record, the narrative component should ideally provide an integrated and coherent story of what is actually going on, one that is not easily obtained from structured records. In some records, poor information design means that data are scattered across multiple record elements, and significant time and expertise are required to conduct a full chart review to arrive at an overview. The narrative is the place where clinicians can quickly get back 'in the loop' without looking at all the structured elements.

The weakness of narrative electronic records is that there can be wide variation in what different individuals choose to record, and key data may be absent. Unstructured text, as the name implies, puts no bounds on the way data are recorded – and clinicians can use anything from terse shorthand with local acronyms or write in long, complex sentences. For example, it is easy to record blood pressure in a narrative section when it should really appear in a structured part of the record. Using narrative sections instead of templates increases the chance that others will not see the data recorded because their mental model indicates that the data appear only in a structured section. It also makes data unavailable for re-use in other data views or for other automated tasks. Narratives may not conform to expected language structures or may use obscure acronyms or local terminology. Although text-mining methods can extract data from narratives, the lack of imposed ways to record data gives clinicians a license to record information in any way they wish, thus making extraction an imperfect process that may introduce errors.

10.5 Electronic records can have a positive impact on record quality, but this may come at the expense of additional clinical effort

Electronic records clearly have many theoretical benefits over paper, but as we have seen, poorly designed record structures can potentially have negative impacts. Evaluations of EHR impact can look at a variety of different measures such as user satisfaction, the amount of time spent on different clinical tasks, the completeness and quality of the data that are captured and workflow efficiency.

Evaluating the costs and benefits of electronic records is hampered because of the inherent variability in system design and use. An EHR, unlike a drug, is not a singular entity, but it comes as a bundle of software, hardware, workflow and educational elements. Comparing the outcomes of using such an EHR 'bundle' at different sites is challenging because these sites are likely to have implemented different software and hardware, with different features, functions and information structures. Each site is also likely to have differences in the way it uses a system, driven in part by local practices, as well as by the types of patient seen and the nature of the care delivered.

All these variations result in heterogeneity of EHR design, implementation and use that makes it very difficult to generalize the impact of any given EHR from one clinical service. It also makes it difficult to interpret aggregate results from a group of organizations because average results mask this inherent variability – some places may be doing very well indeed, whereas others may struggle to realize benefits. A specific site will always be advised to try to find similar organizations that have picked a similar EHR bundle because this is more likely to predict the benefits and costs they themselves may experience.

Electronic records do not have a uniform impact on time efficiency

Many studies have examined the impact of EHRs both on the time spent in documentation and on the proportion of time clinicians spend on different tasks, including direct patient care. There are clear differences in the time that different clinical professionals spend on tasks such as documentation and patient care, and it is therefore perhaps unsurprising that the impact of EHRs also varies by clinical role. In one systematic review, nurses appeared to save about 24 per cent of the time spent on documentation with computerized entry compared to paper. In contrast, doctors increased documentation time by around 17.5 per cent when using electronic records at the point of care and by more than 230 per cent on average when ordering medications or tests via central stations (Poissant *et al.*, 2005).

These stark differences may reflect the different tasks undertaken by different professional groups. The effective bandwidth or rate of data input time may contribute to time costs. Nursing records appear to make greater use of structured templates. Well-designed templates can be fairly quick to complete, but narrative records take much more time. In such circumstances, the hardware used to input data could also degrade data capture rates. If a clinician is a poor typist, then writing a narrative with a keyboard can be a very labored affair compared with writing on paper. Alternate input modalities, such as speech capture systems, may improve the time efficiency of narrative generation. There are also non-technical workarounds that can increase input data rates, such as the use of scribes, sometimes called the Geneva solution (Coiera, 2000). The role of these individuals is to be expert at data input, to work side by side with clinicians and to enter the data that clinicians tell them to input. Use of scribes appears to be an effective and feasible way of reducing the time doctors spend documenting (Bank *et al.*, 2013).

Documentation time can also increase with time after initial implementation (Poissant *et al.*, 2005). This may reflect clinicians' use of more elements of the system as they become familiar with it. It may also reflect the intense training in system use that happens at system implementation. With time, fewer resources may be deployed to training, and new users may not be as well trained in EHR use and may thus be less efficient than early adopters.

The completeness and quality impacts of the electronic health record are challenging to measure

The many in-principle benefits of electronic records often lead to an expectation that patient records will naturally be more complete and of higher quality than paper records and also that these improvements will directly translate into improved service delivery and patient outcomes. However, as we have seen, each specific implementation of an EHR is often a unique bundle of processes and technologies. This means that trying to measure overall impacts of the EHR on record quality is a challenge, and the impact of records on outcomes is also likely to vary widely.

Underscoring the challenge of linking record quality directly to the quality of care by using aggregate data across multiple institutions, several studies have shown that there is little direct correlation between the use of EHRs and improvements in the quality of care (Edwards *et al.*, 2014; Linder *et al.*, 2007). A foundational question that is often overlooked when trying to associate record quality with the quality of care is the causal mechanism that connects record quality to outcome quality. It is naïve to assume that one naturally leads to the other because the quality of care is affected by multiple variables aside from documentation. For example, it has been shown that clinicians who use an EHR appear to document more appropriate clinical decisions compared with clinicians who use paper (Tang *et al.*, 1999). This does not necessarily mean, however, that better documentation leads to better decisions. For example, paper users may still be making the right decisions, but just not documenting them.

Record quality can be measured against many different dimensions (Box 10.1), and one of the most commonly assessed is record *completeness* – the degree to which data that are expected to be in the record actually have been entered. However, the wide variation in the way assessments of record completeness are conducted, as well as the heterogeneity across EHR bundles, makes even this metric a challenge to measure (Hogan and Wagner, 1997).

Record completeness seems to vary among different parts of the record and different data types (Pringle *et al.*, 1995). Completeness also seems to vary with the clinical role of

Box 10.1
Measuring the
quality of a patient
record

Patient record quality can be assessed using multiple dimensions. Any quality evaluation thus needs to decide which of these dimensions are most relevant for the purpose at hand. If we wish to demonstrate that electronic records improve patient outcomes, we would first build a causal hypothesis that links some dimensions of the record to the outcomes of interest. For example, if we want to test whether clinical errors are reduced in electronic versus paper systems, we may be interested in the number of data errors in the record, as well as the number of critical data items that are missing.

Important dimensions of patient record quality include the following (American Health Information Management Association, 2012):

- *Accuracy* – The extent to which data report the state of affairs truthfully and are free of identifiable errors.
- *Accessibility* – Easily found data items, with robust mechanisms in place to limit access to only those individuals who are legally entitled to see the record.
- *Comprehensiveness* – Inclusion of all required data items.
- *Consistency* – Recording of data in the same way and with the same meaning across records.
- *Currency* – The degree to which data are up-to-date.
- *Definition* – The clarity of understood meaning of any given data type (e.g. contrast the ambiguity of the data item labels 'systolic blood pressure' with 'pressure').
- *Granularity* – The level of detail with which attributes and values of data are defined.
- *Precision* – Related to accuracy, the degree to which data values truthfully record the state of the world.
- *Relevance* – The extent to which data are useful for the purposes for which they were collected and do not provide unneeded information.
- *Timeliness* – Whether the data are available within a useful time frame.

the individual making the record (Haberman *et al.,* 2007; Luna *et al.,* 2013), possibly reflecting cultural differences among professions, as well as the types of record used. For example, we could expect template records to encourage specific data items to be recorded and narrative records to therefore be more incomplete. Physician notes indeed are often missing data that are required for quality care, including items such as the reason for the visit or a medication list, but these data can often be found in the template sections of the EHR (Edwards *et al.,* 2014). Nursing records, in so far as they are more template based, may encourage completeness.

Several studies have demonstrated that the move to electronic records from paper is associated with an improvement in record completeness, although not uniformly so across all record elements. When record completeness is looked at in more detail, paper and electronic systems appear to have their own strengths and weaknesses, with some data elements more likely in one or the other (Hamilton *et al.,* 2003). In one study, problem lists and medication lists were more complete in the EHR compared with paper, whereas allergy lists were similar in both (Tang *et al.,* 1999). Sometimes improvements in completeness can be quite modest (Jang *et al.,* 2013), and sometimes paper records appear to be more complete than their computerized counterparts (Pringle *et al.,* 1995). Remember in all these high-level evaluations, we may be comparing 'apples and oranges' because the systems in questions have differences both in physical implementation (paper or computer) and information structure. Most studies do not separate these two components, yet as we now know, the choice of information structure can be quite independent of technology.

One surprising determinant of record completeness is the patient. Patients who die have higher rates of comments and vital sign documentation in their nursing records, compared with similar patients who survive (Collins *et al.*, 2013). Documentation rates for medication orders and laboratory results in physicians' records also increase with decreasing well-being of the patient (Weiskopf *et al.*, 2013). This relationship between acuity and documentation rates makes sense because the requirement for documentation increases with the clinical measures undertaken to manage a patient. Clinicians do not document randomly, nor are missing data randomly distributed across records. The paper records of chronically ill patients are notorious for their volume, weight and unwieldiness. This has a profound implication for any attempt to measure the completeness of records. Simply averaging record completeness across all patients without correcting for patient acuity in some way will provide a distorted picture.

10.6 The electronic health record can actively participate in clinical care

Up until now, the EHR has been considered as if it were simply a repository of clinical data, which is either added to or looked at, as the situation demands. One could characterize the EHR's role in this case to be a passive supporter of clinical activity. This is the traditional way in which the record has been used during care. The transition from paper to computer record brings with it many costs, and as we have seen, and there are great challenges in measuring, let alone demonstrating, the benefit of computer records on their own. However, as discussed earlier, the motivations for computerization of records extend far beyond record keeping. EHRs can be active agents in the clinical care process, by shaping the way data are input or visualized. Perhaps the greatest role of the EHR is as a foundational platform or infrastructure; nearly all other informatics functions and services either sit on top of the EHR or have far greater value when they are connected to it. The most common 'value added' functions that depend on the EHR include:

- *Documentation functions* – The EHR can be designed with software features that increase the ease of documentation, including predefined data templates, lists of standard phrases and paragraphs and automatic data insertion (e.g. populating a template with data drawn from other parts of the record) (Kargul *et al.*, 2013). Copy and paste features are also likely to improve documentation rates, but they do come with risks of their own, such as introducing documentation errors (Hammond *et al.*, 2003). Templates that automatically fill in data elements run the risk that this default information is not an accurate representation of the current patient encounter (Bowman, 2013). Computer alerts that suggest adding a problem to a problem list, based on data already captured in the record, appear a very effective mechanism to increase the completeness of this record element (Wright *et al.*, 2012).
- *Task-specific views of data* – One of the basic roles of any information structure is to provide a specific 'view' of patient data, and EHRs have an inherent flexibility to vary information structure to suit different clinical contexts and tasks. Studies of clinical cognition show that information needs do vary with task and that providing task-specific views should be of value (Fafchamps *et al.*, 1991; Tang and Patel, 1994). The EHR must thus possess models of different clinical tasks to allow it to select, present and even interpret data in a way that is clinically useful (Figure 10.3). Task-specific data displays

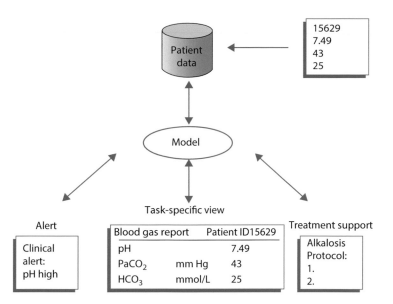

Figure 10.3
Using models of clinical tasks, the electronic medical record can actively participate in clinical care, for example, by generating task-specific views of clinical data, by sending alerts or by invoking models of treatment protocols.

assist in decision-making by presenting views of only the data that are directly relevant to a decision, thus reducing the cognitive effort spent in finding data, as well as focussing attention on important data that may otherwise be ignored (Wickens *et al.*, 2012). One common task when reading a record is to summarize the patient's current state. *Summary care records* (SCRs) are special views onto the clinical record that are designed to provide a high-level or helicopter view of the EHR (Figure 10.4) (Laxmisan *et al.*, 2012). The challenge with this type of task view is that there is no universal 'summarization' task, and different clinicians may highlight different information as being important at different points in the care process. Summarization is an active sense-making act. It requires purpose-driven data synthesis, not simply aggregation (Coiera, 2011). This may explain why demonstrating the impact of an SCR is sometimes problematic. The SCR is often not designed to support a specific clinical task, and in attempting to be a 'universal summary', an SCR may inadvertently achieve very little and may even introduce errors into the summary (Coiera, 2011; Greenhalgh *et al.*, 2010).

- *Computerized provider order entry (CPOE) and electronic prescribing systems* – These systems automate the task of requesting tests (e.g. laboratory or imaging tests) and prescribing medications (see Chapter 25). Prescribing medications is an increasingly difficult task with the large number of drugs available and the ever-present risk of drug-drug interactions, dosage errors and misinterpretation of handwritten medication orders. Indeed, the single most common cause of adverse clinical events is medication error, and the most common prescribing errors can be reduced with better information (Bates *et al.*, 2001). CPOE can check the integrity of an order set, for example, by looking for errors in dosage or for drug interactions. CPOE can use the EHR to detect allergies or pre-existing medical conditions that may contraindicate a new order.
- *Alerts, reminders and decision support* – Computer-generated alerts can notify clinicians of errors in their medication orders, important new laboratory results or changes in the physiological status of patients attached to monitor equipment. Even simple alerts and

Figure 10.4
Different views of
patient data can be
constructed to
support distinct
tasks. A summary
care record takes
what are considered
to be core record
elements that are
most likely to assist a
clinician understand
the current
circumstances of a
patient, but they
may not actually
meet the specific
needs of any defined
clinical task.

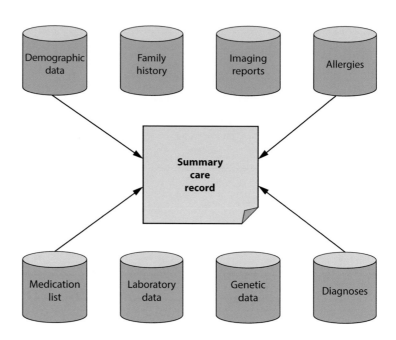

reminders can have a positive impact on care. Computer-generated reminders of the appropriate length of stay for a particular diagnosis have been shown to reduce the median length of stay in hospital (Shea *et al.,* 1995), and they have reduced orders for duplicate tests (Bates *et al.,* 1999). Reminders in ambulatory care can improve the rate of preventive practices such as breast and colorectal cancer screening, cardiovascular risk reduction and vaccination (Shea *et al.,* 1996). Other forms of decision support, including infobuttons, diagnostic aids, risk assessment tools and clinical process support are explored in greater detail in Chapter 25.

- *Protocol-guided care* – The problem-oriented medical record is based upon the assumption that care can be best delivered when the record focusses on the management of specific problems. With the EHR, this notion of record structuring around problems can become more active when the EHR has models of the management of different problems. Clinical protocols or guidelines can provide such models, and if integrated into the EHR, they could support a rich variety of new functions. Guidelines can be used to ensure that specific data are gathered and to suggest tests that need to be ordered or treatments that could be contemplated (see Chapter 15).

- *Clinical audit and population surveillance* – Patient records do not just contribute to the immediate care of individual patients. They can also be pooled to assess the efficacy of particular treatments, determine cost benefits or audit the performance of individual care centres (see Chapter 29). To do this, data often need to be condensed and only key concepts extracted. It may, for example, be necessary to record only a patient's ultimate diagnosis for some purposes. Much of this data condensation is done through the process of *coding* (see Chapter 22). The treatments and diagnoses of a specific patient are assigned a code out of a predetermined list. For example, the World Health Organization (WHO) has a set of epidemiological codes called the International Classification of Diseases (ICD), which is used to track broad global health patterns.

Conclusions

This chapter has presented a broad survey of the rationale for and potential of the EHR. It should now be clear that the role of a computer-based information system in healthcare extends significantly beyond the simple storage and retrieval of patient data. Many of the aspects of the EHR introduced here are returned to in subsequent sections. In particular, protocol-based care, clinical coding and classification, decision support, population surveillance and the support of communication in a clinical setting are all examined in much greater detail in later chapters.

Chapter 14 looks at the way clinical information systems are designed, implemented and evaluated. By understanding the constraints of these processes, we can better understand how information and communication systems fit into the clinical workplace and work more comfortably with some of their inherent limitations.

Discussion points

1. What is the purpose of a paper health record? What is purpose of an electronic health record (EHR)? Are these just the same thing expressed in a different medium?

2. Do you think clinical practice will ever be 'paperless'?

3. What do you think could be lost when a clinical practice changes from a paper to an electronic system?

4. 'Paper record systems can never be better than electronic ones.' Do you agree? Discuss from both a physical and an informational perspective.

5. How have the affordances of paper influenced the design of digital systems?

6. Compare the different contributions that the medium and the message make to the effectiveness of paper and computer record systems. If you wish, use Chapters 4 and 5 as your template.

7. Do you think the problem-oriented medical record is better suited to the paper or electronic medium?

8. A system vendor explains that their computer record system improves the quality of care and patient outcomes because this vendor can demonstrate that use of the system results in patient records that are more complete than those of competitors. Is this a reasonable argument?

9. Two hospitals are comparing their record quality, including record completeness. One sees mainly routine and day-only surgical patients. The other treats complex and chronically ill patients. Do you think that they can learn much from this comparison?

10. The clinical staff members at a hospital complain that ever since the new computer system has been in place it takes longer to record patient data, it is more difficult to find what they want and they are worried that patient care may be suffering. How likely is this, and what do you think could be the reasons for their complaints?

11. What is the purpose of a summary care record?

12. Is copying text from other parts of a record and pasting it into a new record entry a legitimate time-saving trick to improving time efficiency when working with a computer record?

13. A clinical service provider decides to install a basic EHR to save money, but this provider will not purchase some additional modules including computerized provider order entry. What do you think of this decision?

Chapter summary

1. At its simplest, the electronic health record (EHR) is the computer replacement for existing paper record systems. It provides mechanisms for capturing information during the clinical encounter, stores it in a secure fashion and permits retrieval of that information by those with a clinical need.

2. For many, the EHR represents the totality of information and communication systems that could be made available in the support of clinical activities. Systems for ordering tests and investigations, digital image archiving and retrieval and the exchange of messages among different workers in the healthcare system, through to the automated coding of patient data for administrative purposes, may be components of the EHR's function.

3. There are two quite separate aspects of record systems. The first is the physical nature of the way individuals interact with it. The second is the way information is structured when it is entered into or retrieved from the system.

4. Advantages of the paper-based medical record include its portability, its support of informal and formal data capture and its familiarity and ease of use.

5. Disadvantages of the paper-based medical record include its poor use of storage space, its fragility, its limitation to a single user at any one time, the ease with which records can be misplaced or lost and the effort required in searching for information either in large single records or in collections of records.

6. Advantages of computerized records include the great volume of data that can be stored in small spaces and the ability to create and distribute multiple copies and to search across large volumes of data by using complex queries.

7. Disadvantages of computerized records include the rigidity often encountered in the forced and structured designs used to input data and the lack of support for informal information exchange.

8. The information design of a computerized system has a significant impact on its utility – a well-designed paper record can easily outperform a poorly designed computer record.

9. Although it is difficult to measure, and sometimes to demonstrate, the value of computerized records alone (functioning as a passive repository of data), they are a foundational information platform that enables many other systems.

10. Active uses of the EHR include electronic prescribing, the generation of clinical alerts and reminders, decision support, task-specific views of clinical data, protocol-guided data entry and action suggestion, population surveillance and clinical audit.

11. Active use requires the EHR to contain models of care, thus permitting some degree of interpretation of the data contained in the record.

CHAPTER 11

Designing and evaluating information and communication systems

> In creating tools we are designing new conversations and connections.
>
> *Winograd and Flores, 1986*
>
> In the next fifty years, the increasing importance of designing spaces for human communication and interaction will lead to expansion in those aspects of computing that are focused on people, rather than machinery. ... The work will be rooted in disciplines that focus on people and communication, such as psychology, communications, graphic design, and linguistics, as well as in the disciplines that support computing and communications technology. ... Successful interaction design requires a shift from seeing the machinery to seeing the lives of the people using it.
>
> *Winograd, 1997*

There are many examples of well-conceived information and communication systems that can deliver considerable benefit in healthcare. The history of health informatics is also littered with examples of information and communication systems that were ill-considered in design, in purpose or in the resources needed to build and run. Just because something is possible does not mean that it is either desirable or practicable (Coiera, 1995).

So, how does one choose which clinical problems are good candidates for a technological solution? Further, how should one design an information system in a way that maximizes the likelihood that it will actually solve the problem it is intended to solve?

These are complex questions, with many technical ramifications. This chapter examines the process of system conception, design and evaluation and explores how the evaluation process helps shape what is built, as well as tells us how effectively it is working.

11.1 What is the problem that we are trying to solve?

The process of informatics system design, build and evaluation always starts with a definition of a purpose for the project. The difference between a project's success and failure usually comes down to how well we have defined this purpose. There are essentially two ways in which technology is applied to solve a problem. The first approach is *technology driven*. Here one asks 'What problems will best be solved by using this new technology?' Inevitably, whatever the problem, the answer typically is that the technology is the solution. This approach is useful when trying to demonstrate the potential applications of a new technology.

The second approach is *problem driven* and asks the question 'What is the best way to solve this particular problem?' All kinds of solutions are explored, from changes in process to the introduction of new technologies. Sometimes the answer to a problem is that new technology is not the best solution.

Informatics, because it is focussed on supporting healthcare systems, is fundamentally a problem-driven endeavour. It should first and foremost be concerned with understanding the nature of information and communication problems in healthcare. Only then should informatics try to identify whether it is appropriate for technology to solve these problems and, if necessary, develop and apply these technologies.

Sadly, however, it is not uncommon for all the effort to go into technology development, without first seeking to explore alternative solutions to the problem at hand. Clinical information systems may thus end up not being designed to meet the needs of the clinicians who will use them, but instead be designed to solve someone else's problem in administration. Despite the best advice, managers can still be persuaded to purchase expensive technical solutions because that is quicker and easier than finding out what the real problems are. Yet technology cannot fix problems of organizational culture, ill-defined business models or ineffective models of care. Equally, sometimes informatics research explores exotic new technologies that solve problems that could be more easily solved with simpler existing technology or, indeed, in non-technological ways. Sometimes, a paper and pencil truly provide quicker and cheaper answers to a problem than complex technology. Using the simplest and most effective non-technical solutions frees up scarce resources to focus on problems where informatics can truly make a difference.

11.2 Information and communication systems are sociotechnical systems

Once it is clear what the problem is, different solutions are explored. From an information science point of view, we are able to create four different classes of system, each one nested within the next, like a Russian doll (Figure 11.1):

1. *Algorithm* – At the most detailed level, we specify exactly how particular information tasks are to be executed. Algorithms may specify how to calculate the dose of a drug based on renal function and the patient's weight or the type and order of tasks that are to be executed in a care pathway or protocol.

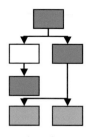
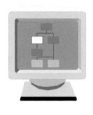
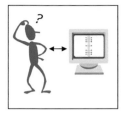
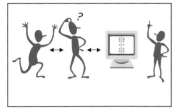

1. Algorithms   2. Computer   3. Human–computer   4. Sociotechnical systems
               programs   interaction

Figure 11.1
There are four levels of informatics system that nest each within each other.

2. *Computer program* – For an algorithm to be executable in a computer, it must be rewritten in a programming language that explicitly instructs the computer how to carry out each step of the algorithm, by defining the data inputs and outputs and the functions that will be used to manipulate the data. The translation from formal algorithm to computer program brings many additional tasks with it that solve problems arising at the software level but are not visible at the algorithm level. For example, if an algorithm requires a specific datum at a decision point and it is stored on another system, then the software needs to comply with a variety of interoperability standards (see Chapter 19).

3. *Human–computer interaction* – Recognizing that the success of a computer system often depends upon how acceptable it is to its human users, the human–computer interface and task flow of the system need to be carefully designed. Human–computer interaction methods provide us with the physical and metaphoric ways that an individual user can interact with a computer. Keyboards, mice, haptic surfaces and eye tracking are all physical ways that human intentions are transduced into something a computer understands. Icons and windows are examples of metaphors for actions and structures in the information space that are easily understood and operated by humans. The use of interface elements such as icons is intended to make user interaction as natural as possible. In the early days of programming, computer interface design was shaped more by what the program needed to function rather than what humans wanted.

4. *Sociotechnical system* – The user of a computer system does not sit in isolation. Users are affected by the people around them and by any other tasks they must also accomplish at the same time they use a computer system. Consequently, the ultimate usefulness of a system is determined by how well it fits organizational structure and workflow, and not just by how well it accomplishes the specific tasks for which it was designed in isolation. Sociotechnical systems analysis thus focusses on the way interactions among humans restrict or shape interactions between humans and technology. Our willingness to adopt a system, or adopt safe usage practices, or educate ourselves in system capabilities, is modified by the attitudes of others to these behaviours. Our capacity or willingness to allocate cognitive resources assumed by human–computer interaction design at level 3 is determined by what is happening at the social level.

Therefore, in the final analysis, people are part of any new information and communication system. The web of interactions needed to make anything work in a complex organization always involves humans solving problems with limited resources and working around imperfect processes.

We know empirically that the value of any particular information technology can be determined only with reference to the social context within which it is used and, more precisely, with reference to those who use the technology (Berg, 1997; Lorenzi *et al.,* 1997). For example, in one early study the strongest predictor of e-mail adoption in an organization had nothing to do with system design or function, but with whether the e-mail user's manager also used e-mail (Markus, 1994). Indeed, we know that people will treat computers and media as if they *were* people (Reeves and Nass, 1996). We superimpose social expectations on technological interactions.

Consequently, the design of information and communication systems does not stop with software and hardware, but it must include the people who will use them, as well as those in the larger group who will influence use. The largest information repository in most organizations sits within the heads of those who work there, and the largest communication network is the web of conversations that binds them. Together, people, tools and conversations – they comprise the 'system' (Coiera, 2003). We therefore are never really designing a technical system, but rather we are trying to engineer *sociotechnical systems* that reflect the machinery of human organization, thought, communication, influence and action.

11.3 Interaction design helps model the way technology embeds within a sociotechnical context

As we have already seen, information system design often occurs with a single task assumption, that the user is going to be wholly focussed on interacting with the informatics system. Such '*in vitro*' laboratory assumptions do not translate '*in vivo*' when individuals use systems in working environments. Individuals in an organization are working in a complex environment and may at any one time be carrying out a variety of tasks and interacting with different agents to help them execute tasks. With the exception of environments with rigorous workflow control, this means that we cannot predict what interactions will actually be occurring at the same time as any interaction we specifically design.

Although we cannot predict every specific interaction that will occur in the real work environment, the design process can model the typical *interaction space* within which any new system will be introduced (Coiera, 2003). The interaction space can be modelled to include the most important interactions that will be competing with the newly designed interactions. *Interaction design* focusses on constructing the ways people interact with objects and systems (Winograd, 1997).

An interaction occurs between two agents when one agent creates and then communicates a message to another, to accomplish a particular task. A *mediated interaction* occurs when a communication channel intermediates between agents by bearing the messages between them (Coiera, 2001). For example, e-mail can be used to mediate an interaction between two individuals, just as can an electronic health record (EHR).

The first step in modelling the interaction space is to note which other agents will be local to a new interaction. The next step is to examine the likely effects any interactions may have

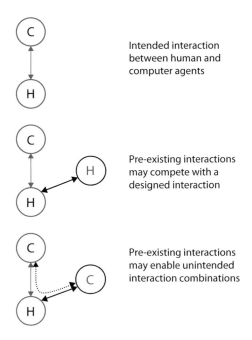

Intended interaction
between human and
computer agents

Pre-existing interactions
may compete with a
designed interaction

Pre-existing interactions
may enable unintended
interaction combinations

Figure 11.2
When a new
interaction is
designed, it does
not exist in isolation
but is placed within
a pre-existing
interaction space.
Other interactions
that exist in the
interaction space
affect the new
interaction in a
variety of ways, and
if they are ignored in
the design process
they may have
unexpected
consequences when
the new interaction
is implemented.

on the new interaction. For example, the introduction of a computer on a doctor's desk changes the interaction space from a dyadic one between doctor and patient to a *triadic relationship* involving doctor, computer and patient (Scott and Purves, 1996). The triadic relationship sees fundamental changes in the doctor and patient interaction. The doctor's attention is now split between computer and patient. As a result, less time is available for the patient, and responses to the patient's questions may be delayed as the doctor shifts attention from computer to patient. The patient may wait his or her 'turn' to interact with the doctor, by waiting for appropriate cues or pauses in the interaction between doctor and patient, and may use the computer to challenge statements made by the doctor (Pearce *et al.*, 2011).

In general, the impact of one interaction on another may be as follows and as shown in Figure 11.2:

- *Compete with another interaction as a direct substitute.* A telephone conversation is often a substitute for face-to-face discussion. People sometimes work around designed interactions by finding quicker and easier substitutes to accomplish the same goal (often to the frustration of designers). The designers of a difficult to use drug database should not then be surprised if they find clinicians using the telephone to call a colleague and ask for the same information. The human–human interaction mediated by the telephone competes with the database as an alternative path way to meet information needs.
- *Compete with another interaction for the resources of an agent.* Both human and computational agents have limited resources. If they are expended on one interaction, this may be at the expense of another. For example, an information system may be well received in '*in vitro*' laboratory tests, but when it is placed in a work environment, we may find that users have insufficient time to use the system because of competing tasks. The new system is then rejected not because it does not do what was intended, but

because the impact of the real world interaction space on its intended users was not modelled. Concurrent interactions can also subvert the execution of a designed interaction. For example, a user may be interrupted in the workplace, take up a new task and not log off the information system, creating a potential breach of security.

- *Create new information transfer pathways through a combination of interactions.* Each interaction connects agents, and each new interaction enables novel conversations between agents. If these combinations are not factored into system design, then the introduction of a system may produce unexpected results. For example, consider the interaction between a human agent and an EHR. Computational agents that co-exist with the EHR could include other applications such as e-mail or a word processor. If the design process fails to include these additional agents, then unintended interactions made possible through these agents may subvert the original design. For example, it may be possible for a user to copy a section of text from the patient record to a word processor, where it can be edited, and then re-inserted into the EHR. However, because this interaction with the word processor is not part of the original design, it may introduce problems. A user could inadvertently paste the text into the record of a different patient, and no formal mechanism would be in place to prevent this context-switch error. Similarly, text may be copied from an EHR that has been designed with powerful security features to prevent unauthorized access and then copied into an e-mail message, which is insecure. In both cases, the co-existence of unmodelled computational agents introduces interactions beyond the scope of the original system design and permits behaviours that would be prohibited within the designed interaction but are permitted in the interaction space.

- *Support a new interaction by providing resources that are critical to its execution.* The designer of a patient record system usually focusses on sculpting the interaction between a single clinical user and the record. However, other human agents also populate the EHR interaction space. The EHR user is often not the sole author of the content that is captured in the record, but is recording the result of a set of discussions with clinical colleagues, for example during a ward round. If the goal of designing an EHR is to ensure that the highest-quality data are entered into the information system, then it may be even more important to support the collaborative discussion among clinicians than it is to engineer the act of record transcription into the system. Failing to model the wider EHR interaction space means that we may overengineer some interactions with diminishing returns, when we could be supporting other interactions that may deliver substantial additional benefit to our original design goals.

Based upon cognitive psychological models, we should be able to say something about the cognitive resources available to human agents, the cognitive loads they will typically be under in a given interaction space and the types of errors that may arise because of these loads. Consequently, it should be possible to craft information or communication systems that are tolerant of the typical interaction load our users will experience. There is a rich literature connecting cognitive psychology and systems engineering (e.g. Wickens *et al.,* 2012). A strong understanding of cognitive informatics, or the cognitive aspects of interaction design, should lead to a deeper, more nuanced interaction experience for users, fewer errors and more effective system outcomes (Patel *et al.,* 2013).

11.4 A value chain extends from system use to health outcome

Given the complex organizational space within which any informatics intervention must co-exist, it is not surprising that getting design right or demonstrating success is non-trivial. The evaluation process is nevertheless crucial in creating informatics interventions that work.

There are two basic goals to evaluating an information or communication system. First, the evaluation can help determine whether a system is fit for purpose (i.e. Does it do what it is meant to do?). Second, we may want to decide whether a system is the best choice among the alternatives (i.e. Which solution should we pick to solve the problem at hand?).

Neither of these goals is easy to achieve because there are many ways to measure success and not every measure tells us the same thing. For example, imagine that a government has built a national summary health record for every citizen. The system is classed as a success because large numbers of citizens have records created for them, and there is a regular stream of record updates every month. What if, however, we look not at how much data are uploaded into the system but at how often clinicians queried the data? If the system was not actually often used to support clinical care, perhaps the evaluation would be very different. Evaluation could reveal that the system was not easy to use by clinicians (who therefore were abandoning it), that the information within the records was not useful or even that the systems in place to access the records were not mature compared with the data upload arm of the system. Finally, one could look at the downstream impact of system use on the cost and quality of care delivered. What changes to care result from accessing the record? Do these changes translate into better decisions that improve patient outcomes or create service efficiencies? It could prove very difficult for a government to answer these final questions and very easy to provide data about record or usage numbers. There is, however, no logical reason to assume that usage of a system translates into changes in end outcomes.

We can imagine that there is an information value chain that connects use of a system to final outcomes (Figure 11.3). The chain begins with a user interacting with a system, and some of these interactions will provide information. Some of this information may lead to a change of decision and then a change in the process of care. Some (but not all) process changes may affect the outcome for a patient (e.g. avoiding a decision that may be ineffectual or harmful, or improving a decision so that a patient will benefit from longer survival or better quality of life).

Evaluation can take place at each of these steps in the value chain, but it is not possible to assume that a good result at one step translates into a good result at the next. For example, a new telecommunication system between a primary care physician and patients may allow a doctor to talk to patients without the need for a physical visit. We may demonstrate high utilization and user satisfaction with this telehealth system but may be surprised to find that there is no significant change to the survival or quality of life for patients who are engaged in this way. This could be because the quality of normal care is already of a high standard, and

Figure 11.3
The information value chain starts with a user interacting with an information system, but it must go through many steps before changing clinical outcomes.

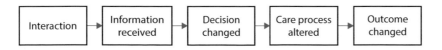

all we are doing is replacing face-to-face interactions with online interactions. If the goal of this system was only to reduce the need for a patient to travel to the office, then demonstrating a cost-effective reduction in such visits (once we add in the costs of the telehealth system) would be a success. Evaluations for information and communication systems are thus potentially needed at every step of the value chain, and the measures used vary with the type of system being developed (Table 11.1).

The value of information can be quantified

Value chain analysis makes clear that creating and accessing information does not always lead to a change in process or clinical outcome. We know from Shannon's information theory that not every additional piece of data is as informative as another (see Chapter 4). The amount of Shannon information is a measure of how 'surprising' new data are compared with our expectation. If data do not tell us anything new, they bring little or no new information. Another way of thinking about this is to ask how many times information must be read before there is a measureable impact on clinical outcomes. Metrics such as the *number needed to read* (Toth *et al.*, 2005) and the *number needed to benefit from information* (Pluye *et al.*, 2013) are attempts to correlate the rate of access to information such as clinical guidelines with their ultimate impact on process or outcome.

Decision theory perhaps provides us with the most powerful and theoretically robust way of estimating the *value* we place on receiving a new set of data. For example, if a new diagnostic test result changes a patient's treatment and saves the patient's life, then instinctively the

Table 11.1 Examples of measures that can be used to evaluate systems at different stages of the interaction value chain for information retrieval systems that search for documents, for electronic health records that allow records to be stored or retrieved and for telehealth systems that support the communication of patients' information

	Interaction	Information	Decision	Care process	Outcome
Information retrieval	Number of queries made, number of query reformulations	Number of documents retrieved, precision and recall, document relevance	Number of correct or incorrect decisions, decision velocity	Number of and type of tests ordered, medications prescribed, cost of care	Morbidity and mortality, QALY
Electronic health record	Number of steps in creating or retrieving a record, time per interaction, number of queries to record, number of alerts created or dismissed	Number of records in EHR, number of records viewed, record completeness and accuracy	Number of correct or incorrect decisions, decision velocity	Number of and type of tests ordered, medications prescribed, cost of care	Morbidity and mortality, QALY
Telehealth system	Number of conversations, call time, user satisfaction	Quality and quantity of patient level data shared	Number of additional correct or incorrect decisions	Health service utilization rates, travel costs	Blood pressure, HbA1c, blood glucose etc., morbidity and mortality, QALY

EHR, electronic health record; HbA1c, glycosylated haemoglobin; QALY, quality-adjusted life-year.

value of that information is high. If a diagnostic test allows a patient to avoid a risky treatment and follow a less risky but equally beneficial option, then information value is based on those avoided risks. If a new diagnostic test result is only confirmatory and triggers no change to treatment, then the information it provides may have a relatively low value.

This *value of information* (VOI) can simply be defined as the economic value we place on receiving particular data before making a decision (Howard, 1966). We could calculate such a value in financial terms such as money saved or earned, or as patient-expressed utilities. In other words, VOI is the *difference* between the value of persisting with the present state of affairs and the value to us of being able to embark on a new decision, influenced by new data. VOI is by definition zero whenever obtaining new data would not change decisions or outcomes.

We have already encountered this concept in a different guise in Chapter 8, where we created a decision tree for different treatment outcomes based on the data reported in a blood test result. For each outcome, we calculated an *expected utility,* which is the likelihood of the outcome multiplied by its utility (see Figure 8.6). Expected VOI is calculated in a similar way, with each branch of a decision tree structured to represent decisions or actions that are enabled by the arrival of data. The VOI is defined as the difference in the expected utility of different decision tree branches (Downs *et al.,* 1997; Fenwick *et al.,* 2008), as follows:

$$VOI = Expected\ utility\ (option\ 1) - Expected\ utility\ (option\ 2)$$

For example, the arrival of new data before choosing a course of action may alter the probabilities of outcomes and may change which course of action can be chosen.

The key idea here is that for new data to have value, the information must be *actionable* in some way. It is not enough that data, for example, provide us with a new diagnosis; the diagnosis must then trigger some action in the world (Braithwaite and Scotch, 2013). The action needs to result in a change in morbidity or mortality or in some other way increase a patient's quality-adjusted life-years (QALYs). VOI can be negative if the proposed data collection cannot lead to an actionable decision with potential benefits but gathering the data has greater costs such as risks of complications or pain.

The value of events along the information value chain can be quantified

An interesting property of the information value chain is that there is typically an asymmetry both in the *number of events* at each step and in the *value* of these events as we progress down the value chain (Figure 11.4). For example, the number of times a clinician reads a patient's record is always going to be greater than the number of times that reading leads to a change in decision. Similarly, not every computer alert results in a change in decision. The number of times a decision is changed is also going to be greater than the number of times any such change leads to a measureable improvement in patient care.

We can say in general that there is a transition probability for moving from one class of event in the chain to the next. For example, there is a probability (but not a certainty) that interacting with an information system will yield information or that the information will lead to a decision change.

In contrast, the value of events early in the value chain is often lower than for events later in the chain. The time saved in optimizing a user interaction with an EHR is likely to be of

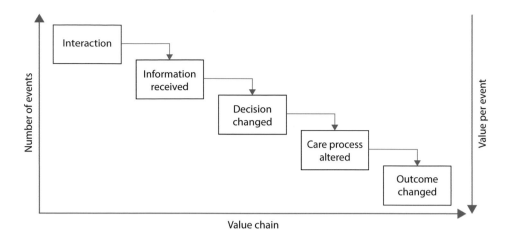

Figure 11.4
The number of events is typically higher earlier in the value chain, whereas the value of individual events tends to be higher further down the chain. Combining event frequency (or probability) with event value (or utility) provides the expected utility at each point in the chain.

lesser value than improvements to the way medications or tests are ordered, and these are often of lesser value than patient outcome changes such as improved survival or QALYs.

Recall that by combining event frequency (or probability) with event value (or utility), we arrive at *expected utility*. This means that we can calculate the expected utility of events at different steps in the value chain. The resulting profile of expected utility is not necessarily constant across the different steps. For example, a telecare system may be designed to maximize expected utility at the interaction stage by reducing face-to-face interactions, but with no expectation of changing clinical outcomes. A decision support system would be designed specifically to improve decision-making and outcomes, whereas an EHR is typically designed to improve record keeping, and process improvement goals are reserved for other functions such as computerized provider order entry (CPOE). Different systems have quite different *value profiles* for their expected utility at different stages of the information value chain (Figure 11.5).

11.5 The design and construction of a technical system moves through discrete stages from conception to test

Early in the development of a system, we typically focus on measuring its performance at the beginning of the value chain. As we grow in confidence that the system is performing well, we move along the chain to try to demonstrate improvements in process and clinical outcomes. The life cycle of an information system that stretches from conception through to final implementation is traditionally broken down into a set of key stages (Figure 11.6), which directly map to the model creation and technology build cycle introduced in Chapter 1 (Figure 11.7):

- *Requirements analysis* – This is the problem definition stage, in which the particular need that is to be met is clearly articulated. The expected measurable outcomes of creating and implementing the informatics system are also explicitly identified. At this stage, one tries to understand the specific context within which the system will be used, including the

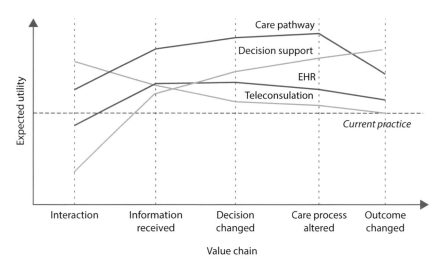

Figure 11.5   The value profile of expected utility for an intervention varies across the steps of the information value chain, depending on the primary purpose of the system. Hypothetical utility profiles for four different classes of informatics intervention illustrate that an intervention (1) may be designed to provide value by improving the quality of interactions in a health service but may provide little additional information compared with current practice (teleconsultation), (2) may optimize the quality of information capture (EHR), (3) may be designed to improve the quality and efficiency of clinical processes (care pathways), or (4) may be intended to intervene in the decision-making process to improve clinical outcomes. Some downstream benefits may even incur an upstream cost (e.g. interacting with some EHRs requires more time than normal practice). The actual benefits for these intervention classes may be very different, depending on the specific bundle of services offered.

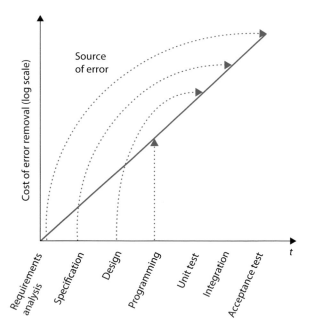

Figure 11.6
The cost of removing an error in the different stages of software development increases logarithmically. Errors introduced at the beginning of the specification phase are likely to be detected only during the use of the product. (After Cohen et al., 1986.)

Figure 11.7 The cycle of designing and building an informatics system such as software is one of building a model, which is captured in a functional specification, and then building and integrating a system that is based on the model into a working environment. (compare with Figure 1.2.)

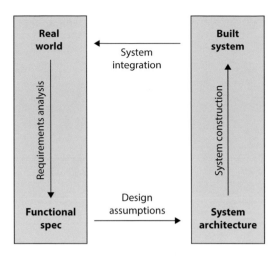

abilities and constraints of any system users. System designers often undertake interviews of different stakeholders to make sure that they understand their needs and expectations. *Use cases* are a powerful way of documenting requirements, and these cases describe typical situations in which a system will be used. A use case contains a definition of what users are doing in a given situation and with which other parts of the organization's systems any new system will need to interact. One should not exit this first stage without a clear answer to the question 'How will we know we have succeeded?'

- *Functional specification* – The user requirements gathered in the previous stage are translated into a formal functional description of the system to be built. These 'specs' are typically produced as a formal document, which represents to the problem owners what the technologists have understood the new system needs to do. The spec does not define *how* the system will achieve its goals, only *what* those goals are. The data inputs and outputs of any particular information process are defined, as are any performance requirements, such as the speed at which a process must be completed or the allowed system downtime in a 24-hour period. User interfaces for software systems are often mocked up at this stage to make clear what the user experience will be like.

- *Architecture design* – The functional specifications are next translated into a system architecture, which defines the individual components and subsystems of the overall system and the rules for how they will interact with each other. This conceptual model thus captures both the system's structure and its behaviour. Typically, one defines a separate architecture for software, hardware and for the overall organizational processes (sometimes known as the enterprise architecture). For example, the software architecture may define which databases will be needed and the information model within those databases, as well as the flows of data within the system. Good architecture tries to separate the overall system into components and subsystems that are as self-contained as possible and minimally interact with other modules. This makes it easy to test each component later on, and it minimizes unexpected problems across the whole system when changes are made to one component. Well-designed architecture also makes clear how user requirements map to it.

- *System build* – In this stage, the conceptual architecture is translated into a working system, much as an architect's plans are translated into a building. Software architecture, for example, is implemented as working software. This requires hardware to be selected, along with software tools such as programming languages, and components such as databases, so that the detailed software architecture is translated into 'code'.

- *Unit test* – Once a system has been implemented, it must be tested to see whether it contains errors or whether its use can lead to harm (see Chapter 13). Errors may be introduced at any of the previous stages, and any software will need to be tested for such 'bugs'. For example, software engineers may have made mistakes in the programming, the software architecture may have had design flaws or the original use cases were based on incorrect assumptions. Debugging is more difficult when the system modules are very dependent on each other because it is easier to identify the source of a bug if it can be isolated to a particular component. When bugs are the result of an interaction among system modules, it can be very difficult to isolate them. *Test cases* can be created in which the expected behaviour of the system is defined, and the behaviour of the system can be checked against them to see whether it performs as expected. *Safety cases* set out potential risks that could be associated with system use and identify any changes that can be made to mitigate such risk. *Load testing* checks to see whether the system can handle the number of users or transactions expected at peak times once it is in the real world.

- *System integration* – Many new information systems are added to a pre-existing and complex environment where there already are working information and communication systems. Interfaces thus need to be built between new and pre-existing systems so that they can interact and share information. For example, a new EHR may need to be connected to a pre-existing administrative database containing patients' names and demographic details, and both systems will need to share data elements such as patients' identification numbers. Interfaces are typically identified at the requirements stage and are defined in the functional specs, but they truly are tested only when actual integration is attempted. Data sharing is easier when both systems are built to conform to pre-existing technical standards for data exchange (see Chapter 19).

- *Acceptance test* – Once integrated, the new system needs to be tested by the system's users for acceptability. It is checked to see whether it performs as expected and whether there are any unanticipated problems now that the system has been placed in a real working environment. Acceptance testing should ideally involve typical users working in conditions that are as close to real conditions as possible and should also use individuals who were not necessarily involved in the original specification because these workers are less likely to have bought into the project and may be less forgiving of system problems. If typical users are not involved at this stage, and user problems are not ironed out, then a fully deployed system may create significant backlash from its users, who complain that it does not work as expected or makes their work less safe or less efficient.

- *User training* – Before a system can go into widespread use, significant investment of resources needs to be made in training the user population. Failure to do so can cause the system to be poorly used, underused or used in unsafe ways (see Chapter 13). In the worst case, frustrated staff may reject a system and cause the implementation to be a failure, not because the system is poorly designed or built, but because the intended users do not know how to use it.

- *Outcomes assessment* – Once a system has been introduced, its performance against the original design objectives can be measured. For example, is the organization more effective or efficient than before? For a new technology, it may be necessary to carry out formally designed evaluation trials across multiple sites, to see whether there is a significant difference between sites with and without the system.

In the *waterfall model* of software development, each of these stages is carried out in a linear sequence (Royce, 1970). Waterfall has its origins in the construction and manufacturing industries, where the cost of change at the end of the process is high and there is thus a strong imperative to ensure absolute clarity at every stage in the build process. Indeed, the best time to modify software is early in the development cycle. In Figure 11.6, the cost of error removal is shown to grow exponentially during the development of software.

Unfortunately, the times at which errors are introduced and detected are likely to be different. An error introduced during the initial requirements of a program is likely to be detected only when the system is completed and in regular use. At this time, the users may suggest ways in which the system's actual functionality differs from the functionality they expected. Introducing changes into a mature system is expensive (Littlewood and Strigini, 2000).

A linear approach to design is thus really sensible only when a highly structured process is meaningful, for example, when manufacturing a mass commodity such as a consumer electronic appliance. However, there are drawbacks when building software that is going to operate in a complex environment such as healthcare. Different health service organizations are likely to have different workflows and cultures, and what works well in one organization may not be well received in another. It is also often difficult to obtain a robust set of initial requirements (Parnas and Clements, 1986). A hospital, for example, is a highly complex entity, and it is difficult to specify all the ways in which a new system may interact with existing systems until it is actually in place; by then it may be too late and too expensive to change the system.

To avoid these risks, a *spiral model* of software development is often used in which rather than working linearly one step at a time, one works through several cycles of system design and development (Boehm, 1988). *Agile software development* takes this idea even further and provides a clear alternative to the waterfall model (Larman and Basili, 2003). In agile development, we still have the same stages, but progress is not linear (or cyclical, as with the spiral model). The idea is that one works on all stages in parallel, incrementally building up an understanding of each of them through small rapid cycles of system build and test. At the end of each short cycle, a working version of the system is shown to the eventual users, and their feedback is incorporated into the next cycle of development. This contrasts with waterfall, in which testing happens at one particular time in the overall process. Agile development is less focussed on producing the heavy requirements and functional documents used in the waterfall approach and instead emphasizes having a working prototype of a system at every cycle of development. This is possible because agile software developers use methods such as object-oriented programming, in which high-level software modules (corresponding to the functional architecture) can be built, even if the details of their internal operation are not yet fully specified. Using such a modular approach, software always can "work" at every stage of its development, and simply evolve in sophistication over time.

Design and evaluation are linked processes

Consequently, for most healthcare applications that involve constructing systems to be used in a health service, evaluation and development of an informatics system are intertwined and concurrently executed. Allowing users to work with or react to simple prototypes can reveal flaws in the initial user requirements or in the architecture or implementation. This iterative approach to system development avoids overinvestment in immature systems and last-minute 'surprises' when a system is actually deployed in a working environment.

System evaluation thus has two very distinct roles:

- *Formative evaluation* is focussed on shaping the design of an intervention such as a technology or process. The design of a technology undergoes testing and the results of such testing are used as input for another round of system design.
- *Summative evaluation* is concerned with rigorously determining whether a technology or process, once in use, actually makes a difference to measured outcomes in the way expected. Clinical trials are a good example of a summative process.

Formative assessments tend to be lightweight, inexpensive and quick, and they focus only on improving a specific design. Summative assessments tend to require a rigorous approach to outcomes measurement and need significant funds and time to run a trial at the scale needed to detect the differences expected. Because we usually compare the performance of a newly designed system against either standard practice or a competing system, a summative evaluation is usually a *comparative effectiveness study*.

It is probably a mistake to combine formative and summative goals into an evaluation study because it will be difficult to generalize any results from the summative evaluation if further redesign occurs at the same time, thus 'shifting the goal posts' (Lilford *et al.*, 2009). It is thus likely that technology will undergo many formative rounds to shape design, before undergoing a summative trial, which itself may discover things that further affect design (Figure 11.8).

This view of systems development holds true of most systems destined for use in complex environments, not just information systems. For example, drugs go through a period of drug discovery and testing in which many versions of a compound are developed and tested in laboratories. This stage is equivalent to the formative assessment cycle. Once a drug is ready for

Figure 11.8   The process of building an information or communication system may require many short cycles of modifying system design informed by user responses to prototypes and then fewer and more expensive technology trials that measure the actual impact of system use.

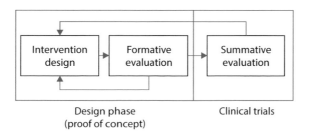

Design phase   Clinical trials
(proof of concept)

the system development cycle, once there are clear ideas about the role and design of the system.

11.7 Summative evaluations attempt to determine the measurable impact of a system once it is in routine use

Information and communication systems can be considered a health intervention designed to improve the care delivered to patients, just like a new treatment. Using summative methods, we should be able to identify the effects of the intervention on outcome measures and to measure the size of the effects (Talmon *et al.*, 2009). Such evaluations can be made in three broad categories – user experience with the intervention, outcome changes resulting from using the intervention and the economic benefit of the intervention.

User experience studies measure how well users respond to a technology

User experience studies can take several forms. User satisfaction studies try to determine whether users are happy with an intervention and do not necessarily try to compare intervention with others. Satisfaction is necessarily a very subjective measure, and many variables may affect it. Consequently, simple assessments of satisfaction may not reveal much about the underlying reasons for attitudes to a service. Satisfaction surveys are also prone to positive biases. For example, patients may rate a service positively simply because of the novelty factor associated with new technology or because they wish to please those asking the questions (Taylor, 1998).

Information systems researchers have thus developed more robust scales of how well a technology 'fits' with user tasks and have validated these task–technology fit instruments to show that they repeatable identify robust effects in the world. The best known of these is the *Technology Acceptance Model* (TAM), which is a family of related instruments – typically questionnaires – that can be administered to users of a technology (Davis *et al.*, 1989; Holden and Karsh, 2010). TAM attempts to measure the *perceived usefulness* of a technology as well as its *perceived ease of use*. The Unified Theory of Acceptance and Use of Technology (UTAUT) brings together different technology acceptance models in the TAM family and reportedly outperforms these models as a measurement instrument (Venkatesh *et al.*, 2003). Despite the widespread use of TAM, it has many critics. First, TAM seeks to measure factors that are statistically associated with the concepts of usefulness and ease of use. It is not, however, a theory but rather an empirically assembled and statistically validated set of factors. This means that it may shed little light on why one technology has a higher task–technology fit value than another. Another significant problem is that TAM-like measures focus on the individual system user and do not see technology use from a broader organizational or social perspective (Bagozzi, 2007; Chuttur, 2009). Yet, this broader perspective is crucial to understanding why some technologies work and others do not. *Team climate inventories* come some way to fixing this gap by helping us understand how teams shape the way a technology is adopted and accepted (Gosling *et al.*, 2003).

Clinical trials are designed to measure process and patient outcome changes following the introduction of an intervention

System outcomes typically require large randomized trials to demonstrate statistically significant changes. Outcomes are usually either *process measures* (which capture how work practice changes in some way, such as the time to write a record or the average length of stay for patients in a hospital) or *patient outcomes* (which capture the end effect of the system on patient level measures such as survival times and death rates). Some patient outcomes may have a subjective utility value associated with them, and various methods such as calculation of QALYs may be carried out. When final outcomes are difficult to measure, process variables can act as proxy indicators of the quality of care being delivered. For example, when assessing a prescribing decision support system, we can measure an improvement in patient safety through a reduction in medication errors and adverse events, even if it is too early to demonstrate improvements in patient health or survival. If we wished to assess the impact of asking clinicians to follow a computerized protocol that guides management decisions, we could measure process variables such as an improvement in the quality of clinical documentation, changes in a clinicians' available time for direct patient care and increased adoption of recommendations in the clinical guidelines.

Clinical trials can take many forms (see Figure 7.7). In health informatics, the most common study designs are described in the following paragraphs.

Observational studies

When a system has been in use for a while, it is possible to collect historical data and compare patterns in the data from periods of system use, matched to similar earlier periods without the system. Equally, we can compare two sites, in which one has a new system in place and the other does not. Given that health organizations are complex enterprises, it is important in an observational study to try to adjust data for variables that are known to influence the outcome measures being compared. For example, patterns of illness and rates of patient presentations vary between summer and winter. Testing a system in summer and comparing it with a period in winter that may have a higher death rate is not a fair comparison. The data selected for any comparison would need to be closely matched to the trial period to make it meaningful. Adjustments are typically made for differences in patient diagnoses, illness acuity, demographics and clinician variables such as experience and staff numbers. One powerful method of adjusting for these confounding variables is known as a *case-control study*. Here we randomly select patients from one period and match them to as similar a patient as possible from the comparison period. Observational studies can reveal statistical associations, but they are not formal trials in which we set out to test whether use of a system causes an outcome change – 'association is not causation'. This means that any associations between system use and changes in outcome that are uncovered in an observational study still need to be tested in a prospective trial.

Before-after studies

Before a system is installed, data can be collected for a baseline period and then collected again after installation for comparison. As with observational studies, statistical adjustments would need to be made for known variations that could affect what is being measured, and the periods being compared would ideally be matched to ensure that, as far as possible, similar periods are being compared. Clinical trials need to run long enough to ensure that genuine and stable system usage patterns are being measured. Short trials run the risk of falsely reporting benefit in the early stages of system use that is not sustained in the longer term. The *Hawthorne effect* is a well-known risk in such studies in which system users temporarily perform at a higher than normal level because either they know that they are being studied or they are influenced by the novelty of the system change. After a time, performance drops to normal levels. Equally, some system benefits really become apparent only over a longer period, as system users slowly become proficient in operating a new system and make it a routine part of their work practice. Before-after studies typically involve one site, and as such they also suffer the weakness that any results may not easily generalize to other institutions if the same thing was done there. Multisite studies are thus more likely to demonstrate a generalizable result, but they would be conducted only once there was confidence from a single-site trial that the intervention was meaningful.

Randomized controlled trials

There are so many possible ways for a study to be biased, and for researchers to influence the outcomes of a study unintentionally, that much effort has gone into developing RCTs as a gold standard for research studies. RCTs are prospective in the sense that they require a clear hypothesis and then carry out a study to test that hypothesis. Trials have at least two arms where an intervention is tested side by side with a control (Figure 11.9) – which is typically either current standard practice or a previously studied competing intervention. If none of the

Figure 11.9
A two-armed randomized controlled trial first assesses likely subjects against inclusion criteria and then randomizes suitable subjects to either arm. We record which subjects actually receive or use the intervention and who drops out or is otherwise lost, and we analyze outcomes by noting who was excluded from the final analysis. As far as is possible, an intention-to-treat approach is used. (Adapted from Schulz *et al.*, 2010.)

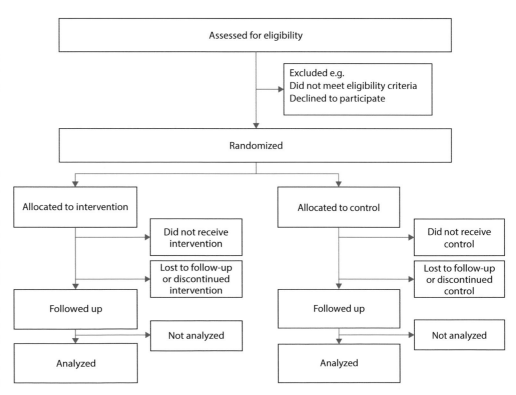

arms of the study contain a previously measured and understood intervention, then we do not strictly have a control condition. The conditions for both trial arms are also controlled and should be as similar as possible. This is in contrast to a before-after study, which has only a single arm, and the comparison periods are not the same. For example, we could conduct a trial of a new clinical information system in general practice and would seek to make sure the practices in each arm of the study were similar, for example, all coming from an urban setting and seeing a similar case mix of patients. Randomization sees patients or system users assigned in random order to either one or the other arm, so that there is no risk that the investigators could accidentally skew who goes into either arm, or that individuals of a particular type could self-select to one or the other arm of the trial. RCTS are of great value in informatics, but they can be very expensive to run.

In healthcare settings it is extremely difficult to guarantee that the conditions in both arms of a trial are similar, and it is difficult to randomize truly so that subjects are blinded to the arm of an intervention to which they have been assigned. In such cases, we accept such flaws and carry out a *pragmatic RCT,* accepting the daily variations of normal clinical practice, and that there may be contamination in the way participants are selected. A common flaw in informatics RCTs is that they are statistically underpowered, meaning they do not collect enough data from both arms to show a difference statistically. This may be because the study does not run for long enough or does not enrol enough subjects. When a study's sample size is too small to detect a difference, it is important not to jump to the conclusion that there was no difference between the two arms of the study. Rather, the study was not designed in a way that it could see a difference even if there was one – 'absence of evidence is not evidence of absence'.

Failure to follow *intention-to-treat* principles when calculating results is also a common flaw when reporting trials. Over the period of a trial, subjects may drop out for any number of reasons. If we calculate outcomes only for those who do not drop out, we can end up with a biased analysis because those who dropped out may have done so for significant reasons. For example, if half of the users of a system stop using it in a trial, and the study reports only those who used it for the whole period, then the results will not reflect the potentially poor results from those who did not find a reason to continue to use the system. It is always better to report, as far as possible, against the whole population you intended to 'treat' at the start of the trial.

Cluster randomized controlled trials

RCTs work in part because both the investigators and the participants are blinded to the trial arm to which they have been assigned. A patient in a drug trial will not know whether he or she is receiving a tablet with a new medication or an identical placebo tablet, and the investigators will also not know who is receiving what. Such blinding can quickly be undone in an informatics trial, and one arm can contaminate the other. For example, if a hospital ward is conducting a trial of a new clinical pathway system, and half the clinicians are randomized to use it while the others carry on as normal, participants will quickly know which arm they are in. Worse, if the new system results in improved compliance with care pathway recommendations, this is likely to change the practice of the unit as a whole, and we may see the subjects in the control arm change practice to keep in line with what they see others doing. To avoid unblinding and contamination, sometimes the unit of randomization is not an individual patient or clinician, but a group or an organization. In a cluster RCT, different groups are randomly assigned to different arms. We thus may see a whole general practice be assigned to one arm, so that all its clinicians are given the same intervention and by definition cannot unblind or contaminate each other. One drawback of cluster RCTs is the statistical dependencies among subjects in one group requires a larger sample size to compensate. These trials are also larger, more expensive and more complicated to run and so are unlikely to be done often.

Health economic analyses attempt to estimate the cost benefit of using a system once it has been deployed

Economic analyses determine whether there is any additional cost benefit from using a new way of delivering a health service compared either with standard practice or perhaps another competing solution. Cost-effectiveness is assessed by first measuring the outcomes of an intervention and then assigning these a benefit. For example, we can estimate the benefit of the additional number of years that patients will live because of an intervention compared with current practice. We can also calculate any QALY gains associated with a new intervention. For example, if a patient has fewer complications from treatment, then he or she can assign a utility to the improved quality of life, and a price can be placed on this value (see Chapter 8). If patients are healthier or there are fewer adverse events and errors, there will also be savings to be made through reduced use of health services, including investigations and medicines, and time may be freed up for clinicians to attend to other tasks.

Economic analyses also look at costs. The cost of an informatics intervention typically includes software design, maintenance and upgrading, hardware and communication costs, help desk and user training costs. The cost of technology, as with most information technology, is never the major component of total lifetime costs.

Rapid changes in the cost and capability of technologies may make it difficult to predict future cost benefits from the present. *Opportunity costs* are benefits forgone because of a decision to use one solution over another. For example, if the purchase of an EHR is predicated on the system's being in place for 10 years before there is a cost benefit payoff, then the organization is locked out of buying innovative new systems for that 10-year period. If a new generation of technology arrives that is substantially better than the system in place, the opportunity cost measures the additional benefits that could have come if newer technology been introduced.

Once costs and outcomes benefits have been estimated, they are typically extrapolated to estimate an intervention's effect over a longer time period and across a larger population. Statistical analyses are often needed in this process to estimate the impact of different variables, such as rate of intervention uptake and effectiveness, adverse event rates, changes in technology, people costs and utilities over time.

Informatics interventions are typically a bundle of technological and process changes

A significant challenge in evaluating any informatics intervention is the way we define what the intervention actually is. Typically, an informatics intervention is not a singular entity like a medicine, but rather is a *bundle* of technology, process and workflow changes. For example, an EHR bundle includes different software modules from record keeping through to CPOE, the user interface design and the particular information structure chosen for the record (e.g. SOAP). The bundle also includes the local workflow and procedures for accessing the system, any interfaces to other clinical systems and the training, help desk and maintenance programs. Together, all these elements define what the intervention actually is.

Failure to account for all the bundle elements when describing an evaluation may lead to falsely assuming that two different implementations of an intervention are similar enough to be lumped together or compared. For example, if the same EHR is studied at two different sites, but the workflow at each site is different, then the changes that need to be made to workflow to fit around the EHR are different. These workflow changes may mean that the impact of the new EHR is very different at the two sites. The reason for the difference is not the EHR, but rather the workflow changes.

Technology bundles also make causation difficult to attribute. A clinical information system is likely to have many different features, and some of these features may be the reason a system does well or poorly. Small changes in the features offered, or the design of individual features, may yield different results. Some of these nuances can be detected during formative evaluation, as detailed feedback is given on system design and interaction. However, at the summative stage it is very difficult to associate specific bundle items with the overall outcome.

One approach to untangling such bundle effects is to log user activity over a trial and identify which features are being used, how often they are used and in which settings or for which patients. It is possible to stratify data according to feature usage and statistically estimate which features are most closely associated with which outcome changes (e.g. Lau *et al.,* 2013).

The bundled nature of technology sometimes leads to poorly designed studies, with only a loose causal connection between intervention and outcome. A causal hypothesis for a trial should directly link the function of an intervention to its hypothesized outcome further along the value chain. For example, because a care pathway is intended to remind clinicians which tasks should be completed, it is reasonable then to try to measure compliance with pathway as an outcome measure and to expect that there may be a demonstrable benefit.

However, studies often simply test an informatics intervention in the hope that something may happen, but without an underlying causal explanation of the way system use translates into downstream value (e.g. testing to see whether generic use of social media will lead to increased exercise rates). Unless there is a clear explanation for why the intervention will lead to a change in the care process or patient outcome, it is unlikely that it has been designed to effect that change, and it is thus unlikely that any change will be seen.

Electronic records are an excellent case in point. As shown in Chapter 10, electronic records clearly have a causal story between record use and improved record quality. It is much more difficult to link record use to clinical outcomes such as reduced death rates because so many other factors can intervene to shape that outcome. Unsurprisingly, the research literature shows that electronic records do very well at what they are designed to do, which is improve record keeping, but when studies try to show more downstream clinical outcomes, they struggle.

11.8 Designing for change

One of the greatest challenges for any designer is arriving at ways of coping with change over a system's lifetime. As the world changes, the design assumptions become outdated. As environmental changes accumulate over time, a system becomes increasingly out of tune with the environment for which it was built. There are countless examples of this process of system 'decay' (Hogarth, 1986). Political systems arise out of the needs of a society, only to become increasingly inappropriate as society changes around them. Antibiotics become increasingly ineffective through overuse, as the bacteria they are intended to attack change their pattern of drug resistance.

The rate of obsolescence of a human artefact is thus directly related to the rate with which its design assumptions decay. Because building an artefact such as a hospital or an information system is often an expensive affair, coping with the inevitable process obsolescence is frequently critical. This is especially so if the costs of building need to be recouped over an extended period. If a system becomes obsolete before it has paid back the investment in it, it will fail financially. Consequently, its builders may not be in a position to design and build the next generation of system to replace it.

An information system is particularly susceptible to the effects of change in:

- The users' problems, needs or patterns of illness that define the initial purpose of the system.
- The model of user workflow and practices around which a system is designed.
- The technologies available to construct a system.
- Organizational resources, including finance and staff availability.

A change in any one of these elements will affect the performance of the system as a whole. For example, when the original need for a system changes, irrespective of how advanced the technology is, the system as a whole has become obsolete. Equally, technology can change rapidly, and a well-designed system may become obsolete because newer technologies make it seem slow by comparison.

Once it has been built and implemented, an information system is probably already obsolete in its modelling of user needs, its definition of organizational structures and processes or the technology used to implement it. Informal systems are less susceptible to this sort of obsolescence because they avoid modelling specific attributes of an organization and consequently are much more permissive about the information that is being stored or transmitted within them. The telephone system in an institution such as a hospital may thus undergo little change, whereas information systems may go through several generations of change. Indeed, informal systems are often used increasingly during the period that a formal information system becomes out-of-date, thereby bridging the gap between the deficiencies of the formal system and the actual situation (see Figure 9.3).

Part of the solution to the problem of designing for a changing world is to construct a system with the assumption that its design will be altered over its working lifetime. Design modularity in particular creates a system whose different components, or subsystems, are cleanly separated. In a car, for example, the braking system is designed to be a separate set of components from the suspension. When change demands that a component be redesigned, the effects can hopefully be contained within that component module without affecting the performance of other modules. A well-designed functional specification is thus crucial to longer-term adaptation of system design. The decision to separate a system into particular subcomponents will never be completely right, however, and interactions among modules mean that sometimes changes in one module require more extensive changes elsewhere.

What modularity does achieve is that it allows a system's design to degrade over time more gracefully.

Conclusions

We have seen that the design and evaluation of informatics interventions are deeply entwined processes. The nature of evaluation changes as systems become more mature, but the changing nature of the working environment probably means that evaluation never stops. Indeed, in recent years it has become clear that system implementation – the process of bringing a working system into a complex organizational setting and making it fit – is a major factor in explaining a system's success. The technology bundling needed to make a system work in the real world is thus not an add-on process at the end of technology design. Rather, it is central to shaping what the technology is and what it ultimately does in the hands of its users. Chapter 12 looks at system implementation and implementation science, among the most important topics in health informatics.

Discussion points

1. Find two recent evaluations of different health informatics interventions in the research literature. Using the STARE-HI (statement on reporting of evaluation studies in health informatics) guidelines for reporting health informatics evaluation studies (Talmon et al., 2009), make an assessment of the quality of the study and how strong you think the reported evidence is.

2. What is the expected VOI for the human immunodeficiency virus blood test in Figure 8.6?

3. A new computer system has just been introduced into your organization, but it immediately causes problems. The users decide that they do not want to use it. What may have gone wrong?

4. A clinical colleague asks you for your views on whether to buy the latest augmented reality headset for use in their clinical practice. How do you respond?

5. What is extreme programming all about? How does it compare with other models of software development such waterfall, spiral and agile?

6. Why do we evaluate information systems?

7. What is the difference between a formative evaluation and a summative evaluation?

8. A senior administrator comes to you to discuss a pet informatics project; which he or she designed and has now been in operation in the organization for a year. The administrator is very pleased with how it has gone and wants you to conduct an evaluation to show how good it is. What are your thoughts about this request?

9. Why may clinical workers not know what type of information system function they need, when asked in an interview or in a focus group?

10. How do social or organizational issues affect the successful deployment of new technologies?

11. Why may an information system that works beautifully when tested with real users in a controlled trial still fail when it is eventually introduced into a working environment?

12. In what ways can the existing interactions in a work environment affect a new interaction introduced through a computer system?

13. What is a workaround, and what does it say about system design when it happens?

14. A working party at a hospital consults widely for 2 years before producing the blueprint for a new hospital information system. Two more years pass, and the system is finally put into routine use. What kind of problems do you think this delay will produce, and how could they be minimized?

15. You read a paper that reports a before-after trial of a new decision support system to aid clinicians diagnose abdominal pain. The trial ran for 1 month following system installation and showed an improvement in diagnostic performance. Do you have any concerns about the results of this study?

16. Pick a clinical information system you are familiar with and describe all the components of the bundle.

17. The government decides that a clinician in the emergency department must see all patients within 10 minutes of presentation. One hospital meets this measurement target only 70 per cent of the time, whereas a second hospital meets it 90 per cent of the time. Which hospital delivers better clinical care? If the two hospitals initially met the target 70 per cent of the time, what factors could contribute to the 'improvement' in the second hospital's score?

Chapter summary

1. Technology can be applied to a problem in a *technology-driven* or a *problem-driven* manner. Information systems should be created in a problem-driven way, starting with an understanding of user information needs. Only then is it appropriate to identify whether and how technology should be used.

2. Information and communication systems are ultimately socio-technical systems and can be described at four levels including algorithm, program, human-computer interaction and socio-technical.

3. Interaction design is concerned with shaping the human–computer interaction component of an intervention, and in healthcare such interactions compete with pre-existing ones in the sociotechnical environment of healthcare organizations.

4. A pre-existing interaction can compete with a new one for user attention or resources, substitute for it or work with it to create unexpected interaction pathways.

5. There is a value chain extending from system use through to clinical outcomes. Benefits at one step in the chain do not imply benefits at the next. The number of events typically decreases along the chain but their value typically increases. Different classes of system have different value profiles over the value chain, depending on their intended purpose.

6. The value of information quantifies the economic benefit or utility of information should it result in a changed decision with a different outcome and can be calculated as the difference in expected utility of two different decision options made with and without information.

7. The design and construction of a technical system has discrete elements: requirements analysis, functional specification, architecture design, system build, unit test, system integration, acceptance test, user training, and outcomes assessment.

8. In the waterfall model of software development, each of these elements is carried out in a linear sequence. In the spiral model one works through several cycles of design and development. In agile development, a working version of the system is always available, and is refined through small rapid cycles of system build and test.

9. The formative assessment cycle defines clinical needs, and many methods are available: anecdotal or individual experience, asking clinicians, non-participatory observation and formal experiments.

10. Whilst formal experiments answer only narrow questions and are relatively expensive to conduct, qualitative research methods relying on non-participatory methods are formal enough to allow robust statements to be made. They also have the advantage of being grounded in the realities of the clinical workplace.

11. A summative evaluation can be made of a user's satisfaction with an informatics intervention, the clinical outcome changes resulting from using the intervention and the economic benefit of the intervention.

12. Outcomes can be measured with observational, before-after, randomized controlled trials and cluster randomized controlled trials.

13. Informatics interventions are typically a bundle of technical, process and workflow changes, and assigning causality to change can be challenging.

14. An information system is susceptible to the effects of change over time at several levels – the user needs that define the role of the system, the model of user needs and system design, the technology used to construct the system and organizational resources, including finance and staff availability. A change in any one of these affects the performance of the system as a whole. Aiming for modularity in design helps minimize these effects.

working systems are actually implemented. For example, most computerized provider order entry (CPOE) implementation outcomes data are derived from a very few leading academic teaching hospitals in the United States (Classen *et al.*, 2007). However, the evidence from these studies is difficult to generalize because it comes from home-grown systems that had evolved over many years and closely fit the specific work practices of these organizations.

Yet such studies set expectations about what may be achievable by implementing 'off the shelf' commercial systems into a wide variety of different settings, including community hospitals, and different countries with quite different approaches to health service delivery. Although there is an expectation that the impact on quality, efficiency and safety of care of commercial systems will be similar to these home-grown lead institutional experiences, there are so many differences between the two that it seems difficult to equate them.

Such variations in implementation outcome indeed seem to be the norm. After introducing two different commercial electronic prescribing systems into similar hospitals in the same city, one series of studies found significant variations in performance, including both the types and frequency of prescribing error rates (Westbrook *et al.*, 2012; Westbrook *et al.*, 2013). In a study of 62 hospitals that had all implemented CPOE, a comparison was made of the capacity of the implemented systems to detect medication orders that could cause serious harm (Metzger *et al.*, 2010). The study found wide variation, even among hospitals using the same electronic health record (EHR). Indeed, only 27 per cent of the variation in performance was associated with using different EHR products. The results for hospitals using the same CPOE software product varied by 40 to 65 per cent.

Why does the same information or communication technology sometimes perform so differently when implemented in a different organization? It seems that the local context of an organization is a major determinant of post-implemented performance and user acceptance. Differences in clinical context appeared to shape how positively clinicians view new systems (Niazkhani *et al.*, 2010). Differences between medical and surgical specialties, for example, can result in a disparity in their medication prescribing needs and hence their CPOE requirements. Compared with surgical users, medical specialties have a significantly greater medication ordering burden, with greater and more diverse interactions with the system. As a result, the same CPOE system is much more likely to affect medical rather than surgical workflow and yield very different user responses and outcomes.

As a result of all these variables, many large health information systems are implemented at great cost, but they sometimes perform well below expectations. Indeed, sometimes they may even be withdrawn. In a now famous example, in 2003 the Cedars-Sinai Hospital in Los Angeles, California withdrew its $34 million CPOE system only 3 months after implementation because of significant concerns from clinical staff (Connolly, 2005). The CPOE system had been created in-house and was 'clunky' and slow. The previous system was based on pen and paper, and so the new system represented a major change in work practice. Yet few clinicians were involved in system design, and there was insufficient training in its use. One consequence was that the CPOE system generated what was perceived to be an excessive number of medication alerts during the medication ordering process. The actual implementation of the system saw it turned on across all the hospital at once (a 'big bang' implementation) rather than gradually introducing the system, one ward at a time. A more gradual approach would have allowed problems to be identified with smaller, more engaged groups, and those formative assessments could have guided further changes in the implementation process or the technology.

Implementation represents the third stage in translation of research into practice

In Chapter 11, we saw that formative evaluation (T1) and then summative evaluation (T2) represent the first two stages in the translation of research into practice. Implementation (T3) can now be seen to be the next critical stage in what is seen as a four-stage process (Figure 12.1 and Box 12.1).

Demonstrating that an intervention is effective in T2 clinical trials is not the end of the matter. It is the next stage of local implementation that substantially shapes outcomes. A feature of T3 is the impact that local context variables have on implementation outcomes. In Chapter 11, we were introduced to this idea through the lens of sociotechnical systems. The ways in which we organize ourselves and interact with each other create that local context in which a technology must operate. Changes in the sociotechnical context from one place to another alter how technology is received and used, as well as how well it fits the needs of any given organization. Because of this heterogeneity that we find across health services, a one size fits all, 'cookie-cutter' approach to implementation is unlikely to succeed. Implementation must be sensitive to local context, and changes in technology or process cannot proceed without due attention to the needs and concerns of those who will be affected by an implementation or who may have to use it once it is in place (Box 12.2).

Recall from Chapter 1 that when a new technology is placed in a working environment, its success depends very much on how well the design assumptions that are implicit in the technology match the reality of the new environment. When information and communication technologies are designed, we make many assumptions about the types of workflow they will be slotted into and the skills and resources of those who will both carry out the

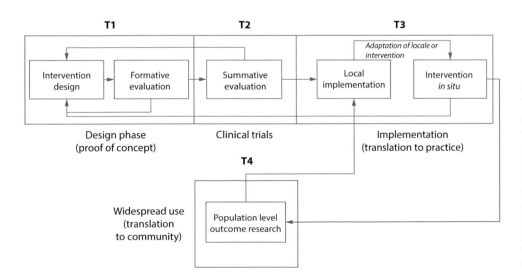

Figure 12.1 There are four stages in the translation of research into practice. Implementation represents the third stage, where tested interventions are now adapted to work in varied real world contexts.

Box 12.1
The four stages in
research translation

Proof of concept (T1) – Using findings that come from basic research (e.g. user needs analyses) new system designs are proposed, and formative studies test the performance of the emerging concept (e.g. with cognitive walkthroughs or laboratory experiments). This stage corresponds to phase I clinical trials in medicine.

Clinical trials (T2) – New interventions are tested using summative methods to demonstrate whether they have the expected impact on organizational processes or patient outcomes. As much as possible, we try to control the setting and adjust for confounding variables, to obtain as unbiased an estimate of effect size as possible. Such research provides the evidence for the benefit of a new design and may be used to formulate evidence-based guidance. This stage corresponds to phase II and III clinical trials in medicine.

Implementation (T3) – Tested interventions are now translated into practice. Studying this phase generates knowledge about how an intervention works in real world settings and how one must adapt T2 recommendations or guidelines for them to work in routine practice. Much health services research occurs in this stage, and it corresponds to phase IV clinical trials in clinical medicine.

Population studies (T4) – Once an intervention is in widespread use, researchers can study its impact on the health of whole communities or populations and explore reasons for variations in population outcome, such as social determinants of health and access to and quality of healthcare delivery. This stage corresponds to population outcome studies in clinical medicine.

implementation and use the system after implementation. From this perspective, variations in the outcomes of a specific implementation arise directly from a mismatch between system design assumptions and the working environment.

12.2 Implementation is a process of mutual adaptation between technology and organization through defined interfaces

When a new informatics system is placed within a working environment, the system needs to become coupled or 'hooked up' to existing organizational technologies and processes. If we think of the new system simply as a black box that either inputs or outputs data, then each input or output must be connected to the inputs and outputs of existing information elements. These connections happen at the *interfaces* between the old and new parts of the system. If an organization exactly meets the design assumptions of the technology, then this process is straightforward because every input or output will just plug in as designed. More often, there will be local variation that requires several adaptations so that these connections can be made.

For any information system element, there may be a need to modify how data are input or output from one information component so that it can interoperate with others. Such adaptions are also required for organizational processes. Workflows may need to be adapted to fit around a new informatics system, perhaps because it is now automating something that previously was done manually or it is creating workflow steps that did not exist before. Clinical information systems often have some capability to be customized, so that the adaption burden does not sit solely with those whose workflow is being changed. Customizations allow software workflows to be modified to suit existing work practices better.

The promoting action on research implementation in health services (PARiHS) framework proposes that the successful local implementation *(SI)* of evidence is a function of three major variables – the nature of the evidence *e*, the implementation context *c*, and the presence of active facilitation *f*. This is summarized in the relationship *SI = f(e, c, f)* (Helfrich *et al.*, 2010; Stetler *et al.*, 2011).

Evidence in this model is characterized by its nature, strength and potential for implementation. Evidence comes from research, as well as from the tacit knowledge or expertise of practitioners, the community in which the change is to be implemented and data about the local context and environment.

Context is the setting in which a proposed change is to be implemented and is subdivided into three elements – the prevailing culture, leadership roles and the organization's approach to evaluation.

Facilitation describes the type of support provided to help people to change their work practices, attitudes, habits and skills. Facilitators are those individuals who can assist people to understand what has to change and how these changes can be made to achieve a desired outcome.

PARiHS tries to make clear that for any implementation to be successful, the quality of the summative evidence is not enough. We also have to take account of the setting in which implementation is occurring as well as how implementation is being done (facilitated into practice). PARiHS incorporates many recurrent themes from the implementation science literature, including:

- Implementing research into practice is an organizational issue.
- Research evidence must be strong (e.g. a systematic review of methodologically sound studies) before any implementation is justified.
- Strategies for implementation must address the need for education, audit and the management of change.
- Criteria for evaluating an intervention must be agreed on before implementation commences.

Other key features of the PARiHS model include:

- Implementation involves negotiating and developing a shared understanding about the benefits, disadvantages, risks and losses of the new practice over the old among all concerned parties.
- Some organizations are more likely to have successful implementation than others, perhaps because they have transformational leaders or elements of learning organizations.
- Appropriate facilitation should improve the likelihood of implementation success. Facilitators work with individuals and teams to enhance the implementation process.

PARiHS is a very useful empirical model of the pragmatic issues faced when implementing a change in a complex healthcare (or indeed any) organization. Its emphasis on the importance of leadership, culture and the need to engage all the key stakeholders in an organization is strongly backed up by many decades of research in organizational science and health services research.

PARiHS is a qualitative theory of implementation, and it is what could be called a middle level theory in that it assembles important factors but does not provide deeper causal explanations for why or how they relate to each other, nor does it provide theory-based mechanisms for the causal prediction of outcomes based on the values of particular variables during an implementation.

Box 12.2
PARiHS – promoting action on research implementation in health services

Implementation is thus an adaptive process that may require both *construction* – building necessary components to allow new and old elements to interoperate – and *customization* – the localization or tuning of components and processes to the special needs of an organization or process. Given that both technology and organizational process are themselves bundles of individual elements, specific functions such as creating a report or admitting a patient will require the coupling of several different bundle sub-elements into what we can call an *implementation network* (Figure 12.2).

We saw in Chapter 11 that there are four different classes of system that we may design and then implement, from algorithm through to sociotechnical system (see Figure 11.1). We can identify three different types of interface that are needed for their implementation:

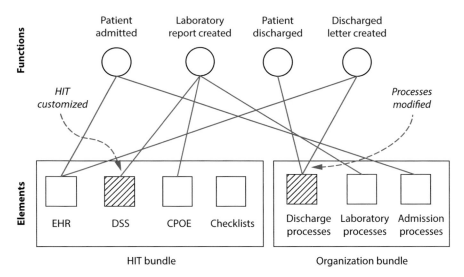

Figure 12.2   An implementation network. Any health information technology (HIT) is typically a bundle of separate elements, such as the electronic health record (EHR), decision support systems (DSS) and computerized provider order entry (CPOE). Each of these may need to interface with pre-existing organizational and technical elements to contribute to a function, such as creating a laboratory report or discharge letter. Such interfaces may require modification of either the technology or the organization to ensure a clean functional fit. In this example, functions such as patient admission or discharge depend on coupling between different process and technology elements.

- *Technology to technology (TT)* – Sometimes a special software adaptor called a *wrapper* is built as a *mediator* between two elements to translate the output of one into a form that is understandable by the input of the other. A common strategy to minimize the need for such local adaptation and maximize the likelihood of interoperability between components is to design every information element with the assumption that it conforms to a publically accepted standard. Standards exist, for example, for the way a message should be structured, such as the Health Level 7 messaging standard (HL7; see Chapter 19), as well as for which words should be used to described a concept such as a disease, such as the tenth International Classification of Diseases (ICD-10; see Chapter 23).
- *Technology to human (TH)* – The human–computer interface is perhaps the most ubiquitous example of this interface class. Every human sensory modality (seeing, hearing, touching) can be used as an interface with machine, and the interaction design of such interfaces is based upon finding readily understood metaphors or workflows that make interacting with machine as unobtrusive as possible. Poor human–computer interaction (HCI) design, of course, leads to poor human–technology coupling and unsatisfactory, sometimes unsafe outcomes (see Chapter 13).
- *Human to human (HH)* – Many clinical processes are designed to allow different individuals to 'interoperate', including clinical handover and morbidity and mortality (M & M) meetings. Communication technologies such as audio and video channels, when acting as a simple pipe connecting individuals, can also be thought of as an HH

interface. HH interfaces work best when they comply with good communication practices such as Grice's maxims, when they do not introduce unnecessary noise or loss of data and when they follow agreed structures for content sharing such as SBAR (situation, background, assessment, recommendation; see Box 5.1).

Many interfaces couple more than two elements. A social media application, for example, is not a simple HH interface because the social medium sits between the interacting humans. There are thus two human–computer interfaces, where the nature of the dialogue that can occur between individuals is constrained by the application's design. We can think of a social media application as an HT–TH interface, or because the technology in the middle is identical in this case, HTH.

12.3 Adaptation continues after implementation

Adaption does not cease once a new informatics system is implemented and enters routine use. The individuals working with technologies such as a clinical information system continue to adapt their own workflow and physical environment around the technology over time. They may also make *change requests* to those supporting the technology, by asking for elements of the technology to be further customized or even to be removed.

Workarounds are one organizational response. They are routines, behaviours and processes created by people to bypass or augment a design element of a technology such as an information system (Cresswell *et al.*, 2012; Ferneley and Sobreperez, 2006). Workarounds are probably a universal feature of organizational work, and they arise for a number of reasons. A technology or process may not allow a particular function, either by blocking it or simply not being designed to support it. A workaround may trick a system into doing what is needed or to bypass it. Workarounds can also be new procedures or processes, invented locally, to perform tasks that an information system cannot support. Putting a sticky note with the password to log onto a clinical system on a computer terminal may be a workaround designed to allow casual clinical staff members to use the system because they do not have their own account to access the clinical system. A software patch may be a quick workaround for a design flaw in software, to prevent triggering a specific behaviour in a situation the initial design did not anticipate.

Workarounds, software patches and system upgrades, local customizations of workspace such as annotations with notes and signs and changes to process all arise after implementation for a number of basic reasons:

1. The current implementation is performing sub-optimally and needs to be modified so it can function as intended. For example, the human–computer interface may provide *insufficient information* on how to complete a task or use a tool for the current users of a space (e.g. a computer workstation is annotated with the meaning of software icons because their function is not obvious) (see Figure 10.2).
2. There is a need to *support local variations* in workflow by customizing the implementation to fit local practices better.
3. There is a need to *restrict local variation* in workflow by 'patching' the implementation to prevent unexpected user behaviours or to encourage behaviours that are not happening

despite the design's intent (e.g. a sign to remind users of a clinical information system to log out after they have finished).
4. The implementation is *repurposed* for uses not initially specified by their designers. For example, the progress notes component of an EHR that is meant for free-form text begins to be used in a structured way, to communicate information not captured formally in the EHR database.

Every adaption thus appears to make an implemented system more suitable for someone's purpose. We may think of *adaptations as repairs* to an implemented system, thereby improving its fitness for current purpose, fixing inadequacy in design or meeting emergent or unanticipated needs. Adaptations may contain *missing information* needed for tasks to be executed in a specific work environment by its current occupiers (Coiera, 2014).

Adaptations thus help make visible the gap between work that is done with an implemented system and the capability of the system to support that work. The notes, manuals and instructions that can annotate a computer workstation make explicit the gap between the information system workflow and the needs and capabilities of those who use it. The gap repaired by adaptions is a measure of task–technology fit (Dishaw and Strong, 1999; Goodhue and Thompson, 1995). Put another way, adaptions represent the gap between the mental models of a technology's users and those of its designers (which are captured in their design assumptions). They are *gaps in common ground* (Coiera, 2000).

Implementation has long been seen as a process of mutual adaptation of technology and organization (Leonard, 1988). The act of adaptation or repair is therefore one of unfolding or emergent design (Rice and Rogers, 1980), which occurs after implementation, for example, through user customization (Bogers *et al.*, 2010).

Post-implementation adaptions may introduce new errors or reduce system performance in unexpected ways

By the time a system is ready for implementation, it should have passed through numerous technical tests, as well as its summative evaluation. Given the complicated nature of information and communications systems, such testing involves running new technologies through a variety of different test cases to make sure every component works well in isolation, as well as ensuring that every interface between internal components is also well-behaved.

It is in the nature of post-implementation adaptions (especially workarounds) that they often are not tested in the same way. Although a local workaround may improve a particular task, the inventors of the workaround can often be surprised to find that the workaround has created unanticipated consequences elsewhere. This is usually because the inventors have not realized that the thing they have tinkered with also interfaces with multiple other elements, and they have not taken account of what happens because of their workaround at these other interfaces. So, some adaptations may lead to local improvements but can be maladaptive globally.

Software developers are well aware of the challenges of making changes to working systems, for example through the installation of updates, the alteration of configuration settings or through patches to a system. *Regression testing* is the process that is instituted after such software changes to try to find whether new and unexpected faults (or previously fixed problems) emerge elsewhere in the system. Testing usually involves rerunning a previously defined set of tests for each system component and each earlier system revision, which are designed to make sure that all are operating as expected. The nature of software allows such testing to often be automated, although manual tests may be needed in addition. Non-software adaptions are no less important to an organization, but they are not dealt with in the same rigorous way. Their negative impacts may not be detected until a specific case emerges, such as when a patient is harmed (see Chapter 13).

12.4 Healthcare is a complex adaptive system

Sociotechnical environments such as healthcare can now be seen as dynamic and evolving ecologies in which implemented systems and organizations both adapt to each other, as well as adapt over time around each other, in the same way that any human–machine system is ecological (Gaver, 1996; Vicente and Rasmussen, 1992). Healthcare is a CAS that exhibits the same basic properties of all such systems:

- It is *complex,* in that there are many interconnections among the different elements of the system, and complexity increases with such interconnection. In health services we, by definition, are dealing with complex interventions within complex organizations. (Shiell *et al.,* 2008).
- It has a purpose, and its *fitness for purpose* can be measured, either explicitly though outcome measures or implicitly, in the sense that some individual organizations or services within the overall ecosystem can be seen to be unfit and fail. This fitness can be represented mathematically as a *fitness function,* and the fitness function can be used to select adaptions that lead to increased fitness.
- There are mechanisms for generating *variation* in the population of health services. In biology, genetic mutation introduces such variation. In healthcare, variation can either be teleological (explicitly designed) or accumulate in a notionally random way (in the sense that any object changes with time accumulates minor damage or change from its interaction with the physical environment).

Fitness for purpose can be represented using a fitness landscape

Biology provides perhaps the classic example of a CAS in which organisms adapt to survive in an ecosystem and in doing so change that ecosystem. Biologically inspired models of the evolutionary adaptation process can be used to help us understand the process of organizational adaption through implementation.

In biology, we know that the fitness of an organism in a given ecosystem changes as the organism evolves. Evolutionary processes have the effect of both introducing variation and selecting the variation that has greater fitness for longer-term survival in a species. So, changes in genetic structure lead to changes in the phenotype or physical make-up of the organism. Some of these mutations lead to improved fitness, and some have the reverse effect.

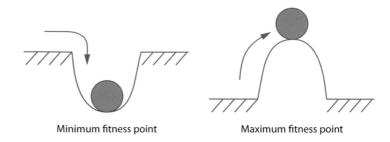

Figure 12.3
As an organization
changes, it moves
over a fitness
landscape and can
end up improving or
worsening its fitness
for purpose.

We can theoretically model a notional fitness value for any specific phenotype with respect to a given ecosystem. The phenotype can then be mutated by one 'step' or distance (e.g. by changing one DNA base pair), and the potentially modified fitness of the revised phenotype is calculated. We can continue to make such calculations by making step-by-step changes to DNA, with some of those changes affecting the phenotype and some of these altering the fitness of the phenotype (see Box 30.2).

Once we have calculated the fitness for every possible variation of DNA, we have actually created a space that maps how variations in genotype lead to variations in fitness. This can be visualized as a surface, just like a landscape (Kauffman and Levin, 1987; Kauffman and Weinberger, 1989). On this *fitness landscape,* mountains represent areas of higher fitness that every species would like to adapt into, and lower areas are regions where phenotype configurations have poor fitness. Therefore, the process of adaptation can see a biological species evolve into low-lying areas of poor fitness by making maladaptive changes or climb peaks to maximum fitness by making improvements (Figure 12.3). It is in the nature of fitness landscapes that they are typically *rugged,* exhibiting a varying surface of peaks and troughs (Figure 12.4).

Fitness landscapes can also model the fitness value of stepwise changes to organizations. We can think of making a sequence of changes in an organization as the organization 'walking' across the landscape. A bundle of changes implemented at the same time would have the same effect as making a jump across the landscape to a new organizational phenotype.

Fitness landscapes provide many intuitive lessons about the nature of sociotechnical system adaptation that occurs through implementation. For example, to find a region of higher fitness than a current one, an organization may need to traverse the landscape, first going through regions of lower fitness and then approaching a new and higher fitness peak.

It is also the case that if the ecosystem changes, then the fitness landscape will change. Changing the fitness landscape means that a particular organizational configuration may have its fitness value altered. Consider, for example, what happens to a health service set up to treat a disease surgically once a cheaper and more effective medical treatment becomes available. The service's fitness with respect to the health system as a whole changes dramatically, even though it has not changed. This means that if an organization finds itself operating in a changing world, then it may need to adapt simply to 'stand still' in terms of fitness. Adaptation thus is a prerequisite for individuals (or organizations) living in a changing world. Without adaptation in a dynamic environment, any change in an individual's fitness is out of that individual's control.

Although organizations may have a sense of how fit they are for purpose currently and may even understand some of the fitness implications of changes occurring in the

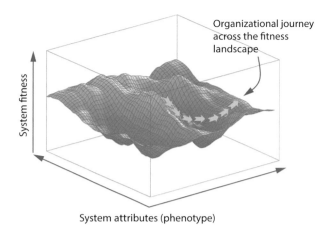

Organizational journey
across the fitness
landscape

System fitness

System attributes (phenotype)

Figure 12.4   A
fitness landscape is a
rugged surface that
describes how the
performance or
fitness of an entity
such as an organism
or an organization
varies as it changes
the way it is
configured in terms
of structure, process
and the
interdependence of
these. As changes
are made to
organizational
configurations, we
can trace a path that
the organization
makes as it 'walks'
across the
landscape. Fitness
values vary
according to the
height of the
landscape at any
particular point.

ecosystem around them, they do not have the 'big picture' of the fitness landscape around them. They, for example, do not know whether they have reached peak fitness or are merely half-way up a peak, locked in a local minimum and missing the opportunity to reconfigure and improve further (Figure 12.5).

Fitness landscapes also can give us an intuitive understanding of why the implementation of the same technology in two different organizations can yield different outcomes. Even though two organizations occupy the same ecosystem, they as *individuals* have different configurations or phenotypes. That means each organization is on a different spot on the same landscape, with a different fitness value. Asking both organizations to make the same set of phenotype changes will not move them to the same spot on the landscape unless they become clones in every way.

It is also possible that the 'ecosystem' that two organizations such as hospitals inhabit are different. A rural hospital and an urban hospital, for example, inhabit different environments, and so their fitness landscapes are different as a consequence. This helps us understand why asking two nearly identical organizations to implement the same system may yield very different results. Both make the same phenotypic changes, but for one organization the changes result in a higher fitness outcome than for the other because they are on a different landscape in which the changes work better (Figure 12.6).

It should now also be clear that organism and ecosystem both change around each other in a bi-directional process. Individual organisms or organizations adapt themselves in an effort to improve their performance on a given landscape. In doing so they affect their ecosystem and change it. Fitness landscapes are thus dynamic as are the different entities that traverse them.

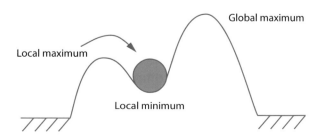

Local maximum

Global maximum

Local minimum

Figure 12.5   Organizations may become stuck in suboptimal configurations, even though higher fitness values are possible on the fitness landscape. A local maximum value appears to be the best solution because every direction a short distance away is of lower fitness. Higher fitness peaks require leaving the local maximum, traversing a local minimum and then ascending a better and hopefully globally maximal peak.

people are lost to the organization because there is no way of recognizing the fitness penalty of such losses until much later.

Middle-out change strategies may be ideal for organizations

Attempts to change the health system are sometimes characterized as top-down, with central control of new initiatives, or bottom-up, in which local practices aggregate to have global impact. Top-down strategies have come in for criticism, and there is increasing interest in bottom-up reform (Braithwaite *et al.*, 2009). An alternative middle-out approach sees government and local providers mutually agree on goals, and then each implementing the things for which they are best suited. This approach seems well suited to undertaking large-scale health information technology implementations (Coiera, 2009).

NK modelling of centralized and decentralized organizations shows that both suffer deficiencies when it comes to finding optimally fit solutions on the landscape (Kauffman and Macready, 1995). An intermediate form of co-ordination, equivalent to a middle-out strategy, gives agents exclusive control of only some elements (their 'patch'). Patching is very similar in effect to creating modularity in design. It can often outperform bottom-up processes and leads to discovering better optima on the landscape than centralized processes, along with a major reduction in search time and cost.

12.6 Excessive system complexity may explain why change fails to improve organizational performance

Despite great efforts to implement a wide variety of health system changes to improve the safety, quality and efficiency of service delivery, many observers have noted that progress is often painfully slow. Safety and quality initiatives often struggle to make care delivery safer for patients (Braithwaite and Coiera, 2010). Evidence-based recommendations and standards pile up, unheeded or poorly enacted (Grimshaw and Eccles, 2004).

Seeing healthcare as a CAS allows us to explore the reasons that change is often difficult and not sustainable. We have already seen that when an organization is reaching the top of its fitness peak, much greater change is required to achieve a diminishing amount of benefit. What this does not explain is why organizations that are nowhere near the optimum also struggle to lift their performance.

Competing demands create decision complexity and force the acceptance of suboptimal solutions resulting in clinical inertia

The reluctance of clinicians to change their practice and adapt it to evidence-based recommendations is a good example of an implementation science challenge. Translation of clinical research into new guidelines that are then disseminated may have less impact than desired (see Chapter 17). This *clinical inertia* to change is defined as a failure by healthcare providers to initiate or intensify therapy when indicated (Phillips *et al.*, 2001). It has been documented for many conditions, including diabetes (O'Connor, 2005), hypertension and dyslipedaemia (van Bruggen *et al.*, 2009).

One compelling explanation for clinical inertia is that clinicians are, in fact, making the best decisions they can in the presence of multiple *competing demands* (Jaén *et al.*, 1994; Parchman *et al.*, 2007; Stange, 2007). Clinical encounters are constrained by time and by uncertain or absent data (Grant *et al.*, 2009), and clinicians juggle multiple problems, prioritizing some over others (Hofer *et al.*, 2004). As the number of patients' problems increases, any decision to change therapy becomes more likely to be put off until the next encounter (Parchman *et al.*, 2007). The decision to increase hypertensive therapy when faced with high blood pressure may be delayed if the clinician believes that other clinical priorities must be dealt with first.

Managing competing demands thus requires compromise. We satisfy some demands at the expense of others. Competing demands have been demonstrated to shape decision-making in diabetes (Parchman *et al.*, 2007), mammography (Nutting *et al.*, 2001), depression (Klinkman, 1997) and smoking cessation (Jaén *et al.*, 2001). In decision theoretical terms, making a suboptimal decision to satisfy competing demands is called *satisfycing* (Simon, 1956). When resources are limited, humans choose a 'good enough' solution that meets a number of goals.

Organizational inertia appears common in many sectors including healthcare

Clinical inertia alone cannot explain resistance to change across the health system. Inertia is not seen only in therapeutic decision-making, but probably in part it underpins the slow progress with patient safety initiatives and the limited effectiveness of health service restructuring. Clinical inertia is thus probably just one manifestation of a more general phenomenon. We can define *system inertia* as a failure by a human organization to initiate, or to achieve, a sustained change in behaviour despite clear evidence indicating that change is essential (Coiera, 2011).

Organizational inertia has long been studied, and the blame for inertia was initially assigned to slow administrative and political decision-making (Purola, 1972). The *structural inertia* thesis contends that organizational inflexibility is an outcome of poor adaptation to change (Hannan and Freeman, 1984). Although the external environment is constantly changing, humans apparently favour organizations that are structurally static, possibly because they are believed to be more reliable or accountable. Unfortunately, static organizations become increasingly out of step as the surrounding environment changes around them.

For a time, the only solution to stasis was believed to be a dramatic or catastrophic organizational shift – a 'big bang' theory of organizational adjustment. Such ruptures temporarily opened the window for major institutional change, only to be followed by a period of further inertia, until the next crisis. Parallels have been drawn between this type of dramatic human system change and punctuated equilibrium in evolutionary biology (Krasner, 1984). Clearly, however, system changes do occur, and crisis is not at the centre of them all. Rather, change is typically hard won, erratic and difficult to reproduce. This process of more erratic change

4. Implementation is an adaptive process that may require both construction – building necessary components to allow new and old elements to interoperate – and customization – the localization or tuning of components and processes to the special needs of an organization or process.

5. When a new informatics system is placed within a working environment, the system is coupled to existing organizational technologies and processes through interfaces connecting technology to technology, technology to human and human to human to create an implementation network.

6. The individuals working with technologies continue to adapt their own workflow and physical environment around the technology over time. Workarounds are one example of post-implementation adaptation. Post-implementation adaption may introduce new errors or reduce system performance in unexpected ways.

7. Healthcare is a complex adaptive system for the following reasons:

    a. It is complex, in that there are many interconnections among the different elements of the system.

    b. It has a purpose, and its fitness for purpose can be measured and used to select fitter configurations.

    c. There are mechanisms for generating variation in the population of health services.

8. Fitness for purpose can be represented using a fitness landscape. Organizational fitness landscapes model the fitness value changes associated with stepwise changes to organizations.

9. As organizations adapt, they affect their ecosystem and may change the fitness landscapes.

10. *NK network models* can demonstrate the impact of complexity on fitness. N is the number of elements in an entity (e.g. genes, structures or processes), and K is the number of dependencies that exist among these elements.

11. The ruggedness of a fitness landscape for an entity with N components depends on the number of dependent connections K between those components. With no interdependencies, the landscape is smooth, with a single point of maximum fitness. When the network is fully connected, the landscape has no obvious structure but becomes randomly peaked. In between we find regions of grouped or correlated peaks with flatter areas between them.

12. When the rate of mutation exceeds a certain point, it is possible for an organization to evolve into areas of the landscape that are of lower fitness (the error catastrophe).

13. Organizational inertia appears common in many sectors including healthcare. One of the effects of increasing K (number of dependencies) is a flattening in the height of increasingly uncorrelated local maxima, and this may explain why little improvement is possible in overly complex organizations.

14. Methods for reducing system complexity should improve the likelihood that change will result in improved fitness, and these methods include the use of modular designs such as care bundles and the retirement of older interdependencies and system elements.

CHAPTER 13

Information system safety

> I will prescribe regimens for the good of my patients according to my ability and my judgement and never do harm to anyone.
>
> *Hippocratic Oath, fourth century BC*
>
> *Primum non nocere.* (First do no harm.)
>
> *Thomas Sydenham, 1624–1689*

13.1 Although information technology has the potential to improve safety, it can also contribute to harm

Information technology (IT) has repeatedly demonstrated its capacity to improve the safety and quality of healthcare. It does this by shaping the information that is collected or seen at the time of decision-making or using that information to automate clinical processes. Indeed, there is probably no more foundational way of intervening in the practice and delivery of healthcare than to alter its informational and decision substrate. When the consequences of such an intervention are as intended, then we have a powerful tool to alter practice for the good. When it goes awry, there are unintended consequences, and these may distort information, misguide decisions or trigger actions that can lead to harm to a patient (Ash *et al.*, 2004). Recall from Chapter 1 how errors in the design of the software and hardware of the Therac-25 radiotherapy machine harmed multiple patients, some of whom died as a result of radiation overdoses (see Box 1.1).

That IT may sometimes be unsafe should come as no surprise. There are many other well-known sources of risk in healthcare delivery. The drugs we use can have side effects that hurt patients. The diagnostic and therapeutic procedures that are performed on patients sometimes go wrong. So-called *iatrogenic harm* is unfortunately common and widespread across healthcare delivery, affecting all types of practices and all nations. In the developed world, about 10 per cent of admissions to hospital are associated with some kind of adverse event. Half of these adverse events are deemed to be preventable, and one in five results in permanent disability or death (Thomas *et al.*, 2000). Indeed, we see similar safety issues across all areas of technical human endeavor, affecting transport sectors such as aviation, rail and motoring, as well as activities such as mining or energy production.

Recognizing that whatever we do should be as safe as possible is therefore core to any technical endeavor. The existence of a mature approach to safety is a non-negotiable requirement for any sustainable technical enterprise. In this chapter, we review basic principles of patient safety and then explore the different sources of risk associated with health IT. Approaches to detecting, minimizing and managing these risks complete the chapter.

13.2 Not all hazards lead to a safety incident, and not all incidents lead to harm

The anatomy of any particular set of events that leads to harm to a patient is likely to be somehow unique. Different individuals, contexts and circumstances all have their part in shaping the unfolding of any process that leads to the harm. An analogy often drawn is that harm events have both a phenotype (the specific local circumstances that led to the event) and a genotype (the underlying root causes of the event). A number of core concepts can help understand the genesis (or genotype) of most unintended harms (Figure 13.1):

- *Hazards* are potential sources of risk that exist in any environment. They do not themselves cause anything to happen, but their presence increases the likelihood that an accident will occur. An object left on the floor is a hazard that increases the risk that someone will trip over it and fall. A password written on a sticky note attached to a computer monitor increases the risk that an unauthorized person will access a clinical information system.
- *Events* such as a human taking an action, or a machine changing state, are the means by which any organizational process is enacted. An *adverse event* (or critical incident) occurs when an event (e.g. equipment failure or a human action) leads to an unwanted and potentially negative outcome. The existence of hazards increases the probability that the event will be adverse. A drug side effect and a laboratory report with the wrong

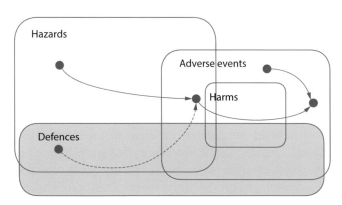

Figure 13.1   Hazards make adverse events more likely, and some but not all adverse events lead to actual harms. Harms often have more than one contributing event or hazard at their root cause. System defences seek to interrupt the causes of harms, whether through hazard reduction or adverse event detection or disruption.

patient identity are examples of adverse events with clear opportunity for harm. Not every adverse event leads to harm, however, and not all harms are severe (Box 13.1). If an adverse event does not have a negative consequence because it did not reach the patient, it is called a *near miss*.

- *Errors* (or mistakes) arise when a planned sequence of events is not executed accurately. Errors may occur because (1) the wrong plan is selected, (2) the right plan is not carried out correctly (e.g. omitting steps or carrying steps out in the wrong order), or (3) a particular step is not executed as directed. Some errors are *latent,* in that they are not discovered until a later time. For example, a software bug may not be noticed because it is triggered only in a special set of circumstance. *Active errors,* in contrast, are felt immediately. When an error occurs because an intended action is not executed, it is known as an *omission error.* When an error occurs because an action is wrong, this is called a *commission error.* We can think of an omission error as a false-negative result and a commission error as a false-positive result.

Box 13.1
Assigning a severity score to a safety incident

Incidents vary in their severity and the likelihood of recurrence. In health, as in any safety-critical sector, a risk rating is applied to grade the seriousness of an incident to help prioritize the investigation and response to of high-risk events. The Severity Assessment Code (SAC) is an internationally accepted rating system, developed by the US Veterans Administration. One of four risk ratings (1, extreme; 2, high; 3, medium; 4, low) is assigned based on the severity of the *consequences* of an incident and the *likelihood of recurrence* (DeRosier *et al.,* 2002).

Likelihood	Consequence				
	Serious	Major	Moderate	Minor	Minimum
Frequent	1	1	2	3	3
Likely	1	1	2	3	4
Possible	1	2	2	3	4
Unlikely	1	2	3	4	4
Rare	2	3	3	4	4

Consequence

Serious – Incident is likely to lead to death.
Major – Incident is likely to lead to a major permanent loss of function.
Moderate – Incident is likely to lead to permanent reduction in bodily functioning (e.g. leading to increased length of stay or surgical intervention).
Minor – Incident is likely to lead to an increase in level of care (e.g. review, investigations or referral to another clinician).
Minimum – Incident is likely to have little or no effect on the patient.

Likelihood

Frequent – Incident is expected to occur again either immediately or within a short period of time (likely to occur most weeks or months).
Likely – Incident will probably occur in most circumstances (several times a year).
Possible – Incident possibly will recur at some time (every 1 to 2 years).
Unlikely –Incident possibly will recur at some time in 2 to 5 years.
Rare – Incident likely to recur only in exceptional circumstances (every 5 to 30 years).

- *Harms* are the measurable negative outcomes of an adverse event. For example, an overdose of radiation from a radiotherapy machine may lead to skin burns, organ damage or death.
- *System defences* are the procedures, tools and practices that are created within an organization to detect hazards, errors and adverse events before they can lead to harm. *Redundancy* in system defences means that there is more than one way to detect or prevent an adverse event or error. Defences decrease the probability that an adverse event will occur or will lead to harm.

Given the complexity of clinical work, there are clearly multiple ways in which hazards and events can come together to create harms. More often than not, system defences are present to catch adverse events just before or after they happen, so that harm does not result.

Information errors can affect data, knowledge and inference

The currency of information systems is the data they store, manipulate and communicate. *Information errors* occur whenever a datum is incorrect, absent, only partially present or delayed in its arrival (Box 13.2). For example, in a medication ordering system, information errors would occur when:

1. *Data are wrong* – If a clinician orders the antibiotic *flucloxacillin* but the antimetabolite *methotrexate* appears in the pharmacy system, then an error has occurred somewhere in the process between clinical order and pharmacy receipt of the order.
2. *Data are missing* – If a patient's medication record does not display that the patient has a penicillin allergy that has been documented, then this missing information creates a hazard that may lead to harm.
3. *Data are partial* – If a patient's discharge medication list includes a medication's name but not its dose, this creates a hazard in which the primary care physician may reorder the medication at the wrong dose.
4. *Data are delayed* – Should a hospital clinician order a new medication urgently, but the medication fails to appear on the patient's medication list immediately, it may not be dispensed in a timely fashion.

Information errors are adverse events, and they may be caused by hazards (e.g. in system design or implementation) interacting with normal clinical behaviors. Often information errors interact with human errors (or use errors) to trigger the adverse event.

Recall from Chapter 2 that for an information system to support decision-making, it requires three elements – a *database*, a *knowledge base* and an *inference procedure*. Information errors can occur in any of these, with varying levels of impact. An error in the data of a particular patient is most likely to affect only that individual patient's care. An error in decision rules, for example, checking for drug–drug interactions or in an order set, may affect many patients. Several studies have identified that inconsistencies in drug interaction rule sets are common, and medication order entry systems from different manufacturers often generate very different alert responses for the same combination of medications (Fernando *et al.*, 2004; Sweidan *et al.*, 2009). Should errors occur in the basic inference procedures of an information system, their effects could be nearly universal across the system. For example, if a

Box 13.2
Examples of
information errors

Wrong information

- A hospital electronic medical record (EMR) wrongly displays patient A's medications in patient B's record, and this leads to prescription of an incorrect medication.
- An x-ray is stored the wrong patient's folder; the results are an incorrect diagnosis and subsequent unnecessary intubation, contributing to the patient's death.
- Cancer is not detected because a doctor is wrongly shown an image that he or she believes is the current image but in fact is 2 years old.
- The left and right markers used to orient a digital x-ray image are swapped and cause a surgeon to operate on the wrong side of a patient's head.

Missing information

- A prescribing system fails to alert a clinician about a potentially fatal drug interaction because the system's interaction rule base is not up-to-date and is missing the necessary trigger rule.
- Incompatibilities between two clinical databases caused by variations in the way data (e.g. patients' allergies) are coded mean that when a hospital migrates from one system to a new one, some data are lost or are changed because the new code system interprets the data differently.

Incomplete information

- The administration time for a blood pressure–lowering drug that needs to be administered at night to reduce risk of falls is omitted, so the drug is given at a higher-risk time of day.
- A picture archiving and communication system (PACS) lists only the most recent results and does not provide information about the existence of earlier investigations that may be needed to evaluate the course of disease.

Delayed information

- An order for a clinical test is significantly delayed because the order message is caught in a queue during computer network downtime and is successfully sent only once the network is restored.
- A clinical note is left open and unsaved on a computer screen because the user moves on to other tasks, and so the text of the note is not uploaded to the medical record until the clinician returns to the screen.

statistical module incorrectly computes average values, then any time other parts of the system request this procedure, an error may occur.

Humans are also a source of information errors, although the cause of the errors may be different. In Chapter 8, we examined how interruptions can lead to failures in working memory. For example, if a clinician is writing a clinical note and is interrupted, when the clinician returns to completing the note, he or she may write down information associated with a different patient because the interruption has disrupted their memory process.

13.3 Information technology–related harms have their origin in system design, implementation or use

The complex and sociotechnical nature of IT use means that the origin of adverse events reflects this union of human and machine–related factors (Sittig and Singh, 2010). Often an event has multiple contributing factors coming from both the human and the technical spaces, and no single hazard or event is uniquely the 'cause' (see Box 13.3).

Classification systems have been developed to assist in understanding the kinds of problem that lead to an adverse event. One of the most widely used classifications divides the problem space into two – (1) human factors and (2) technical or machine-related factors (Magrabi *et al.,* 2012). Within these two causal spaces, we subdivide safety problems based upon the type of information error – whether data are incorrect, absent, only partially present or somehow delayed in their arrival (Figure 13.2).

Within the technical space, the classification tree breaks down problems into hardware and software types, covering everything from computer network issues through to software

Box 13.3 Case study – an adverse drug event	An elderly patient suffering from *hypokalemia* or low potassium (serum potassium was 3.1 mEq/L; creatinine, 1.7) became severely *hyperkalemic* (serum potassium level, 7.8 mEq/L). Wrong, incomplete and missing information in the hospital order entry system resulted in the patient receiving multiple doses of potassium. In total, 316 mEq of potassium chloride (KCl) was administered over 42 hours as a result of the following orders entered into the computerized provider order entry (CPOE) system (Horsky *et al.,* 2005):

1. 40 mEq by intravenous (IV) bolus injection.

2. 80 mEq/L by IV drip in 1 L of 5 per cent dextrose solution at the rate of 75 mL/hour. The order ran for 36 hours, delivering 216 mEq before it was detected (36×75 mL = 2.7 L; 2.7×80 mEq).

3. 60 mEq by IV bolus injection.

The first order for 40 mEq KCl was placed on a Saturday morning by clinician A, who correctly diagnosed the patient as hypokalemic. After placing the bolus order, clinician A realized that the patient already had an IV fluid line inserted and decided to change the order to use the IV line. The clinician made several attempts to enter this order, intended to specify the rate and concentration and wanted to limit the total volume of IV fluid to 1 L. The user interfaces for entering drip and IV injection orders were visually very similar, but there were inconsistencies in the use models. Whereas injections could be specified by dose, IV drip orders were specified by duration, with a default stop time of 7 days. Clinician A was not aware of this difference. After several attempts to limit the total fluid volume to 1 L, the clinician tried to work around the system by using the free-text comments field. However, this information was not used by the system, and the IV drip ran until the adverse event was detected on Monday morning.

These commission errors by the clinician were compounded by an error of omission. The clinician intended to delete the original order for 40 mEq/L but mistakenly deleted a similar order that had been placed 2 days before by another clinician. Thus, the initial order remained in the system, and the medication was also given to the patient. These events have a remarkable similarity to those of the Therac-25 events, in which multiple radiation doses were delivered (see Box 1.1).

One system defence that failed was automated dose checking by the pharmacy. Although the system could detect an out of bound concentration (i.e. 100 mEq/L), it could not detect the overdose delivered by 80 mEq/L running for 36 hours (Figure 13.3).

Care of the patient was transferred to clinician B on Sunday morning. When asked to check the potassium levels by clinician A, clinician B failed to notice that the latest test result (3.1 mEq/L) was 24 hours old, even though date and time of the result were displayed by the system. The previous KCl drip was still running, but this information was missing because drips were not displayed on the screen used by clinicians to review patient medications. Thus, believing that the patient was still hypokalemic and untreated, clinician B ordered a further 60 mEq KCl to be given as IV injection. Just like clinician A, clinician B had problems with the CPOE user interface and made multiple attempts to enter the order. This adverse event was eventually detected on Monday morning, when laboratory test results were checked and the patient was found to be severely hyperkalemic.

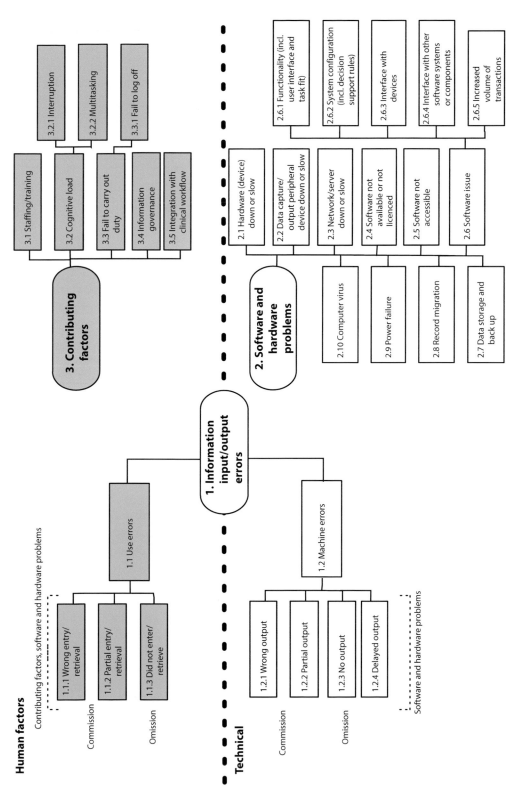

Figure 13.2   A classification of the contributing human and technical problems associated with information systems that can lead to an adverse event and potentially harm a patient. (From Magrabi *et al.*, 2015.)

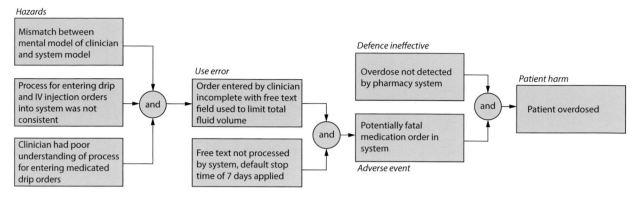

Figure 13.3   A simple accident model of the events that led to a patient being overdosed through multiple doses of KCl.

viruses. Within the human factors space we find a matching set of problems that contribute to human errors. The amount of cognitive load and attentional resources available to complete a task, distractions through interruption and cognitive biases all can contribute to how well we perform tasks (see Chapters 4 and 8). The degree to which human workflows match the workflows embedded in an information system, the level of training in system use attained by individual system users and the safety defences or governance structures put in place around the use of technology are also all major contributory factors to the likelihood of adverse events.

This classification does not imply that an adverse event has only one cause, and when an adverse event is investigated, it often has multiple labels assigned to it from the classification. For example, a network failure may cause the computer network to respond more slowly than normal, thus contributing to a delay in an urgent medication order from a medication ordering system arriving at a pharmacy in preparation for dispensing. At the same time, the ordering clinician may have failed to notify nursing staff about a forthcoming urgent order (which would have been a useful system defence) because the clinician was distracted by an interruption on the telephone during the ordering process and so did not remember to communicate the urgency of the order verbally.

13.4 Information technology may be unsafe when its design does not meet quality standards or fails to account for how it will be used

We saw in Chapter 3 that information systems are machines constructed with a purpose in mind. When the model on which they are based is flawed or does not match the context of use, then these systems can cause harm. In this section we explore why clinical information systems sometimes behave in such unexpected ways. It also may be beneficial to reread Chapter 1, to recollect how mismatches between a system as designed and a system as implemented can shape outcomes.

System design may not reflect how it will be used

When designers have a poor understanding of clinical work, they may make incorrect assumptions about how a system will be used, the tasks it must support and the clinical workflow in which those tasks need to be executed. Problems with system design include:

- *Incomplete or incorrect assumptions about clinical tasks or system users* that a system should support. This is one of the most important sources of error. Patients may continue to receive medications because an order entry system incorrectly assumes that orders will not need to be changed once made and thus does not support discontinuation or modification of orders. Errors are also generated when there is a mismatch between the system and the mental model of users. For example, an electronic health record (EHR) that displays weight in pounds when clinicians work in kilograms is primed to cause errors.
- *Inadequate or poorly designed user interfaces* increase cognitive load and the probability of use errors. Poor usability can also make a system hard to learn and difficult to recall after a period of not using a system, and it can make completing tasks inefficient (Nielsen, 1993). Consider a prescribing system that requires users to scroll through a list of options in a drop-down menu. If there are too many options, or they are counter-intuitively arranged, patients may be prescribed the wrong drug or dose through a 'pick list error'. Risks are also increased when systems do not facilitate recovery from use errors (e.g. when an order entry system does not allow clinicians to modify or cancel an order once it is placed).
- *Mismatches between system workflow and clinical workflow* can also lead to use errors. For instance, a nurse might be prevented from reviewing medication lists at the time of administration because the system is accessible only from a central workstation and is not accessible at the patient's bedside. Errors also occur when system design does not match the sequence in which clinical tasks are carried out. For example, prescribing decision support can be ineffective if users are not asked to complete allergy information before medications are entered.

Quality issues in build are a potential source of hazard and harm

Defects introduced during software construction can cause systems to behave in unexpected ways. The chance that defects will persist in working systems increases if software is not adequately tested by a manufacturer. There are scant public data about the rate of software errors in clinical systems or their impact on patient safety. Such data, when they are actually collected, are likely to be commercial and kept confidential. There appear to be no uniform formal mechanisms for enforcing the recording or reporting of software error rates. One now old data set was generated from three releases of a major commercial US medical record system and is illustrative (Hewett *et al.,* 2006; Stringfellow *et al.,* 2002). The system contained 188 separate software components across 6500 files. Release 1 had defects in 58 of 180 components, 7 of which were discovered only after release. Release 2 had 64 defects in 185 components, with 5 discovered after release. Release 3 showed a numerical improvement in quality, with only 40 of 188 components being defective, but still 6 were discovered after release. Such analyses allow us to estimate the defect rate in even good-quality software and help developers decide when to release software, based upon estimates of the number of as yet undetected errors.

Unexpected interactions between modules and systems may lead to errors

Clinical information systems are typically composed of multiple modules. For instance, a general practice system contains modules for record keeping, prescribing and ordering tests. Such systems could also be connected to a medical device such as an electrocardiograph and connect to other systems such as a laboratory information system to download test results. All these different components, devices and systems, often coming from different vendors, need to *interoperate* – that is, to share information in a structured way that is understandable by all. Information errors can arise from communication failures among system components, just as they can manifest when humans communicate (see Chapter 4). Communication failures among system components can manifest in many ways, from a message with an order that does not reach the intended clinical system because it could not be understood by an intermediating component, through to distortion of the information in some way that causes it to be misrepresented when it arrives because the systems use slightly different standards (e.g. in clinical terminology). Formal standards for system interoperability are designed to minimize the chances of such errors (see Chapter 19).

Problems with information technology infrastructure can affect a wide variety of clinical systems and processes

A stable IT infrastructure is critical to the safe operation of clinical software and includes everything from computer hardware to operating systems, data networks and data storage facilities. Problems with IT infrastructure can directly affect the availability of clinical systems and disrupt the delivery of care. For example, if a desktop computer or printer fails, a clinician may not be able to access the EHR or generate a prescription. A network problem in a hospital may cause a picture archiving and communication system (PACS) to be inaccessible for many hours, thus preventing image files and reports from being read or created. As a result, surgery could be cancelled and clinics rescheduled. Failures with back-up facilities and computer viruses can similarly disrupt care delivery.

13.5 Human factors and system use practices are major sources of risk

It is not only the machines we use that can lead to harm to a patient. System safety can compromised by *human factors* – when humans are the source of adverse events, or when machine designs do not fit well either with our bodies or our cognitive abilities. The *knowledge and skills* of users are particularly fundamental to safe operation, and inadequate knowledge about how to use a system can lead to harm to a patient (Box 13.3). When users are unaware of system limitations, then errors of omission may occur. For instance, a clinician may inadvertently prescribe the wrong medication, by wrongly assuming that the system would have alerted them if a mistake had been made. This type of *automation bias* is further discussed in Chapter 28.

Training programmes are thus essential for safe use of clinical information systems, and they must be appropriately tailored to the needs of clinicians in different roles or with different experience levels. For example, training in the use of a prescribing system that will be used by doctors, pharmacists and nurses should be tailored to the different needs and tasks of each group.

Adverse events can also occur when the *cognitive resources* devoted to using a system are inadequate. For example, if a clinician is already heavily cognitively loaded, and he or she is distracted or interrupted, then that clinician may make errors because they do not devote enough attention to the information system in use. For example, after being interrupted by a telephone call, a physician might complete a medication order but give it to the wrong patient because the physician returned to the wrong patient's record after the call.

System use can also be compromised by our built-in *cognitive biases* (see Chapter 8). For example, both clinicians and consumers can misinterpret data presented to them by information retrieval systems because they interpret new information through the lens of prior belief (anchoring effect). Other factors that shape how information is viewed include the order in which documents are accessed (order effect) and the amount of time spent on documents (exposure effect) (Lau and Coiera, 2007). One consequence of these effects is that clinicians or consumers who would otherwise make a correct decision are swayed by information presentation effects into switching to an incorrect decision (Lau and Coiera, 2009).

Deficiencies in *organizational policies and procedures* for system use are another threat. For example, although setting up training in the use of clinical systems is commendable, the lack of a policy to enforce completion of such training before systems are used is a significant weakness. Policies that require all permanent clinical staff to have a secure system password while failing to require the same of casual staff simply creates loopholes that anyone can use to gain unauthorized access to clinical records. Similarly, restricting access rights to information that could help manage a patient creates its own risks (see Chapter 19). For example, making the results of a human immunodeficiency virus test visible only to the ordering clinician and not to those engaged in subsequent care may expose others to risks of harm, but this may be necessary to protect patient privacy. Some EHRs have a 'break the glass' feature to get around this problem (Ferreira *et al.*, 2006), in which unauthorized clinicians can access patients' records in an emergency but must identify themselves to the system so the access can be audited and, if needed, justified later.

13.6 System implementation and transitions can introduce safety risks

In Chapter 12 we reviewed the process of system implementation, when an information or communication system is installed 'in place' to become a routine part of an organization's work processes. The degree to which built or adapted software, hardware and their associated workflows fit the needs of an organization determines both their likely effectiveness and their safety. Information errors can easily be introduced during the implementation process and can create hazards or trigger adverse events. The likelihood of new safety problems increases as the quality of the implementation decreases. For example, undue haste in system implementation, failure to provide adequate resources and time for user training or insufficient

Box 13.4
Case study —
implementation of
an order entry
system at two
pediatric hospitals

Two US hospitals, in Pittsburgh and Seattle, implemented the same electronic health record (EHR) and computerized provider order entry (CPOE) in their pediatric intensive care units (ICUs) (Del Beccaro *et al.*, 2006; Han *et al.*, 2005). At 5 months after implementation, the mortality rate in Pittsburgh increased from 2.8 to 6.6 per cent, whereas there was no significant change in Seattle (13 months after implementation, non-significant decrease, 4.2 to 3.5 per cent). The disparity in patient outcomes reflects the sociotechnical nature of computer systems and was most likely the result of differences in implementation processes:

1. *Speed of implementation* – Implementation at Pittsburgh was a 'big bang' approach, occurring hospitalwide over a 6-day period and thus not allowing staff enough time to adapt to new routines and responsibilities.

2. *User training* – In Seattle all clinical staff members were required to attend role-specific training programmes for 2 to 4 hours and were supported by a peer group of superusers during and after implementation. Users were also provided with 24 hour a day support during implementation.

3. *User interface* – The system in Seattle had been locally adapted to reduce the time taken for doctors to enter orders. Specific order sets were created for the ICU, including frequently used orders. No such adaption occurred in Pittsburgh, thus resulting in delays in initiating treatment.

4. *Poor integration with workflow* – Unlike the old paper-based system, the Pittsburgh CPOE did not allow entry of orders prior to arrival of critically ill patients, delaying life-saving treatment. The new workflow also caused a breakdown in doctor–nurse communication. In contrast user interface changes in Seattle facilitated rapid processing of patients who were transported to ICU.

5. *Changes in other processes* – In parallel with the order entry implementation, Pittsburgh made changes to policies and procedures for dispensing and administering medications that also delayed treatment. For instance all medications including ICU vasoactive drugs were relocated to a central pharmacy.

effort expended on the often expensive and time-consuming process of localization all can affect the fit between existing processes and a new system (Box 13.4).

Implementation effects are felt at many points in an organization's development, and system transitions are often the riskiest because these are the times when new hazards and errors are most likely to be introduced:

- *The transition from paper to computerized systems* – The greatest change for most organizations is the initial switch from paper to electronic systems. It is a time when old processes are abandoned, when new tools and systems need to be learned and when many hidden informal systems that have served the organization well for many years are disrupted – only later to be rediscovered as unexpected events occur. Only rarely do organizations have the abundant resources, time and expertise for a new system to be built from scratch and closely meet their needs. More often, when software is built to order, resources and timelines are fixed, which means that the desired system and the one eventually delivered are not the same. Expected features may have been cut or quality sacrificed. Most organizations thus take a different route, which is to buy 'off the shelf' systems that are close enough to their needs. The process of localization allows such systems to be configured to match local needs better. It also involves changing local practices and processes where such reconfiguration is not possible. For instance, implementation of an order entry system involves configuration of system alerts to match local antibiotic guidelines. If the system cannot be configured to display different brand names of medications, then clinicians may need to change their work practice to prescribe generic drugs.

- *Hybrid systems* are created when the transition from paper to computer is only partial. For example, processes such as order entry or prescribing are computerized, but others are left on paper. Hybrid systems are a pragmatic staging strategy because 'big bang' implementations that completely abandon paper all at once may be very risky, leaving little opportunity to learn about how well new systems fit existing processes. Hybrid systems may also be created when electronic systems cannot adequately meet clinical needs. For instance, a paper chart may be used when variable-dose medications are not supported in a new order entry system. However, hybrid systems have their own unique safety risks to patients (Sparnon, 2013). Clinical data are now stored in multiple places, some on paper and some electronically. Clinicians thus need to look up patient data from several sources when making a decision. For example, using CPOE in an otherwise paper-based unit creates a hybrid workflow that requires checking paper notes for allergies and history of past drug interactions. This creates an opportunity for information to be missed. Some organizations may choose to implement only sections of the EMR, such as progress notes alone, which creates similar problems.

- *Routine system updates and software patches* – Information systems require regular maintenance, and update delays or omissions can lead to safety problems. For example, failure to update a drug interaction database with a newly reported drug–drug interaction, or failure to update an electronic protocol following the publication of new guidelines for cancer therapy, creates risks for patient care. Local system configurations may mean that when a manufacturer-supplied software patch is applied (e.g. to fix a newly identified system problem), unrecognized inconsistencies between the local software and the version on which the patch was tested result in problems. Updates can also cause local configurations to be overwritten by older default settings. For example, medication alerts tailored to a hospital's medication policy may revert back to the default configuration supplied by the manufacturer.

- *Changes in system function* – System updates sometimes alter the way software appears to a user, through redesigns of the user interface, by moving functions to different locations on the screen or adding or removing functions. If such changes are not explained to users, then users may carry out what they think are reasonable actions (based on their mental model of the older version) but with very different results. For example, changing the units with which the dose of a drug can be prescribed may mean that a clinician orders an overdose or underdose because he or she has not noticed the change in units. Changes may not manifest at the user interface but affect underlying decision rules. For example, rules that generate alerts when a drug is prescribed (e.g. suggesting that a drug dose be reduced because a patient has renal insufficiency) may be turned off, but clinicians prescribing the drug still assume they are there and so do not check for renal failure when they prescribe.

- *The transition from one version of a system to a new one* – New versions of software may require associated hardware updates, and these may not always be planned for or indeed apparent. For example, a radiology department may upgrade its PACS but discovers that its existing monitors do not support the higher-resolution images displayed by the new software.

- *The transition from one information system to an entirely different one* – New systems acquisitions bring with them the opportunities for an organization to upgrade to faster, more efficient and cost-effective technologies, as well as acquire technical innovations unavailable in older systems. The risks in this process very much mirror the transition from paper to electronic in that major assumptions about the way the new system will work and the way it actually works may be only uncovered after implementation, and some of those differences may result in risks to patients. A well-known system change risk is the process of *data migration*, in which clinical records are moved from the old to the new system. Manufacturers often state that they fully comply with a given information standard, and one would expect two systems conforming to the same standard to interoperate easily and allow the exchange of data between them. Unfortunately, the way in which standards are implemented at a software level may differ subtly among manufacturers, and these differences may manifest as information errors and often take some time to be discovered.

Workarounds are post-implementation adaptations that seek to bypass system constraints on workflow

Safety issues may not manifest immediately, and sometimes it is well into the post-implementation period before they are noticed. Some safety issues arise from the post-implementation response of an organization to the system. As we saw in Chapter 12, *workarounds* are one type of post-implementation response. Workarounds, however, carry risks. The password on the sticky note is an example of a workaround designed to fix a problem (no process for providing casual staff with a personal account and password) that also creates a problem (there is now an easy way for unauthorized individuals to access clinical records). Another well-documented workaround comes from a medication administration system that used wristband barcodes to identify patients. A workaround was developed to allow nurses to pick up the medications for multiple patients, and it saved time walking back and forward between medication cart and patient. Copies of patients' barcodes were stuck to desks, scanner carts, doorjambs, supply closets or clipboards or were even affixed to nurses' belt loops or their own arms, thus allowing multiple patients to be scanned at once (Koppel *et al.*, 2008). The risk with this workaround is that the wrong medication will be given to a patient, exactly the opposite of the intent of the system design. Using cut and paste features for copying text from clinical notes and duplicating it in a new entry may be a workaround to save time, but it can also cause significant quality and safety issues, for example, incorrectly recording that patient observations were taken when they were not (Sheehy *et al.*, 2014).

A feature of workarounds is thus that they are not formally designed or tested processes. They may work very well for the specific circumstance for which they were created, but they can cause unintended problems. We could say that workarounds are likely to generalize poorly to other tasks and contexts or that they are brittle processes.

13.7 Safety can be improved by identifying and mitigating hazards

The behaviour of a system emerges from the way its components interact, and safety is one such emergent property. Safety emerges from the collective interactions among all system components, including technology, people, workflow, organization and the external environment. It follows that safety could be improved if we could identify and address potentially unsafe interactions. Unfortunately, all the possible interactions among different system components are not predictable at design time, especially when technology is embedded within a sociotechnical system. Consequently, processes must be set up to detect adverse events and the unexpected system interactions that cause them.

Hazard assessment is based on accident models

By modelling the behaviour of a system, we can identify many unsafe interactions. An *accident model* is a representation of the behaviour of an information system and its interactions that gave rise to an incident. Accident models are formal hazard assessment techniques that can be used to prospectively or retrospectively identify errors, influences and system states leading to an incident.

There are three main approaches for building accident models (Hollnagel, 2004):

1. *Sequential models* see an incident arising from an ordered sequence of events. Although sequential models mainly focus on technical failures, the approach also considers human error as a deviation from standardized operation procedures. Sequential models are thus inadequate for describing human error in complex tasks and system-related variables where direct causal relationships among contributing factors cannot be established. Common hazard assessment techniques such as *failure mode and effects analysis* (FMEA) and *fault tree analysis* (FTA) are based on such sequential models. FTA analyzes incidents using Boolean logic to combine contributing system states or events (Figure 13.4). The probability of the incident can be calculated from the probabilities of contributing events. FMEA is a bottom-up technique that qualitatively identifies how a system may fail and the relative impact of those failures. For instance, FMEA can be used to identify all the possible consequences of a failure in a patient database.

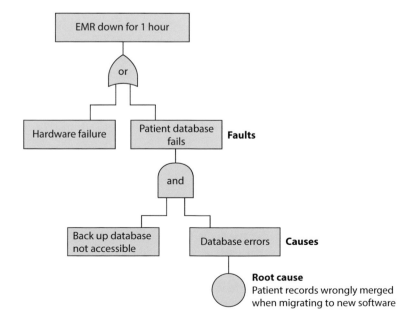

Figure 13.4
A fault tree analysis of the events leading to electronic medical record (EMR) downtime.

2. *Epidemiological models* see the events leading to an incident in a manner analogous to the spreading of an infectious disease. For example, just as pathogenic organisms can lie dormant, so, too, can latent hazards and errors. An incident is thus modelled as the result of a combination of active and latent factors. *Root cause analysis* is perhaps the most common epidemiological technique and considers more than just the immediate events leading to an incident. The events leading to an incident are reconstructed by an expert group by repeatedly asking 'why' until all underlying hazards (root causes) have been discovered.

3. *Systemic models* overcome the limitations of sequential and epidemiological models by attempting to capture the dynamic behaviour of a system. Such models focus on system characteristics and not just the specific events that give rise to an incident, and they are commonly used in domains such as aerospace and nuclear power. Systemic models tend to use more complex representations. For example, Leveson's systemic model considers safety as a control problem (Leveson, 2011), whereas Hollnagel's functional resonance accident model is based on stochastic resonance (Hollnagel, 2004).

Because each of these approaches has its own strengths, they are generally used in combination. Hazard assessment techniques also vary with system life cycle. For instance, FMEA is suitable when designing an EHR, whereas root cause analysis is more appropriate to examine an incident involving use of an EHR.

Hazards need to be prioritized and mitigated

Once hazards are identified, they either need to be eliminated from system design or mitigated (their effects minimized) by a safety strategy (Box 13.5). For instance, if there is a known hazard for human users of an electronic prescribing system, and a design solution is impractical, then a mitigation strategy may create an alert when the specific hazard or error occurs, as a new system defence.

Because it is usually not possible to address every system hazard, there is a need to prioritize the most important or safety-critical problems based upon their risk. Risk is a product of the degree of harm arising from an event (severity) and its rate of occurrence (likelihood) (see Box 13.1). This approach also means that some known risks are not addressed or are given very low priority. Given that no endeavour is free of risk, we thus design and operate systems at an acceptable level of risk. Designers of safety-critical systems use the ALARP principle, which means that safety measures have been applied and the remaining risks associated with the system (residual risks) are *As Low As Reasonably Practicable* (Leveson, 2011).

A safety case explains which hazards have been identified and what has been done to address them

The overall set of processes used to identify and mitigate hazards throughout the life cycle of a system is called a *safety management system* (McLaughlin *et al.,* 2012). Safety management systems evolved in high-risk industries such as aviation, and they formalize and document hazard assessment and mitigation so that system safety can be independently verified. The documents that set out the evidence for how hazards have been identified and managed are called a *safety case*. For instance, a manufacturer may create a safety case when implementing

Box 13.5
Safety strategies to
minimize information
system errors

- *Standardize – A common user interface* can specify basic information design elements such as the position of items on a screen, the use of standardized fonts, terminology and measurement units. Different system creators can all adopt the common interface specification while still adding in their own specific design elements. A common interface helps clinicians who move among different systems because they know how key functions work and where to find important information (Kushniruk *et al.*, 2013). Data entry and retrieval errors can similarly be minimized by standardizing the most common or high-risk processes. For example, a cancer clinic could implement standard best practice protocols for high-risk chemotherapy and common medication regimens in their computerized provider order entry.
- *Reduce complexity* – Another way to reduce information errors is through reduction of cognitive load generated when using a system, by removing some user steps in an overly complex task. For instance, complexity can be reduced by pre-populating data items, such as patient details or drug details such as name, form and dose. Unnecessary switching between different parts of a clinical system such as the electronic health record and an ordering screen can be avoided if the data needed for the order are already available on the order screen.
- *Add redundancy* – Duplication of critical system components or functions provides additional defences. For instance, prescribing errors can be detected when pharmacists independently check medications prescribed by doctors on their own system before the medications are dispensed to the patient.
- *Provide feedback* – System feedback, for example, from an alert or prompt, can be a highly effective way to correct information errors at the point of data entry or retrieval. However, excessive prompting can itself lead to cognitive overload or can cause clinicians instinctively to dismiss alerts without reading them, even when these alerts are important.

a new EHR. The safety case is continuously updated with new hazards identified during deployment or when any changes are made to the system.

13.8 Minimizing information technology–related harms relies on effective surveillance, investigation and response

The environment in which information systems are used is typically dynamic, characterized by variations not only in clinician roles and staffing levels but also in changes to disease patterns, clinical tasks and tools, workflow and organizational structure. All such changes have the potential to create new hazards. This means that hazard reduction is not confined to the design and implementation phases of a technology, but it must extend throughout its lifetime of use. There is thus a continuing requirement for systemwide safety surveillance and for responses to newly identified hazards or events (Sittig and Classen, 2010).

Reports from users can identify new hazards

Incident reports from clinicians and patients are central to safety surveillance in healthcare, are used widely and are not limited to information systems. Clinicians report circumstances in which patients are harmed or were very nearly harmed. Another source of incidents data comprises the problems reported to clinical information system help desks. For example, an excessive number of requests to reset passwords may indicate problems with the usability of an authentication system that may potentially prevent clinicians from accessing the EHR.

Box 13.6
An example of an
incident report

1. Date and time.
   02/03/2014; 10:00 to 10:59.

2. What happened?

   All the computer systems are down in the emergency department. The problem is disrupting work, and clinicians are unable to track patients, admit patients, order tests or review results.

3. What was the consequence or outcome of this incident?

   Manual lists are being used to track patients, and clinicians need to leave the unit to access tests. This is slowing everything down, and there is an increased potential for error.

4. What is the nature of the event?
   ☐ Adverse event.
   ☐ Near miss.
   ✓ Delivery of care affected.
   ☐ Event with no noticeable consequence.
   ☐ Hazardous event or circumstance.

5. Severity Assessment Code (SAC) rating: 4.

A clinical incident report is typically entered into a database within an *incident management system* (Runciman *et al.*, 2006). Each incident report generally consists of a combination of free text and pre-defined fixed data fields that are used to describe the event and its consequences (Box 13.6). Such structured reports could be enhanced with a screenshot of the information system display at the time of the problem or a log of the system state when an incident occurred.

Because incident reports are typically voluntary, it is likely that many incidents go unreported. Thus, incident reports cannot be used to determine the true frequency of adverse events. Users are also more likely to report incidents that appear unusual or interesting or events that are of current interest. Such preferential reporting introduces a bias in the types of events recorded and an under-reporting of minor or routine events as predicted by sample theory (Chapter 8) (Runciman *et al.*, 2005).

For incident reports to be useful as a surveillance tool, there need to be processes in place to review reports in a timely fashion. The large volume of reports received, however, impedes rapid response. To assist collating and analyzing reports, classification systems have been developed for use in incident management systems. They cover the most common critical incident types, to assist with detecting clusters of similar incidents that all point to a common underlying problem, as well as to help identify the places where similar risks need to be dealt with. The classification system described earlier in this chapter for IT incidents was derived from analyses of incident reports in multiple countries (Magrabi *et al.*, 2010; Magrabi *et al.*, 2012), and it is now being used for surveillance and classification of new incidents (Sparnon and Marela, 2012). The US Agency for Healthcare Research and Quality (AHRQ) also includes categories for information systems in its standard 'common format' for incident reporting.

The quality of incident classification depends very much on the expertise of the individual doing the classification, and there is wide variation in which classifications are attached to a given report. Automated classification methods based on natural language processing are a promising alternative and can categorize incidents by type and severity (Ong *et al.*, 2010; Ong *et al.*, 2012a).

Surveillance of clinical information systems can be automated

Because users are not expert in technology, many hazards involving clinical information systems may go undetected or be detected only after an adverse event has occurred. This problem can be addressed by proactively monitoring clinical systems to detect deviations from expected performance, well before they affect care delivery or harm patients. Monitoring of IT system performance can detect hazards associated with infrastructure (e.g. power supply, data network availability) and specific software systems (e.g. availability of the EMR, order entry and PACS).

Automated methods can also be used to detect some types of information errors as they occur, at three different levels:

- *Transaction level* monitoring tracks the delivery of messages among systems and can detect missing or delayed information. For example, the traffic of messages between an EHR and an order entry system can be monitored to ensure that records in the EHR are updated when new orders are placed in a CPOE system. Test messages can also be used to provide a regular baseline performance measure.
- *Systems level* monitoring examines the content of messages between systems and may detect incorrect and partial information. For example, one can over time build up a statistical model of the normal range of values expected for different tests on any given day or time from a laboratory. Similarly, one can build up models of the normal level of duplicate orders expected in any day (Figure 13.5) Deviation from the expected rate is a potential early warning sign that something has changed in the way the system is performing or that clinical actions may be risky. Such techniques are commonly used for early detection of disease outbreaks (see Chapter 29). Syndromic surveillance methods can also be applied to detect patterns across different information types (Ong *et al.*, 2012b). Trigger rules can be embedded within software to generate alerts automatically when specified circumstances are identified. For example, rules that detect suspicious credit card activity can trigger temporary suspension of a card. Trigger rules similarly may detect discrepancies among clinical systems. For example, contradictory drug allergy records in an EHR and a patient's personal health record could trigger a message to resolve the discrepancy at the next patient encounter.
- *Use level* involves monitoring interactions in real time. For example, orders that were retracted within 10 minutes and then reordered by the same clinician on a different patient identified 58 wrong-patient orders per 100,000 orders (Adelman *et al.*, 2013).

Investigation and response to safety incidents builds upon conventional processes for information technology systems

Assessment, investigation and resolution of incidents may be overseen both by a dedicated safety team, which has responsibility for safety across all aspects of an organization, and as a part of routine IT service management. Reports from users and system monitors first need to

Figure 13.5
A time series model
of the expected
number of duplicated
tests in a laboratory
system is used to
detect unusually high
levels of duplicate
orders. (a) A statistical
process control chart
is developed based
upon a baseline
profile of the average
number of duplicate
tests typically ordered
over a day. Alerts are
then triggered when
duplicate values
exceed a pre-defined
threshold (e.g. three
standard deviations
from baseline). (b)
Detection rates using
this model were 70
per cent in the first 6
hours when the
duplicate rate was 5
per cent and greater
than 80 per cent with
a duplicate rate of 15
per cent; a perfect
detection rate was
found within the first
2 hours when the
duplicate rate was 30
per cent. (From Ong
et al., 2012b.)

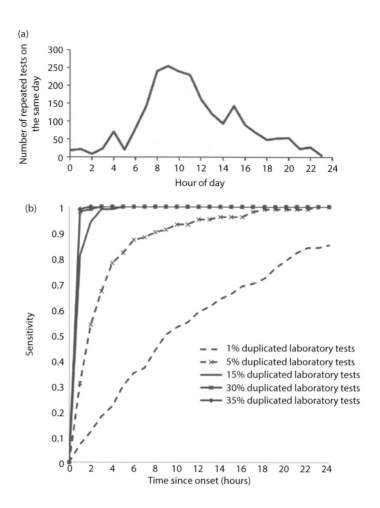

be triaged and prioritized because timeliness of response is especially critical when dealing with a live system. For instance, a clinician with a password issue may receive assistance from a help desk, whereas an error in the display of x-ray images across a hospital would be rapidly escalated for a safety team investigation and response. In the extreme, systems can be taken offline if a threat is serious enough. In such instances there is usually a 'failover' process in which clinicians revert to manual processes, which are well documented and rehearsed. Paper-based back-up processes are an essential component of any EHR implementation, to allow clinicians to create records or make orders while a computer system is down.

Solutions to problems (sometimes called controls) may involve changes to software, hardware, work processes or training. Short-term workarounds may be needed while waiting for a longer-term fix. Once a solution has been found, it should be communicated widely through safety alerts or advisories, so that other organizations that share the potential for risk can also proactively institute controls. For instance, the manufacturer of a clinical system may issue an advisory to all its customers that a software update needs to be applied immediately to correct an error in the display of test results.

For clinical information systems, this process of detection and control builds upon conventional IT service management. Best practice processes, procedures, tasks and checklists widely used in many industries have direct relevance to healthcare; they aim to restore the normal operation of systems as quickly as possible and minimize any adverse effects of incidents. The Information Technology Infrastructure Library (ITIL) is one such best practice approach that is globally recognized (Steinberg, 2011).

13.9 Clinical safety governance introduces rules and processes to maximize whole of system safety

Organizational governance describes all those processes that an organization uses to oversee its own performance. Clinical safety governance is thus the set of processes in place to dictate how patient safety is ensured – whether at the level of an organization, a region or a nation. Safety governance can be self-imposed and voluntary, or governments can mandate it when there is general risk to the public and an organization has responsibilities to minimize that risk. The balance between voluntary and mandated governance varies widely among industries and nations, thus reflecting the maturity of different industries and the differing commitment to the public good amongst nation states.

Information system *standardization* and *operational oversight* are the two main governance approaches that are relevant to health IT (Singh *et al.,* 2011; Walker *et al.,* 2008):

- Many international technical standards can be applied to a clinical information system and to the quality of processes at different points in the technology life cycle, spanning design, build, implementation and use in a clinical setting. However, few standards directly address the safety of clinical systems (Magrabi *et al.,* 2013). In the absence of clear standards, looser guidelines can still offer a mechanism to promote safe design and implementation practices (Singh *et al.,* 2013). Guidelines are generally directed at manufacturers and clinical organizations. For instance, a guideline can be used to provide recommendations for the safe display of patient information within an EHR based upon usability principles. A process guideline may recommend best practices for implementing an order entry system in a hospital.
- *Certification* is a formal oversight process that can be set up at a national or regional level to ensure that an information system meets specific standards. Certification provides independent assurance that an information system is fit for purpose and that it meets specific requirements for functionality, interoperability and security. For instance, the manufacturer of a prescribing system may be required to show that a system provides certain core clinical functions, that it is secure and that it can be integrated with other information systems such as the EHR. Certification can be voluntary, and it requires *regulation* to compel manufacturers to comply with standards or performance targets (Coiera and Westbrook, 2006). For example, a manufacturer may need to submit a safety case that demonstrates that its equipment is safe for use in a clinical setting before it is allowed to deploy the system. Existing regulatory regimens for medical devices such as the CE mark in Europe or the Food and Drug Administration (FDA) process in the United States provide a template for the regulation of clinical information systems. In general, the level of oversight or regulatory control should be proportional to the degree of risk that an information system poses to patients.

CHAPTER 14

Information economics

The diffusion, acceptance and ultimate success of any information technology are at least as dependent upon the social system within which it is placed as on the technology itself. Yet we still lack clear models that explain why some information services are so successful and widely adopted, whereas others struggle even though they seem to be good ideas.

Technology acceptance models provide some insights into the factors that shape the decision to adopt or not adopt a technology (see Chapter 11). Economics is another discipline that can offer us insights into the dynamics of information creation and use. Economics is able to factor in both the specific technical advantages of one product or service over another, but it also captures the preferences and utilities of individuals who chose to use them.

In the specialist field known as information economics, we find theoretical and practical models for creating, diffusing and using information products (Brousseau and Curien, 2007). Information economics focusses on understanding how and why networks of individuals assemble and interact to exchange information and the emergent properties of those interactions. As such, it provides informatics a core set of theoretical results with wide application.

In this chapter, the basic properties of information as an economic good are introduced. Beginning with information production, the economic properties of information are of substantial importance for those creating and publishing information, independently of whether their intent is commercial. Next, the cost of accessing information, whether by clinicians or consumers, shapes the willingness of these clinicians and consumers to use an information service. Innovations in information creation and distribution, such as peer-to-peer file sharing, crowdsourcing and open access (OA) publishing, all of which try to find a balance between wide dissemination and cost minimization, are also reviewed.

14.1 Information has a value

The value of information (VOI) (see Chapter 11) equates the economic benefit of a specific piece of information with it's ability to influence decision making and the events that follow. More broadly, economists consider any information that can be given a market value such as music, literature or a product design to be an *information good*. Consequently, the economic laws of supply and demand can be applied to the trading of information and assist us in understanding how much individuals may be willing to pay for it (whether in monetary the limiting factor is our ability to spend time-consuming information. Our attention is the scarce resource.

7. The costs of searching for, evaluating and then purchasing any good are all transaction costs. Although information on the Internet may ultimately become virtually free to obtain, the transaction costs in obtaining that information will not disappear. The cost of an information transaction on the Internet is related to the amount of information placed on the Internet and is an example of a negative network effect or negative externality.

8. Network neutrality asks that a provider of a common service such as a computer network not impede or block or otherwise disadvantage the information that is transported across it. Failure to support network neutrality sees some information providers offer improved access to customers or better-quality transmission, and it has wide-ranging importance for the carriage of health information.

PART 4

Guideline- and protocol-based systems

CHAPTER 15

Guidelines, protocols and evidence-based healthcare

> But printed flow charts should not be regarded as a problem-solving panacea! They …
> serve as recipes for a mindless cook. They are difficult to write, rigid, may inhibit
> independent thinking, and are often so intricate as to require a road map and a compass.
> … The good physician generates his own flow chart every time he sees a patient and
> solves a problem. He should not need to follow printed pathways.
>
> *Cutler, 1979, p 53*

> Shortly thereafter, I had the last of the 'insights' to be recorded here: a clinician performs
> an experiment every time he treats a patient. The experiment has purposes different
> from those of laboratory work, but the sequence, and intellectual construction are the
> same: a plan, an execution, and an appraisal. Yet … Honest, dedicated clinicians today
> disagree on the treatment for almost every disease from the common cold to metastatic
> cancer. Our experiments in treatment were acceptable by the standards of the
> community, but were not reproducible by the standards of science. Clinical judgement
> was our method for designing and evaluating those experiments, but the method was
> unreproducible because we had been taught to call it 'art' … .
>
> *Feinstein, 1967, p 14*

For those who regard modern healthcare as a rational and scientific endeavour, the fact that many common clinical practices are not supported by research evidence can come as a shock. It is just as disturbing to realize that many evidence-based practices are yet to be widely adopted. For example, the first trial to show that streptokinase was useful in the treatment of myocardial infarction was published in 1958. Convincing evidence mounted in the early 1970s, and the first meta-analysis proving its value was published in the early 1980s. However, formal advice that streptokinase was useful in the routine treatment of myocardial infarction appeared only in the late 1980s (Antman *et al.*, 1992). This was a full 13 years after a close examination of the published literature would have indicated the treatment's value (Heathfield and Wyatt, 1993).

There are many other examples of similar delays in transferring research findings into routine clinical practice. The use of low-dose anticoagulants in hip surgery and inhaled steroids in the treatment of asthma both could have become routine treatments much earlier

Surgical Safety Checklist

World Health Organization | Patient Safety
A World Alliance for Safer Health Care

Before induction of anaesthesia

(with at least nurse and anaesthetist)

Has the patient confirmed his/her identity, site, procedure, and consent?
☐ Yes

Is the site marked?
☐ Yes
☐ Not applicable

Is the anaesthesia machine and medication check complete?
☐ Yes

Is the pulse oximeter on the patient and functioning?
☐ Yes

Does the patient have a:

Known allergy?
☐ No
☐ Yes

Difficult airway or aspiration risk?
☐ No
☐ Yes, and equipment/assistance available

Risk of >500ml blood loss (7ml/kg in children)?
☐ No
☐ Yes, and two IVs/central access and fluids planned

Before skin incision

(with nurse, anaesthetist and surgeon)

☐ **Confirm all team members have introduced themselves by name and role.**

☐ **Confirm the patient's name, procedure, and where the incision will be made.**

Has antibiotic prophylaxis been given within the last 60 minutes?
☐ Yes
☐ Not applicable

Anticipated Critical Events

To Surgeon:
☐ What are the critical or non-routine steps?
☐ How long will the case take?
☐ What is the anticipated blood loss?

To Anaesthetist:
☐ Are there any patient-specific concerns?

To Nursing Team:
☐ Has sterility (including indicator results) been confirmed?
☐ Are there equipment issues or any concerns?

Is essential imaging displayed?
☐ Yes
☐ Not applicable

Before patient leaves operating room

(with nurse, anaesthetist and surgeon)

Nurse Verbally Confirms:
☐ The name of the procedure
☐ Completion of instrument, sponge and needle counts
☐ Specimen labelling (read specimen labels aloud, including patient name)
☐ Whether there are any equipment problems to be addressed

To Surgeon, Anaesthetist and Nurse:
☐ What are the key concerns for recovery and management of this patient?

© WHO, 2009

This checklist is not intended to be comprehensive. Additions and modifications to fit local practice are encouraged.

Revised 1/2009

Figure 15.2   The World Health Organization Surgical Safety Checklist. (From World Health Organization, 2009; copyright World Health Organization, 2009.)

guidelines found that all but 4 studies showed significant improvement in the process of care after the introduction of a guideline (Grimshaw and Russell, 1993). Patient outcomes were assessed in 11 studies, and 9 reported an improvement.

Surgical checklists have also been closely assessed. The first major study of checklist impact on surgical outcomes found a decline in surgical death rates from 1.5 to 0.8 per cent after a checklist was adopted and a decrease in inpatient complications from 11 to 7 per cent (Haynes *et al.,* 2009). Subsequent studies found a similar range of impacts, but with significant variation in adherence to the checklist and observed outcomes (Bergs *et al.,* 2014). In particular, sites with adequate checklist compliance appear more likely to demonstrate a significant reduction in postoperative complications. Such improvements also appear to be associated with improved teamwork and safety climate, potentially independent of the checklist (Haynes *et al.,* 2009).

15.2 The structure of protocols

There are a variety of different ways to represent a protocol, and the chosen structure should reflect the way in which it will be used. Protocols intended for time-pressured or emergency settings are designed very differently from protocols used in routine practice. Protocol content also varies for similar reasons. For example, the level of detail in the description of steps and the choice of language vary with the intended user of the protocol.

Entry criteria define a protocol's context of use

Irrespective of form, every protocol begins with an inclusion, eligibility or *entry criterion* that defines the context in which it is intended to be used (Weng *et al.,* 2010). For example 'patient presents with acute retrosternal chest pain' may be the criterion that starts a patient on a protocol for the investigation and management of suspected myocardial infarction. If entry criteria are insufficiently precise, then a protocol may be used inappropriately.

Protocol form is determined by function

Flowcharts are probably the simplest way to represent a protocol because they are graphical, and they make decision points and the flow of logic explicit (see Figure 15.1). Flowcharts can be built up in great detail, especially in areas in which there is a high procedural content to the work such as anaesthesia.

A flowchart begins with an entry criterion, for example, 'you are a self-managing insulin-dependent diabetic patient on intermediate-acting insulin, and your urine has tested high for blood sugar'. Choice points in the logic are made explicit. Depending upon responses to questions, often with simple 'yes' or 'no' answers, the protocol user is guided through a decision-making process. Actions are usually arrived at on the 'leaf' nodes.

Flowcharts are thus a form of the decision tree introduced in Chapter 8. When the decision process is well understood but complicated, a protocol could be represented as a full decision

Figure 15.4
The three-loop
model describes the
way in which
protocols can be
used to manage
individual patients in
a uniform way and
use the results of
treatment to grow
clinical knowledge.

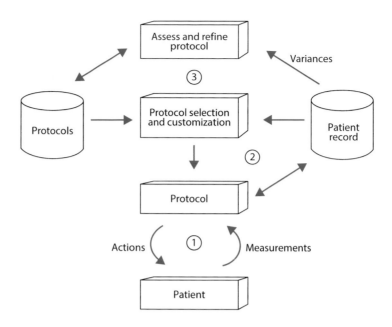

- *Resource constraints* – External factors may contribute to variances. For example, an investigation may be scheduled to occur on a particular day of the admission. If the laboratory carrying out the investigation is overbooked, then the protocol has to be varied.

From a systems science point of view, variances are signals in a feedback loop. Rather than being problematic, variances should be a central part of the way in which protocol-assisted care is given:

- First, variances are signals to the care team to re-assess whether it is appropriate for a patient to be maintained on a protocol, and they may indicate that more individualized care is necessary.
- Second, when variances from a number of patients are pooled, they act as checks on the way in which care is delivered. It may be that recurrent variances suggest that a pathway or protocol is being applied incorrectly, that care delivery is sub-optimal or that changes need to be made in the way staff or resources are allocated.
- Finally, variances offer an opportunity to assess the appropriateness of the protocol over time. In this case, variances provide a measurement of the effectiveness of a protocol and consequently can feed a process of continuing protocol refinement in loop 3.

15.5 The application of protocols is guided by the type of problem being managed

The use of a clinical protocol does not necessarily mean that we will see an improvement either in clinical process or outcome. Indeed, there is significant variation in the impact that guidelines can have on process and outcomes improvements (Darling, 2002). As described in

Chapters 11 and 12, this variation can be attributed not to the content of a guideline, but to the manner in which it is represented and the sociotechnical environment in which it is used. For example, guidelines are more likely to be effective if they take account of local circumstances, are disseminated by an active educational intervention and are implemented by patient-specific reminders relating directly to professional activity. Evaluation of compliance with a guideline, measured by adherence, thus appears as important as evaluating outcomes.

Clearly, it is not always the case that protocols are the best way to improve a decision process. The decision to design or use a protocol to manage a given situation should never be automatic. There are many situations in which protocol application is at the least difficult and at worst meaningless (Box 15.2). Formal decision models (of which protocols are one example) are unlikely to be helpful in many circumstances, including the following (Klein and Calderwood, 1991):

- When clear goals cannot be isolated, and it is dangerous to make simplifying assumptions that would allow a protocol to be applied.
- When end states or outcomes cannot be clearly defined.
- When the utilities of different decisions are not independent of one another.
- When probabilities of outcomes or the utility of individual decisions are not independent of the context in which they are made.

Protocols are thus most likely to be effective if they are applied in contexts where there is strong predictability about the pathway that patients will follow and where the trajectory of progress is going to be similar for most patients (Allen *et al.*, 2009).

Once a decision has been made to introduce a protocol, the next step is to determine the way in which the protocol will be made available. The two main approaches to protocol use can be divided into *passive* and *active*. In the passive approach, protocols act as a source of

Box 15.2
When recognizing is more difficult than doing

It has been argued that there are many situations in which formalized decision models such as protocols are not helpful and are potentially harmful. Indeed, when decision-making is studied 'in the field' rather than in the laboratory, a very different set of human decision problems is observed.

Faced with complex problems, and working under time pressure or stress, people may not evaluate more than one course of action at a time (Klein and Calderwood, 1991). Instead, once a situation has been recognized, individuals may just follow the first acceptable plan they consider. This suggests that the main efforts that go into decision-making are in recognizing and classifying a situation, rather than exploring complex plans to manage the situation.

This result is echoed in work on clinical decision-making, in which the order in which data were presented to clinicians had a significant effect upon the clinicians' reasoning (Elstein *et al.*, 1978). In an analysis of so-called 'fixed-order' problems under experimental conditions, the ability of physicians to generate hypotheses and to associate data with hypotheses was significantly affected by the order in which data were presented. In other words, their ability to assess the situation correctly was influenced by the way data were encountered.

If our goal is to improve decision-making, then the focus of decision support strategies should include supporting individuals to assess situations and not solely on formalizing the decision process that follows once an assessment has been made (Patel *et al.*, 2002). One cannot study decision-making in isolation from other processes, such as situation awareness, problem solving, planning and uncertainty management (Salas and Klein, 2001).

information only and are not formally incorporated into the care process. Thus, clinical guidelines may be consulted only as a check, at the end of a decision-making process or as a reference when an unusual situation is encountered. Healthcare workers may carry them around with them as a set of ready-to-hand prompts.

In contrast, the active use of protocols shapes the delivery of care. The steps in a treatment are explicitly guided by a protocol. Active use of a protocol shapes clinical workflow and may suggest what patient information is to be captured at different stages, what treatment is to be given or what tests are to be ordered.

The introduction of passive systems is unlikely to cause significant difficulty because these systems do not mandate treatment, but rather just add to the information available. This type of decision support is *permissive,* in that it permits all courses of action and exists only as a guide that is accessed as the need arises. In contrast, active systems are *prescriptive* because, by definition, they actively constrain treatment actions in some way.

Unsurprisingly, the introduction of a prescriptive process is organizationally difficult because it inevitably changes the way people work. As we discover in Chapter 16, where we examine computerized protocol delivery, the sociotechnical nature of healthcare organizations means that compromises will always be made between the intent of a technological intervention and the local context, desires, abilities and concerns of those who will have to work with it.

Discussion points

1. 'Using protocols results in the de-skilling of clinicians'. 'Using protocols improves clinical outcomes'. With which statement do you agree, and how do you resolve the conflict between the two?

2. Can every aspect of medical care be controlled by protocols? Perhaps consider your answer by noting that protocols are models of healthcare.

3. Can you think of one clinical workflow that would benefit from the introduction of a checklist and one in which it would not be helpful?

4. You have just championed the introduction of a new guideline, based upon the latest evidence, into your unit. Senior management is concerned about the costs and wants you to demonstrate that the changes are worthwhile. How will you measure the impact of the new guideline?

5. After much expense, your hospital unit has implemented a new care pathway, but after a year there appears to be no improvement in patient outcomes. Some staff members say the process it too much work and want to go back to the old system. What do you say to them?

6. Under what conditions is the use of a protocol likely to cause harm?

Chapter summary

1. The mechanisms that exist for transferring research evidence into clinical practice are unable to keep up with the ever-growing mountain of clinical trial data, thus resulting in delays in the transfer of research into practice.

2. Evidence-based healthcare is an attempt to distil best-practice guidance from the literature into a set of protocols that can be made readily and widely available to practising clinicians.

3. A protocol is a set of instructions. These instructions may describe the procedure to be followed to investigate a particular set of findings in a patient or the method to be followed in the management of a given disease.

4. A protocol can ensure that tasks are carried out uniformly. It can serve as a guide or reminder in situations in which it is likely that procedures will be forgotten, are not well known or are difficult to follow or where errors can be expensive, for example, in the presence of rare conditions, in safety-critical or complex situations, in clinical research, in education and in task delegation.

5. Each protocol begins with an entry criterion that defines the context within which the protocol is designed to be used.

6. Protocols can vary in the form of their structure and their content, depending upon the context of use. Flowcharts make choice points and the flow of decision-making graphically explicit, but they are space consuming. Rules are more compact, but they require more effort and training to interpret. Contextual factors affecting design include the patient, treatment goals, local resources, staff skills, local processes and resources.

7. In a clinical care pathway, a patient's care is broken down into a sequence of days, corresponding to the ideal length of stay in hospital. These pathways have been shown to improve the process of delivering care but appear less likely to influence the outcomes of care, although the research evidence is not of good quality.

8. The creation and application of protocols can be characterized as a model-measure-manage cycle, and their overall use in healthcare can be captured within the three-loop model.

9. Variations in treatment that have not been anticipated in the protocol are termed variances, which can signal the care team to re-assess whether it is appropriate for a patient to be maintained on a protocol. When variances from a number of patients are pooled, they can act as checks on the way in which care is delivered.

10. There are many situations in which the attempt to formalize decision models, such as protocols, is not helpful and may indeed be harmful. These include situations in which distinct goals or outcomes cannot be clearly defined or when probabilities or utilities are not independent of each other or the decision context.

11. Protocol systems can be passive or active. Passive protocols act as a source of information and are not incorporated into the care process. Active protocols shape the delivery of care.

CHAPTER 16

Computer-based protocol systems

The goals of a computer-based protocol system are to provide clinicians with access up-to-date guidelines and to help them apply these guidelines in the management of patients. In Chapter 15, we saw that protocols either can be used as passive resources or can contribute actively in shaping the process of care. In this chapter, we examine the role that communication and computer-based systems can play in the delivery of protocol-based care. Computer-based guidelines are built and executed using specialized representations of clinical processes and are linked to systems such as the electronic health record (EHR). Several of the major competing computational approaches to clinical guidelines are described here, along with a more general description of their typical structure and function. We also review the continuing challenges in studying the effectiveness of such systems in actual use and explore why the evidence for their benefits is mixed and sometimes very difficult to interpret.

16.1 Computer-based systems support both passive and active uses of protocols

Passive protocol systems provide access to best-practice documentation

A passive protocol delivery system acts as a source of information only and is not intrinsically incorporated into the care process. A passive system makes it easier for clinicians to access protocol information during routine care and makes it less likely that steps will be inadvertently forgotten or altered. Although they may be accessed as reference material from within a clinical information system such as the EHR, the protocols are not integrated with other modules of the system such as order entry or results reporting.

Protocol and guideline information can be made accessible through dedicated links to external guideline repositories created by third-party organizations and government agencies. Organizations may have developed their own local guidance documentation and provide direct computer access to these guidelines as part of their clinical information system.

Search functions such as an *infobutton* can be embedded within a specific patient's record to provide anticipatory passive support. By using patient data from the record, a query can automatically be constructed to retrieve clinical guidelines that are likely to be relevant to that patient's care (Cimino, 2008).

Active protocol systems need to integrate with other clinical systems

In contrast to passive systems, in which clinicians have freedom to consult a protocol or not, active protocol systems guide the actions of clinicians (Figure 16.1). Using computer representation of a protocol as a template to action, a variety of clinical activities can be supported or automated. These activities range from assisting with recording events into an electronic patient record to medication ordering or test scheduling (Figure 16.2). Consequently, an active protocol system must be integrated into the wider organizational information system.

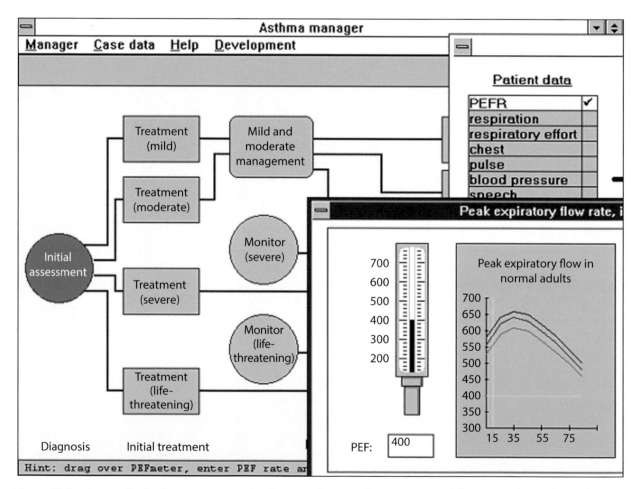

Figure 16.1   A user display from a computerized protocol system for managing adult acute asthma. The asthma manager displays a tree of treatment plan written in the guideline language PRO*forma*. Other panels show the patient's peak flow data and medical record (square = action, circle = decision, round rectangle = plan, connecting line = scheduling constraint). (From Fox *et al.*, 1996.)

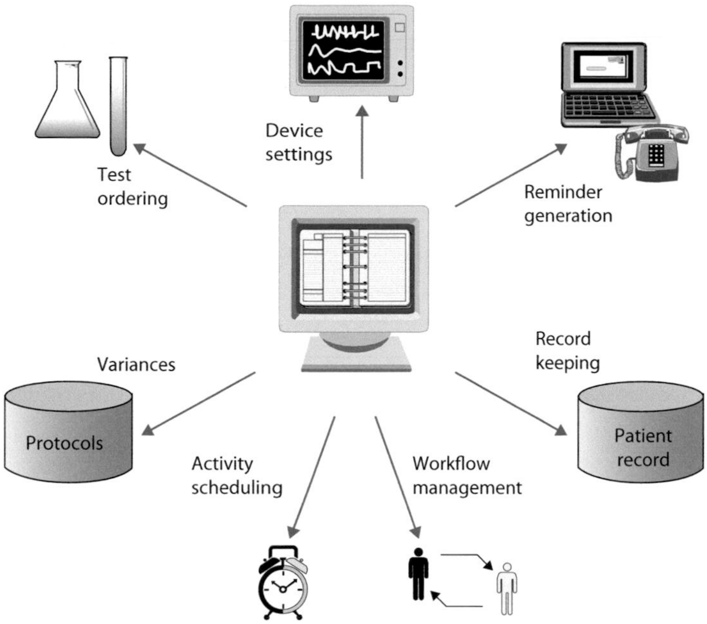

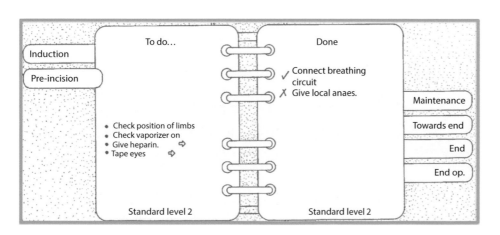

Figure 16.2
Protocol-driven
information systems
can integrate into
many different
clinical systems, with
cumulative benefit.
They can, for
example, guide
record keeping,
prompt alert
generation, trigger
automated order
entry systems and
appointment
scheduling and
provide a
mechanism for
variance capture.

Communication interfaces are needed to allow the sharing of information between active protocol systems and other clinical systems such as the EHR, order entry, pharmacy and laboratory systems (Shiffman *et al.*, 1999).

Record keeping can be semi-automated

A computerized protocol acts first as a memory prompt to undertake a step, as well as to record that it has been done. The act of indicating which steps in a protocol have been done can also automatically create a record that contains the action description and the time it occurred (Figure 16.3). The result should be clinical records that are more accurate, complete and in a more standardized form and language – of benefit for other team members who subsequently read the record, as well as for making the audit of patient populations much

Figure 16.3
Interface design
element for an
anaesthesia record
system. The user is
prompted to check
which items have or
have not been done
at different stages of
the anaesthetic
regimen, thus
automatically
creating a record, as
well as reconfiguring
alarm settings on the
patient monitor.
(From Coiera and
Lewis, 1998.)

easier. There are many clinical situations in which such a template-driven approach to creating a report is valuable. Creating reports for radiological investigations or post-operative surgical reports typically involves repeating the same standard phrases or report elements.

Even if there are variances from protocol for some patients, a protocol system can help by preparing common reasons for variation and supporting variance capture (e.g. Boord *et al.*, 2007). Recording such variations from care and the reasons for doing them makes retrospective audit of care much easier.

Protocol-driven record keeping is a good example of a system function that delivers direct benefit to those who use the system by reducing workload, as well as having long-term benefits because of improved quality of data capture. Systems that are not directly integrated into clinical processes are more likely to require extra work to use, and this can cause the system to be poorly accepted for sociotechnical reasons. There are also downsides to template-driven record keeping, for example, if staff members simply check boxes without looking at a patient or copy yesterday's record (see Chapter 13).

Recommending and reminding can be situational or alert based

Active protocol systems can provide healthcare workers with task recommendations and reminders. The scope of such recommendations includes appropriate tests and treatments, alerts about at-risk states and reminders of appropriate physical assessments and screening activities (Shiffman *et al.*, 1999). Active systems can also provide an explanation function that offers background information including the clinical evidence for a recommendation and the risks associated with not following a recommendation.

There are two typical ways in which an active system can prompt someone to act. First, an alert can be triggered by a computer-detected event such as a clinician's ordering a medication or the arrival of a laboratory result. In one study of an electronic insulin therapy protocol, clinicians initiated a protocol that was linked to the EHR and computerized provider order entry (CPOE). Initiation triggered the CPOE system to generate the corresponding insulin orders and instructed nurses to perform bedside blood glucose testing. The CPOE system then recommended insulin infusion rates based on glucose readings in the EHR. Use of the system was associated with a reduced time from first glucose measurement to initiation of insulin protocol, improved percentage of all glucose readings in the ideal range and improved control in patients on intravenous insulin for 24 hours or more (Boord *et al.*, 2007).

The second form of reminding is situational, in that the protocol itself functions as a reminder of what is to be done because of its visibility. The protocol need not even be electronic to achieve this. A computer generating protocol that was printed and then became the first page of a paper record resulted in a two-fold increase in clinician compliance with care guidelines for diabetes mellitus (Lobach and Hammond, 1997).

Protocols can drive activity scheduling and enterprise workflow management

If an order entry function is linked to a protocol, then order generation can be protocol driven. For example, as soon as a patient is entered onto a protocol, it should be possible to send requests automatically for the tests or procedures that are specified within a care plan. Thus, one could schedule a stress test several days in advance at the time a patient is admitted under a myocardial infarction protocol. *Order sets,* which bundle together a group of medications and test orders, are a common mechanism to implement simple protocols for specific patient groups or clinical situations (see Chapter 25).

The integrated management of task scheduling across an organization is carried out by *workflow management systems.* The goal of workflow systems is to ensure that work processes across the different units of an organization are carried out in the most timely and cost-efficient method possible. Workflow systems use formal descriptions of tasks, the order in which the tasks are to be executed and their interdependencies. For example, a process may require a series of steps to be carried out that involves different departments or individuals. A workflow system would try to balance the work requests that arrive at each point in the process so that the most important tasks are completed or so that each part of the system works to maximum efficiency.

The ability to manage scheduling in a more automated fashion may result in a better use of institutional resources, by avoiding peaks in which facilities may be overloaded or troughs of underuse (Majidi *et al.,* 1993). For example, the preparation of chemotherapy for oncology patients by a hospital pharmacy can be synchronized with the time that the treatment is anticipated to be administered on the hospital ward, and this can result in a significant reduction in wait times (Aboumater *et al.,* 2008).

The degree to which the flow of work across any organization can be automated depends upon the degree to which tasks can be formalized. At one extreme, we have robot-operated assembly plants that require minimal human intervention, given the high degree of regularity of the assembly process. At the other extreme, if every task completed within in an organization is different, then no workflow automation is possible. As in most organizations, healthcare activities sit between these two extremes. As we saw in Chapter 9, for some tasks this formalization is not always possible or even desirable.

The degree to which protocols can integrate workflow across organizational units depends upon the existence of order entry and scheduling components in the organization's information system. The prescriptive nature of some workflow systems can make them complex to set up, and they may be overly constraining on staff. However, simple systems that make sure events and appointments are scheduled automatically or that optimize the flow of 'forms' and 'requests' have the potential to yield considerable benefits, if the organization is willing to formalize its processes sufficiently (e.g. Santibáñez *et al.,* 2012).

Data display can be modified by protocol

The data needed to make a decision vary with tasks, and task-specific displays can be of benefit in complex situations by bringing together the data types needed for a given decision. If a computer system can detect the current step in a protocol, then it can generate a task-specific data display suited to the needs of the current stage in the protocol (Coiera and Lewis, 1998). This is of particular relevance in situations in which large amounts of patient data may need to be filtered, for example, in intensive care or anaesthesia. It is also of value in less critical situations, when a large amount of data has accumulated, for example, when patients have long hospital admissions.

Monitor alarms can be set by protocol

If patient monitoring equipment, such as arrhythmia monitors or oxygen saturation probes, is linked to a protocol system, then this equipment also can have its behaviour configured to the current needs of the clinical context (Coiera and Lewis, 1998). For example, patient monitor alarm settings can be automatically reconfigured, reflecting the changes in alarm limits associated with the different stages of anaesthesia. The computer can detect that a new stage in the protocol has been entered by checking events entered into the patient record or by events detected by the monitor systems, for example, attachment of a device to measure a physiological parameter, or the pattern of measurements across different physiological parameters.

Device settings can vary with protocol stage

Protocols can be used to adjust the settings for biomedical equipment (open-loop control) or control them directly (closed-loop control). For example, protocols have been used to adjust tidal volume and ventilator rate settings for patients with adult respiratory distress syndrome (ARDS) (McKinley et al., 2001; Thomsen et al., 1993). A major application for computer-assisted ventilation is to aid in the process of weaning or discontinuation of ventilation (Haas and Loik, 2012). A review of multiple clinical trials of mechanical ventilation using a weaning protocol compared with usual care found that ventilation duration was reduced by 25 per cent, the duration of weaning was reduced by 78 per cent and stay in the intensive care unit length was decreased by 10 per cent (Blackwood et al., 2011). Closed-loop control systems are likely to need sophisticated signal interpretation capabilities, as discussed in Chapter 28, in addition to access to protocols.

16.2 Computational representations of protocols enable their active use in clinical systems

Unlike passive protocols that are designed for direct human use and can be expressed as human readable text or images, the representation of protocols in active systems requires a rich language that can be interpreted by a computer. Although humans bring much background knowledge to bear when they read a protocol, a computer system typically does not. The more that is required of a computer, the more knowledge it must be given about the task it is to accomplish (see Figure 2.5). As a consequence, computer protocols need to be specified in considerable detail. One ventilator management protocol needed 12 000 lines of computer code for its specification (Henderson et al., 1991).

Protocol representations use a small number of primitives or types that are assembled into longer instructions

Just as decision trees are composed from a small set of components such as decisions, actions and outcomes (e.g. Figure 8.5), protocol formalisms also use a set of primitives (Figure 16.4).

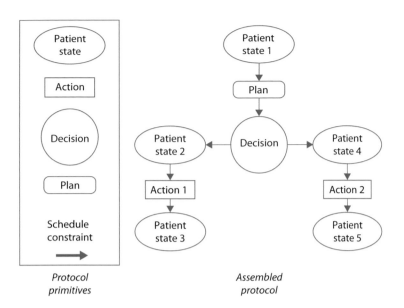

Figure 16.4
Computer protocols
typically are
constructed from a
set of standard
primitives and
assembled to
produce complete
protocols. (Adapted
from Wang et al.,
2002.)

These primitives are assembled into larger protocols and fall into two categories (Peleg *et al.*, 2003; Wang *et al.*, 2002):

- *Actions* – An action is a clinical or administrative task that the protocol recommends should be performed, maintained or avoided, e.g. to give a medication. Actions may also result in the invocation of a sub-protocol, allowing multiple protocols to be nested within each other.
- *Decisions* – A decision is made when one or more options are selected from a set of alternatives based on predefined criteria, e.g. the selection of a laboratory test from a set of potential tests.

Computer representations also need primitives to record intermediate states that track the system's understanding of the current situation:

- *The clinical status of a patient* – A patient's state (sometimes called a *scenario*) is based on actions already performed, decisions already made or data from the EHR. For example, a patient who has received the first dose of an influenza vaccine and is eligible for a second dose could be in the state *eligible-for-the-second-dose-of-influenza-vaccine*. Entry and exit conditions on protocols are also examples of patient states.
- *The execution state of the system* – An execution state records where we are up to with a protocol. For example, a protocol may have entered the execution state *recommend-the-second-dose-of-influenza-vaccine* once a patient has reached the state *eligible-for-the-second-dose-of-influenza-vaccine*.

Finite state machines, introduced in Chapter 15, are one formal approach to the representation of state. State variables determine entry, progression and exit points in a protocol and can also drive the transition from one protocol to another.

Scheduling constraints link each primitive decision or action into a temporal order to construct the specific steps in a protocol. The execution of steps may be a linear sequence, or they

*Knowledge can be represented either **declaratively** or **procedurally**. In the former, we declare how things relate to one another, but do not specify how we use that knowledge to come up with an answer. With procedural representations, we include in the knowledge how the answer may be derived.*

may occur in parallel if more than one set of actions is required. Together the logical connections among the different steps in a protocol are a *process model*.

When there are multiple protocol elements, each specifying a different aspect of care, these can be linked together to specify the overall high-level plan. *Nesting* allows a primitive in one protocol to be expanded into a more detailed sub-protocol, to enable multiple levels of abstraction and different granularities of detail. Nesting thus permits a complex clinical guideline to be decomposed into a hierarchy of component tasks that unfold over time (Fox and Das, 2000).

The nature of the schedule constraints that can connect elements varies with the specific protocol system used. These constraints can simply be deterministic instructions to move or switch from one primitive to the next, depending upon whether a condition is met or not (as in a decision tree). They can also be more complicated, using a formal *decision model* to guide movement along the protocol (see Chapter 26). For example, based upon the current patient state, as well as data from the record, one may calculate a score or a probability, and an action or decision is triggered when a score threshold is exceeded.

For an active protocol to be applied in clinical practice, it will require access to data about a specific patient's state (e.g. allergies or clinical measurements) and clinical context (e.g. medication orders). This can occur when a protocol system is connected to an EHR or CPOE system. At present, there is no one standard approach to the recording of patient data, and several controlled medical terminologies have been developed for this purpose. Given the importance of clinical terminologies and their fundamental relationship with active protocol systems, they are examined in detail in Part 6 of this book.

An *ontology* is often used to support the protocol or guideline authoring process. An ontology defines what is knowable in a domain and how these different concepts may relate to one another. Thus, a protocol ontology would capture all the important knowledge about the things being described in the protocol (Musen, 1998; Noy *et al.*, 2000). An ontology about cardiac surgery may include all the tests and procedures that could be used. It should contain rules about the relationships among these components that could then be used to prevent mistakes when authoring a protocol. For example, an ontology could detect that a test item has been inserted into a draft protocol in the place where a therapy is required. It is this need to create ways of automatically checking protocols for errors that has driven the development of such ontologies (see Chapter 23).

Many different protocol systems are in common use in clinical information systems

Numerous different protocol representation systems have been developed over the years, each adopting slightly different approaches (De Clercq *et al.*, 2008; Isern and Moreno, 2008; Peleg *et al.*, 2003). Some of the more significant guideline representation languages include:

- *Arden Syntax* – Developed originally by the American Society for Testing and Materials (ASTM), the Arden Syntax is a widely recognized standard for representing clinical and scientific knowledge in an executable format. Because it is a part of the HL7 (Health Level 7) standard set, it has wide distribution and can be used across institutions whose systems comply with the appropriate HL7 standards. (Samwald *et al.*, 2012). It can be used to code decisions and actions within a clinical protocol using a set of situation-action rules known as *Medical Logic Modules* or MLMs (Seitinger *et al.,* 2013). The Arden Syntax resembles the Pascal computer programming language and is procedural in its design. The Arden Syntax is agnostic as to the content of rules (or what goes between the 'curly braces'), because there is no underlying ontology. This means that sharing MLMs depends on making sure that variables have the same meaning when used in different systems. Its discrete modular representation means that it is not designed to handle nested or otherwise interconnected protocols, although chaining of modules is possible. The fairly rigid approach originally taken to representing knowledge using rules has meant that Arden Syntax was not always an ideal choice when decisions were not clear-cut. However, the Fuzzy Arden Syntax extends the language to allow a means of representing and processing vague or uncertain data (Vetterlein *et al.,* 2010).

- PRO*forma* – Driven by concerns that poorly designed computerized guidelines may generate incorrect clinical recommendations (see Chapter 13), PRO*forma* is designed to emphasize safe and robust guideline creation (Fox and Das, 2000). PRO*forma* captures both procedural and declarative aspects of a protocol into a set of tasks. Distinguishing features of PRO*forma* are the simplicity and intuitiveness of the underlying task model (see Figure 16.1). Tasks are subdivided into decisions (points at which some choice has to be made), actions (a procedure that is enacted externally such as administering a medication) or enquiries (points in a guideline where information is now needed) (Fox *et al.,* 1996; Sutton and Fox, 2003). Plans are a hierarchical collection of tasks that are grouped together for some reason. PRO*forma* plans can be visualized as directed graphs in which nodes represent tasks and arcs represent scheduling constraints. A guideline itself contains a single root plan, which may be recursively divided into sub-plans. Many PRO*forma*-based systems have been developed. *RetroGram* assists in the interpretation of genotype data and decisions for the management of human immunodeficiency virus–positive patients (Tural *et al.,* 2002). It has also been applied to the management of hypertension in primary care (Sutton *et al.,* 2006). Other applications include *CAPSULE,* a system for advising on routine prescribing; *RAGs,* a system designed to support the assessment of risk of familial breast and ovarian cancer in a primary care setting; *ARNO,* a pain control system for cancer sufferers that was built for St. Christopher's Hospice, London; and *MACRO,* a system for running Internet-based multi-center clinical trials. Objective evaluations of selected systems have demonstrated their potential to improve clinical practice and optimize resource usage (Humber *et al.,* 2001). The commercially available Arezzo system is based on PRO*forma,* as is Tallis, which is a publically available suite of tools.
- *Protégé* – Also structured around tasks, Protégé is a widely used open source tool that allows a user to build a protocol, guided by an ontology (Musen *et al.,* 1996). Once constructed, the protocol is translated into a machine-readable form. A suite of models and software components assists in writing guideline-based applications. These are composed of the following: problem solvers, which use clinical guidelines and patient data to generate situation-specific recommendations; knowledge bases, which contain the machine-readable protocols; and a temporal database mediator that sits between the problem solvers and patient data. The software architecture of Protégé is designed to be extensible, and it allows third-party 'plug-ins' to connect the protocols with other

information system components that run under different standards. Other tools support the collaborative (or crowdsourced) development and verification of the underlying ontology (Tudorache *et al.*, 2013). In both Protégé and PRO*forma,* much effort has been spent to develop a simple graphical interface to allow people to author a protocol. The systems designers have also had to develop mechanisms that translated these high-level descriptions into computer-interpretable code.

- *Guideline Interchange Format (GLIF)* – GLIF is designed as an interchange format that supports the sharing of guidelines among different institutions and software systems (Boxwala *et al.*, 2004). GLIF tries to build on the most useful features of other guideline models and to incorporate standards that are used in healthcare. Its expression language was originally based on the Arden Syntax, and its default medical data model is based on the HL7 Reference Information Model (RIM). GLIF's object-oriented query and expression language for clinical decision support, GELLO, became an HL7 standard in 2005.

Computer-interpretable guideline languages and methodologies are an ongoing and active area of research development, with many different systems beyond those described earlier:

- Some systems are now no longer in use, but they have contributed to the current state of the art. *Prodigy,* for example, was a UK system and was notable for its use of scenarios. It was developed to support chronic disease management in primary care and was for a time the basis of the National Health Service (NHS) guideline representation (Smart and Purves, 2001).

- Some systems are research vehicles that explore advanced issues in protocol representation and execution. *Asbru,* for example, is based on the notion of a skeletal plan, which can be instantiated with data to flesh out what needs to be accomplished at any one time (Miksch *et al.*, 1997; Seyfang *et al.*, 2002). The system is also important for its handling of time in clinical actions, thus supporting temporal abstraction of data. This, for example, allows low-level continuous and dense data such as could come from a patient monitor to map onto a high-level construct such as 'persistent hypertension' (Fuchsberger *et al.*, 2005). Asbru's ability to handle such data streams has also seen it applied to monitoring of activities of daily living through home monitoring devices (Naeem and Bigham, 2009).

- Other experimental systems seek to bring together the different features of existing systems. *SAGE* is one such system, which builds on the contributions of PRO*forma,* GLIF, *Prodigy* and *Protégé* (Tu *et al.*, 2007). One of the foci of SAGE is the development of methods that embed protocol systems more deeply into clinical information system standards and processes.

When these competing representations are compared, most are able to encode guideline knowledge accurately (Peleg *et al.*, 2003). The systems mainly use similar approaches to plan organization, expression language, conceptual medical record model, medical concept model and data abstractions. Differences are most apparent in underlying decision models, goal representation, use of scenarios and structured medical actions. Because all models are essentially task-based constructs, many of the differences among the guideline modelling approaches arise from their intended applications.

16.3 Computerized guidelines and protocols have an impact on the quality of care but are influenced by sociotechnical factors

We saw in Chapter 15 that although clinical pathways have a positive impact on the *process* of care, their impact on the *outcome* of care has been more difficult to demonstrate. The situation with computer guideline systems is the same. Two broad groups of factors help explain this.

The first group is methodological, in that it is difficult to conduct studies to measure impacts on outcomes for a number of reasons. Local circumstances, including culture, work practices, resources and the pre-existing information infrastructure all can affect the outcomes of system implementation (see Chapter 12). What works well in one setting may not work as well in another. In addition, there are many different approaches to representing, authoring and delivering computer guidelines, and these differences introduce further heterogeneity into any attempt to synthesize the results of different studies. Technical differences may have clinical consequences. Finally, if the relationship between practice variation and clinical outcome is small, then very large studies would be needed to demonstrate that a reduction in variation impacts outcomes. Given the large degree of heterogeneity in clinical settings and system implementations, such studies are very challenging and expensive to contemplate.

The second group of factors affecting outcome assessment are contextual, or related to the specific locale in which a system is implemented. The size of any potential improvement in clinical outcomes depends on the local processes already in place. If adopting a guideline means that a harmful or ineffective practice is replaced by a better one, then we may see outcome improvements. If local practices are different from the guideline but of similar effectiveness, then we may achieve process standardization, but not outcomes improvement. If the setting for implementation is a centre of excellence that is working at the cutting edge of clinical practice, it may be the case that this centre is achieving better outcomes than possible by adopting the more standard guideline. Such heterogeneity in the local standard of practice may make it difficult to demonstrate across the board outcome improvements.

Unsurprisingly, when reducing practice variation is the goal, the effort in system design and implementation focusses only on what is needed for variation reduction. In contrast, a focus on outcomes would first ask what the leading causes of poor outcomes were and would then design the protocol system specifically to tackle such causes. If there is no 'headroom' available for real improvement in an outcome measure then there is no likelihood that a new system will make any improvement. If there is no evidence that practice variation is a significant cause of a poor outcome, then it should be no surprise that reduction in variation has no effect on the outcome.

Comparisons of paper and computerized guidelines show variable differences in impact related to task and context

In Chapter 10 we saw that the proposition that computer records were always better than paper records was flawed, and the same logic holds with guidelines. With so many variables involved in making a computer easy or difficult to use, a well-designed paper system can in principle outperform a poorly designed computer system.

In one large randomized controlled trial to compare the effects of computerized and paper-based versions of guidelines, no significant differences in recently qualified primary care physicians' consultation practices were found in more than 3484 patient encounters between the computerized and paper group, perhaps because guideline compliance was already high (Jousimaa *et al.*, 2002). In contrast, a randomized trial examining the impact of computerized and paper guidelines for glucose regulation in the intensive care unit showed improvements in the timing of blood glucose measures (paper, 29.0 per cent, and 40.2 per cent for computer) and in insulin-dosing guideline compliance (paper, 56.3 per cent, and 77.3 per cent for computer), and glucose values fell within target range (44.3 per cent for paper and 54.2 per cent for computer) (Rood *et al.*, 2005).

If we think of a protocol as a message, then we know that the channel of message delivery (in this case a computer) is only one of many factors that affect the ultimate impact of the message on the individual who receives it. The benefits of using the computer channel over paper vary with clinical task and setting. For example, in time-critical, busy or cognitively demanding clinical situations, the speed and interactivity of a computer system should be a distinct advantage. In a primary care or outpatient setting, other design issues, such as the facility to search for supporting evidence or to present evidence to patients, may be more significant.

Guideline adherence is improved with computerized systems

There appears to be consistent and clear evidence that clinicians are more likely to follow the steps recommended in a protocol if they use a computerized system. In one systematic review, guideline adherence improved for 14 of 18 systems in which it was measured, and the documentation of actions in the guideline improved in 4 of 4 studies (Shiffman *et al.*, 1999).

Computer guidelines appear to improve the quality of clinical processes

Linking clinical pathways or guidelines with order entry and results reporting systems has been shown to reduce rates of inappropriate prescription or diagnostic testing. For example, in a randomized trial of antibiotic guidelines, a proportion of clinicians were shown vancomycin prescribing guidelines when they attempted to order this antibiotic through an electronic prescribing system (Shojania *et al.*, 1998). The use of vancomycin dropped by 30 per cent with the guidelines, and the medication was given for a significantly shorter duration compared with the control group.

Providing a structure to guide the way that data are entered into a record has been demonstrated to improve clinical performance. In a study comparing the effect of structured data entry forms for patients with abdominal pain who presented to a hospital emergency department against free-form data entry, it was shown that the diagnostic accuracy of staff rose by 7 per cent over baseline (De Dombal *et al.*, 1991). There was also a 13 per cent reduction in use of acute surgical beds at night.

There are several possible explanations for such results. First, the automatic provision of recommendations to clinicians as part of workflow appears to be a statistically significant predictor of a positive impact on the process of care (Damiani *et al.*, 2010). Providing advice at the right point in a clinical workflow that is easily actionable within the same system must reduce barriers to following that advice. There is also a teaching effect that improves the knowledge levels of individuals using computer systems. Discussing the use of protocols for ventilator setting adjustment in intensive care, the researchers in one early study noted that 'although the protocols were complex, the clinical staff learned to anticipate protocol instructions quite accurately, making it possible for them to recognise that a protocol instruction was based on erroneous data' (Henderson *et al.*, 1991).

It is more difficult to demonstrate the impact of computerized guidelines when adoption rates are low

Many of the challenges to demonstrating outcome improvement were summarized at the beginning of this section, and with such formidable challenges it is perhaps no surprise that at least one large systematic review found no evidence of any effect on patient outcomes when computerized guidelines were used (Heselmans *et al.*, 2009).

It is important to dissect such a headline result to understand the reasons for failure to affect outcomes in different trials. For example, computerized evidence-based guidelines were trial led for the management of adult asthma and angina in 60 general practices in the north east of England (Eccles *et al.*, 2002). The system prompted clinicians to consider management options in the guideline triggered by data in the electronic patient record. No significant effect was demonstrated on consultation rates, process of care measures (including prescribing) or any patient-reported outcomes for either condition. Crucially, however, use of the software was extremely low – the median number of interactions with the computer guideline system was zero for much of the study. It would be difficult to suggest that a medication had no clinical effect if no one took the tablet in a trial, and so the real issue perhaps is to explore what barriers existed to produce such low usages. A number of variables may have substantially reduced this system's use and impact:

- The guidelines dealt with the ongoing management of established cases, rather than initial diagnosis or treatment. Clinicians, however, exhibit *clinical inertia,* which is a reluctance to change the current treatment (Coiera, 2011). The opportunity for affecting care may therefore have been highest at the time of diagnosis, and the imperative to consult with the system in follow-up visits may have been low.
- Staff had limited training in system use, which may have decreased their perception of system value. In a study of paper guidelines and prompts for asthma and diabetes management, the intervention was introduced as part of an educational programme and resulted in significant improvements in the management of diabetes and asthma (Feder *et al.*, 1995).
- The primary care physicians were not the only decision makers, and the system ignored the role of the patient. Patients could present with any clinical problem and, despite having asthma or angina, may not have wished to discuss the issues supported by the guideline.

● Significant problems were associated with the interaction design of the software. Despite being embedded in routinely used clinical software, the guideline had to be accessed through a separate path, and it was not possible to access all other parts of the clinical system from within the guideline. If the guideline was exited, it was possible to return only to the beginning of the pathway.

As we will see in Chapter 17, electronic guideline systems are not simple interventions, but rather function as an embedded component within a complex sociotechnical system. The rate of uptake for electronic guidelines in any specific location is influenced by many variables, some of which are local. Failure to address any one of these variables may have a significantly effect on system adoption and usage.

Conclusions

In this chapter, some of the different ways a protocol system can interact with other components of a clinical information system were outlined. In many ways, protocol-based systems can provide the glue that can connect these different components. Because the goal of protocol-directed care is to improve clinical processes, active protocol systems are richly entwined with the delivery of care. As with any such marriage, costs and benefits result from the union. Poorly designed systems can have a significant impact upon care delivery. Consequently, the emphasis on good design, both of protocols and of the systems that embody them, becomes more critical the more deeply they are used to manage the care process. Striking a balance between prescription and permission, protocol systems need to be only as formal as is necessary to ensure appropriate outcomes without restricting the permission required by clinical workers to vary their work patterns.

Discussion points

1. Redraw the decision tree in Figure 15.1 using the guideline primitives shown in Figure 16.4.

2. Compare the peer review process of a major international biomedical journal with that adopted by a major guideline producer. If there are differences, what explanations can you find for them?

3. How does the representation chosen for a human user of a protocol differ from that used in a computer?

4. Compare the different contributions that the medium and the message make to the effectiveness of paper-based and computer-based protocol delivery systems. If you wish, use Chapters 4 and 5 as your template.

5. How effective would an active protocol system be if it were not connected to an EHR or CPOE system?

6. Why are there so many different ways to represent a protocol in a computer? Why do you think it might be difficult to obtain agreement on a single common representation for computer protocols?

7. The CEO of your hospital wants to cancel the implementation of a new computer protocol system because the research literature she has read says such systems rarely affect clinical outcomes. Do you agree with her decision?

Chapter summary

1. Computer-based protocol systems can support passive and active protocol usage.

2. Using protocols as a central template, a variety of clinical activities can be actively supported or automated. These include recording clinical events for the electronic patient record, reminder generation, adjusting settings on devices such as monitors, ordering tests, capturing variances from protocol specifications, scheduling procedures and guiding efficient and effective workflow.

3. A prerequisite for developing computer guideline systems is the creation of computer-interpretable representations of the clinical knowledge contained in clinical guidelines.

4. All computational representations for protocols share similar features and typically are constructed from a set of standard primitives and assembled to produce complete protocols. Primitives include patient states, actions, decisions, nested plans and scheduling constraints.

5. Computerized protocols and guidelines have a variable impact when studied. They appear to improve guideline adherence and clinical process measures, but it is more difficult to demonstrate impacts on clinical outcomes.

6. The successful implementation of computerized guidelines requires attention to a broad spectrum of sociotechnical issues.

CHAPTER 17

Designing, disseminating and applying protocols

> … many of the diseases to which mankind are subject, particularly fevers, smallpox, and other infectious disorders, might be prevented by the diffusion of knowledge in relation to their nature, their causes, and their means of prevention. …Were general knowledge more extensively diffused, and the minds of the multitude habituated to just principles and modes of reasoning, such fallacious views and opinions would be speedily dissipated, and consequently those physical evils and disorders which they produce would be in a great measure prevented.
>
> *Dick, 1833*

In an ideal world, every clinician has immediate and easy access to all the advice on best practice as well as the supporting research evidence. Clinicians would also have the skills to understand what they find and the technology and resources to implement the best practice within their daily workflow.

In the real world, even if there is a better treatment, not every clinician will know about it or seek it out. When relevant information on best practice is available, it is often not in a form that can be computationally executed. When clinicians are exposed to information about best practice, they are not easily swayed to change their practice. Many forget to follow these recommendations or deviate from them without clear cause. Thus, the uptake of research evidence into actual clinical practice remains slow.

Practising clinicians, conversely, complain of being swamped by a growing tide of information. Systematic reviews and guidelines pile up in their offices and proliferate on the Internet, and there seems to be no hope of ever reading, let alone incorporating, such information into their routine pattern of care (Feder *et al.,* 1995). A further broad area of difficulty lies within the culture of clinical practice. The introduction of a more regimented approach to care is seen by some clinicians, rightly or wrongly, as an intrusion on their clinical freedom to deliver healthcare in the manner they personally consider most suitable. Clinicians often claim that their patients are 'different' and that although their practice deviates from evidence-based recommendations, local circumstances and practices justify such variation.

Informatics has a central role to play in assisting with the problem of assembling the research base needed to formulate evidence-based recommendations, as well as interpreting and synthesizing what the research says. It also has a major role in the dissemination of evidence, and as we saw in Chapter 16, through computerized guideline systems, it can support the integration of guidance into clinical workflow. In this chapter, we first review the barriers to the adoption of evidence-based practices before reviewing a range of informatics approaches to protocol creation and dissemination. The chapter concludes with design principles than can assist in creating protocols that are more likely to be adopted because they better fit the needs of a local context.

17.1 Sociotechnical barriers limit the use of evidence in clinical settings

Guideline adoption cannot be taken for granted. Despite the clear benefits that well-designed protocols can deliver in appropriate circumstances, there is a wide variation in the level of uptake of evidence across the clinical community (Gosling *et al.*, 2003b; Westbrook *et al.*, 2004). Indeed, there are many reasons clinicians provide for not following practice guidelines, and these include (Cabana *et al.*, 1999):

- Clinicians may lack awareness of the existence of a guideline.
- Clinicians may lack familiarity with the content of a guideline.
- Clinicians may disagree with the content of a guideline because they interpret the primary research evidence differently, and they believe that any benefit is not worth the risk or discomfort to the patient or the cost.
- Clinicians may not believe that a guideline is applicable to their specific practice population.
- They may believe that guidelines are oversimplified or 'cookbooks' or that guidelines reduce clinical autonomy.
- Clinicians may not feel able to execute the content of a guideline (also known as low self-efficacy).
- There may be a lack of belief that there will be any outcome benefit if the guideline is used.
- Clinicians may feel constrained and unable to change from a previous practice.
- The guidelines may not be easy or convenient to use or may be confusing.

Unpacking these proffered reasons for failing to adopt or comply with a guideline, we find a number of underlying cognitive as well as sociotechnical reasons shaping clinical behaviours.

The complexity of a guideline appears to shape the likelihood that it will be adopted

Inertia or *status quo* bias sees obsolete technologies and practices persist because of their widespread adoption and the sunk costs of individuals who have put much effort into learning to work with them and shape their practices around them (Box 17.1).

Clinical inertia is a specific example of this bias and is defined as a failure by healthcare providers to initiate or intensify therapy even when it is indicated and the clinician is aware of the need to do so. We saw in Chapter 12 that one explanation for clinical inertia is the number of competing demands in play at the time a decision should be taken. When a decision is constrained by time, uncertain or absent data (Grant *et al.*, 2009) or multiple problems, some

Combining these two measures of expected benefit and frequency of adoption produces a single measure of the clinical impact of the guideline (Coiera, 2001). We have encountered this calculation before because it is equivalent to the *expected utility* associated with using a guideline. Comparing the expected utility of two different guidelines allows us to estimate the value of information (VOI) between the two (see Chapter 11). For example, assume we have a disease in which the baseline outcome with current treatments is 50 per cent recovery. Two new competing treatments are introduced through published guidelines. Treatment A has a 90 per cent clinical success rate, and 1 per cent of patients receive it, based upon the adoption rate by clinicians. If treatment B has only an 80 per cent success rate but a 10 per cent adoption rate, which treatment is the most effective? Based solely on evidence of clinical efficacy, then treatment A is clearly superior. If, however, we measure the impact factor of a guideline based upon its expected utility, then treatment B is 7.5 times as beneficial as A and has a higher VOI (Box 17.2). Thus, a guideline that describes a treatment that does not have the best clinical outcome may nonetheless be the best when we consider its ease of adoption and consequent impact on the health of the population.

The situation is complicated further because the potential benefit seen in a trial may not be the actual benefit obtained in operation. The presence of any number of local variables, from the characteristics of the patients being treated to the constraints of workflow and resources, means that the same guideline implemented in two different locations is likely to produce different clinical outcomes (see Chapter 12). We can thus calculate a more local version of clinical impact by replacing potential (or ideal) efficacy with a measure of local efficacy (see Box 17.2).

The implication for those in the business of creating evidence 'products' such as clinical guidelines is that the notion of the 'best' treatment advice needs to be replaced with a more complex concept that encompasses the likelihood that a published guideline will actually be used, as well as the impact of local implementation on actual benefits realized. Consequently, not only should developers of a guideline think about the scientific contents of a guideline, but also they must consider its usability in practice.

Treatment A gives a 90 per cent success rate, and the guidelines recommending it achieve an adoption rate of 1 per cent within the population of patients. The remaining patients use the baseline treatment with a 50 per cent success rate. The improvement to the population's health produced by treatment A provides us with one estimate of its expected utility:

Impact of treatment A $= 0.9 \times 1/100 + 0.5 \times 99/100$
$= 0.504$

Treatment B gives an 80 per cent success rate, and the guidelines recommending it are used by 10 per cent of the population. The remaining patients use the baseline treatment with 50 per cent success. The improvement to the population's health produced by treatment B is thus:

Impact of treatment B $= 0.8 \times 10/100 + 0.5 \times 90/100$
$= 0.53$

The expected utility of guideline A is thus 0.004 above baseline, and for B it is 0.03. The difference between the two choices is called the value of information (VOI) and is 0.026 utils, and treatment B has an expected utility that is 7.5 times as great as that of treatment A.

Box 17.2
Value of information in a guideline

Box 17.1
The dominant design

It is an interesting feature of the marketplace that the introduction of a new class of product at first usually sees a great variety of competing designs enter the market. Each competing design has new features or different combinations of existing features. After a period, however, such variety almost completely disappears, and most producers end up creating products that have remarkably similar features.

Thus, the first typewriter was produced by Scholes in 1868 and was followed by a host of competing designs. However, 1899 saw the introduction of the Underwood Model 5 typewriter, which became the template for typewriters until they were replaced by computers. Soon after the introduction of the Underwood Model 5, because of its immense popularity, all other manufacturers found themselves forced to approximate the Underwood design. Indeed, the design persisted throughout the first half of the twentieth century. It was not until the introduction of electric typewriters, computers and word processors that radically different sets of designs and functions were introduced.

The evolution of the modern personal computer followed along the same path, with an initial flurry of different designs. Eventually, the marketplace settled upon a set of prototypic features that most people would expect when they bought a personal computer.

This stable design point in the history of a product class is known as a *dominant design* (Utterback, 1996). The dominant design 'embodies the requirements of many classes of users of a particular product, even though it may not meet the needs of a particular class to quite the same extent as would a customized design.'

Further, even though a dominant design may after a time become obsolete, its widespread adoption and individuals' investment in learning to work with it make them reluctant to shift to a better design. Therefore, even though there are probably numerous better designs than the QWERTY keyboard, most people exhibit a *status quo* bias. Those who have learnt to use this type of keyboard are reluctant to shift to using a better design. Thus, once in place, the dominant design remains fixed, not because newer designs do not offer benefits, but because changing to them incurs unacceptable costs. Only when the cost benefit trade-off shifts heavily the other way will a new product class become acceptable. Modern consumer products such as smart phones and computer devices are engineered to quickly become obsolete, for example by degrading in performance as new software is released. This can change the cost-benefit calculation individuals make and drive adoption of newer products or product classes.

decisions are prioritized over others (Hofer *et al.*, 2004). In other words, the more complex the circumstances, the less likely it is that a particular step or decision will be taken. Indeed, when we examine guideline complexity, it does appear that adoption rates are inversely proportional to complexity. Using a measure of document complexity, in one study guidelines of high complexity had a significantly lower compliance rate (41.9 per cent) compared with guidelines judged to be low in complexity (55.9 per cent) (Grilli and Lomas, 1994).

Sociotechnical factors shape guideline adoption and adherence

Organizational, social and professional factors appear to be at least as important as technical and practical factors in shaping the uptake of information technology (Ash, 1997; Kaplan, 1997), and they similarly affect guideline uptake, whether paper or electronic, passive or active. Sociotechnical barriers to guideline use include:

- *Clinical informatics skills* – Studies of the barriers to using online evidence resources have identified a range of factors including insufficient training in database searching and general information technology skills (Hersh and Hickam, 1998).
- *Organizational support* – Lack of organizational support is a barrier to evidence-based practice (Retsas, 2000). Organizational and social factors that promote discussion within

an organization and the existence of 'champions' (people who enthusiastically support an innovation) have been shown to predict the uptake of new innovations (Howell and Boies, 2004), including the access of online evidence sources (Gosling *et al.*, 2003a). Failure to provide support for technological infrastructure or for promoting evidence use and training in searching skills will, however, limit uptake.

- *Professional differences* – There is wide variation in the way different professional groups regard clinical evidence and access it. Doctors appear to emphasise the role of evidence from the biomedical literature in their decision-making culture (Gosling *et al.*, 2003b). In a study of critical care nurses, they appeared to place greater value on policies and procedures and used these to bring weight to their encounters with medical staff (Manias and Street, 2000). Such preferences may on occasion see the continuation of practices known to be potentially harmful (Greenwood *et al.*, 2000).

17.2 The clinical impact of a guideline is determined both by its efficacy and by its adoption rate

Even though there are many barriers to the uptake of innovations such as new treatments, traditional approaches to evaluating the effectiveness of a new treatment consider the costs and benefits of the treatment in isolation, all else being equal. A more meaningful cost benefit analysis reflects the true impact of a treatment once it becomes available and has to compete with other treatment options for adoption. Irrespective of the scientific evidence for a treatment, and the protocols and guidelines that recommend it, if it is not used, it will have no impact in the clinical world.

One way of thinking about this is to consider how many times a systematic review or study report or clinical protocol must be read before there is a measureable impact on clinical outcomes. Metrics such as the *number needed to read* (Toth *et al.*, 2005) and the *number needed to benefit from information* (Pluye *et al.*, 2013) try to correlate access of information with impact on process or outcome. Although they are useful, such measures do not measure the likelihood that the information will be found in the first place. Further, because they are document centric, they do not really unpack the cognitive and sociotechnical reasons behind some information sources having a greater impact on outcomes than others.

When assessing the potential impact of a guideline, there are two broad measures of interest:

- The effect on clinical outcome that a treatment produces if it was to be used, typically estimated from controlled trials that have been conducted under 'ideal' circumstances.
- The actual rate of adoption of a guideline that recommends the treatment. This rate is a function of the following: the *discoverability* of information – the likelihood that the clinical community finds this information; the *utility* of information – does it provide the reader with something useful that they do not already possess? (Magrabi *et al.*, 2004); and the *usability* of the information – the balance of individual cognitive and organizational procedural costs and benefits associated with incorporating a practice into routine care.

17.3 Guidelines and protocols should be designed to reflect the best evidence and shaped to fit clinical context

If we are to maximize the clinical impact of a protocol or guideline and improve the quality of clinical decisions and actions on the ground, three basic requirements need to be met:

- *Protocol utility* – First, guidance must represent an improvement in clinical processes beyond that already in routine practice. As we saw in Chapter 16, the potential for benefit in adopting a guideline is highly dependent on current practice within a particular health service delivery organization.
- *Protocol designability* – Next, it must actually be feasible to prescribe a course of action ahead of time. If the situation in question is novel, constantly changing or in some other way non-deterministic, then it is difficult to see how an explicit recipe for action can be pre-determined. As described in Chapter 15, protocols are more likely to be effective if there is strong predictability about the pathway patients will follow and where the trajectory of progress is similar for most patients (Allen *et al.*, 2009).
- *Protocol usability* – Finally, irrespective of how easy it is to create a protocol, the conditions at the time of decision-making must make it possible to both access and then apply the protocol.

These three requirements mean that a protocol's form and content cannot be separated. A clinical protocol is not an abstract scientific statement about best practice but a tool for clinical improvement. Recall from Chapter 1 that in modelling the world, the processes of abstraction, definition of design assumptions and instantiation all influence the utility of a designed object.

When a protocol is designed, it should be shaped both by an understanding of the best treatment for a disease and by the circumstances in which it will be used. We must, for example, make design assumptions about the level of resource or training of staff available when the protocol is executed. Once a protocol has been developed, it must then be implemented, and this construction of a local workflow is equivalent to the process of model instantiation described in Chapter 1. The overall process of protocol design, creation and application is summarized in Figure 17.1. Protocol creation is also not a single event in time, but rather an ongoing process of assessing protocol performance and refining the design accordingly – the model-measure-manage cycle.

To increase utilization rates, efforts need to be made to increase the immediate benefits for clinicians when using protocol systems, as well as reducing barriers. There thus need to be clear advantages for the clinician beyond exhortations to the public good. For example, embedding protocols and evidence-based guidelines within the electronic health record has the potential to deliver immediate benefits through automation. Selecting a guideline could automatically generate test orders, pre-prepare prescriptions, schedule tests, create elements of the patient record, call up patient educational materials or even see the award of continuing education points. Barriers to system use must also be tackled. For example, the use of mobile computing and smart phone devices offers access to protocols whenever they are needed.

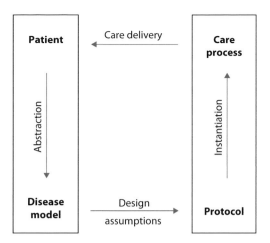

Figure 17.1 Protocols are designed based upon a set of assumptions both about the best way to manage a disease using research evidence and about the context within which the protocol will be used, including who will be delivering care, the available resources and the local goal of care.

17.4 Informatics methods can improve the processes of evidence discovery and synthesis

To maximize protocol utility, clinical recommendations must be based upon the very latest evidence. New research evidence that could substantively change conclusions about the effectiveness or harms of therapies appears often and relatively quickly. In one analysis, there was significant new evidence available at the time of publication for 7 per cent of systematic reviews, or evidence had become available within 2 years for 23 per cent of reviews (Shojania *et al.*, 2007). The median survival time without substantive new evidence appearing was 5½ years. Systematic reviews should thus be re-examined every 2 years and, if necessary, be updated to reflect changes in the research evidence. Such updating occurs only for one third of systematic reviews, however (Jaidee *et al.*, 2010).

This mismatch between the growth in research evidence and the synthesis of research findings into best-practice recommendations means that there is an increasing gap between what is in principle known from research and what clinicians have easy access to through guidelines and systematic reviews (Bastian *et al.*, 2010).

The uniform and rapid transformation of clinical evidence into clinical practice represents not just a major challenge for health, but also a major challenge for health informatics (Coiera, 1996). The process of producing a systematic review of the literature involves steps such as searching for relevant scientific articles, identifying and extracting critical information from the articles, evaluating risk of bias in selected trials and synthesizing and then publishing the results.

Information and communication technologies have a profound role to play in each of these tasks. Where tasks are repetitive and clearly describable, they can be automated, and where tasks require human judgement, tools can be built that assist humans in making the process rapid and efficient (Coiera, 1996; Smith and Chalmers, 2001; Tsafnat *et al.*, 2013; Tsafnat *et al.*, 2014). Indeed, computer systems that can reason from the literature to support clinical decision-making have long been proposed (Rennels *et al.*, 1987).

- *Users* – The skill level of the individuals required to carry out the protocol also affects the form and content of protocols. The words used in a protocol vary if it is designed for patients or members of the public, as may the level of detail and goals of the protocol. In particular, the ability of an individual to recognize that the entry criteria for a protocol have been fulfilled is essential. There is little point in having a set of finely crafted protocols if it is unclear when they should be applied.
- *Local processes and workflow* – Local care processes evolve to reflect not just best-practice knowledge, but also local resources and goals. A protocol has to be designed with an understanding of how it will be used within such existing processes. Will it simply be looked at as a reference after an initial care plan has been drafted, or will it be used to drive every detail of a care process? In each situation, the requirements for clarity, level of detail and availability are vastly different. Context-specific versions of evidence can be created using computerized user models that capture the specific needs of individual groups and permit some automatic tailoring of evidence before it is presented (Elhadad *et al.*, 2005; Pratt and Sim, 1995). Access methods can also be optimized to local needs and contexts in which evidence is used. For example, a clinician faced with an emergency that requires rapid decision-making is unlikely to browse through information in a leisurely way, whereas that may be the perfect solution for less time-critical applications.

Principle 2 – a protocol should not be more specific than is necessary to achieve a specific goal

There is always a trade-off between design specificity and utility. The more closely a protocol (or indeed any model) fits a specific set of conditions, the less likely it is to be useful in others because of 'overfitting'. The converse principle is that general methods can be applied across many different situations, but they will probably have only moderate utility. There are theoretical arguments for choosing intermediate complexity designs (Coiera, 1992). These arguments are supported by experimental evidence that the speed and completeness of information retrieval from medical records are best when intermediate levels of detail are used (Tange *et al.*, 1998).

Excessive formalization for its own sake does not necessarily deliver any greater return and may require unnecessary effort (Martin and American Management Association, 1995). It also may cause disaffection of the staff members who are required to use the protocol. Recall also that overly complex protocols have lower compliance rates than simpler ones.

Protocol designers should thus consider the appropriate level of detail that needs to be coded into a guideline and recognize that widespread adoption requires some sacrifice of detail. One technique to manage this trade-off is to specify a protocol only in general terms and then allow organizations to instantiate it with local data. For example, one could specify a treatment goal rather than a specific action. 'Establish normal blood pressure through intravenous fluid replacement' may be an appropriate goal for a protocol, rather than specifying exactly how much fluid is to be given. The actual amount of fluid given would depend on the specific needs of a patient. This technique is known as *skeletal plan refinement* (Tu *et al.*, 1989), and it can be used to create quite sophisticated protocols that are highly flexible to fit individual patients' needs.

Principle 3 – protocol design should reflect the skill level and circumstances of those using them

The level of description used in a protocol should also match the abilities of those using it. Very simple steps are probably best for use with relatively inexperienced individuals or patients. For example, protocols for first aid resuscitation taught to the public are kept very simple. Protocols for trained paramedical or medical staff in exactly the same circumstance may be much richer and more complex, despite the similarities in overall goal.

Further, different protocol representations make different demands on those who use them. Mnemonic representations such as the ABCs of resuscitation have great value in stressful situations, but they may not permit great detail to be recalled. Flowcharts require relatively little reasoning and can be designed to make the decision logic extremely clear. Thus, one could create a flowchart for situations in which the ability to understand the protocol is limited, such as an emergency situation, or when the user has had limited instruction. The flowchart representation can become too complicated for complex decisions. In such cases, a rule-based representation might be used as a reminder for individuals who have less time pressure or are better trained in the management of the situation.

Conclusions

Throughout this part of the book we have explored one of the foundational challenges facing healthcare, though the eyes of evidence-based practice and protocols. The delivery of healthcare is often at its most efficient, effective and safe when it is a formalized, polished and factory-like affair. Yet patients truly are often unique, both in their personal circumstances and wishes and in their biology. Informatics can provide methods and tools that support both circumstances. Protocols are a tool *par excellence* for automation. When protocols are designed to fit well with workflow, are up-to-date and fit the needs of the population, they become a powerful tool in our armamentarium. In circumstances where we need to embrace variation, then other informatics approaches come to the fore, such as personalized approaches to medicine (see Chapter 31), consumer-focussed systems (see Chapter 32) and case-based reasoning methods (see Chapter 26).

Discussion points

1. You have joined a working party that will produce expert guidelines in your area of clinical speciality. The team has agreed to devote all the working time to arrive at the consensus guidelines and write them up for publication, but it has allocated no time to thinking about design or dissemination issues. What will you advise them?

2. Design a protocol for a short common clinical process that is to be used by clinicians. Next, redesign the protocol while assuming that it is going to have to be read by patients. What issues have guided the design choices you made?

3. Which is more complex – a protocol designed for a human to use or a protocol designed to be used by a computer? Why?

4. Do you think the process of systematic review can ever be fully automated?

5. The protocols designed and used by your local children's hospital, which is a world-class centre of excellence, are now going to be made mandatory for any hospital that sees a mix of acute adult and paediatric patients. Is this a good idea?

6. How does professional culture affect the use of evidence in clinical settings?

7. Can you use the notion of the dominant design from Box 17.1 to explain why clinicians may stick to outmoded practices?

Chapter summary

1. Sociotechnical barriers limit the use of evidence in clinical settings. Cultural differences among professional groupings account for some of these differences, and organizational support through provision of training and infrastructure and the presence of local champions also have an impact.

2. Guideline adoption rates appear inversely proportional to complexity, driven in part by clinical inertia.

3. The true clinical impact of a guideline is determined both by its efficacy and by its adoption rate, and the adoption rate is related to protocol discoverability, utility and usability.

4. Guidelines and protocols should be designed to reflect the best scientific evidence but also be shaped to fit the clinical context of use. Protocol designability is also critical because it must actually be feasible to prescribe a course of action ahead of time.

5. Informatics methods can improve the processes of evidence discovery and synthesis:

   a. Evidence retrieval systems assist in locating the primary research evidence.

   b. Once a document is found, text-processing tools can help in screening for relevance and risk of bias, and then extracting key information such as the Population on which the study was conducted, the Intervention that was studied, the nature of the Control arm and the Outcomes that were measured (PICO).

   c. Once data are extracted from multiple trial reports, the data must be synthesized into a systematic review, and automated statistical methods can conduct meta-analyses on well-structured data extracted from trial reports.

   d. Text generation tools can assist by publishing protocols and guidelines in multiple formats for use in active and passive systems.

6. Design principles for protocols include:

   a. Making assumptions about the context of use explicit.

   b. Creating protocols that are no more specific than necessary to achieve a specific goal.

   c. Reflecting the skill level and circumstances of those who will eventually use them.

PART 5

Communication systems in healthcare

CHAPTER 18

Communication systems basics

> It is through the telephone calls, meetings, planning sessions... and corridor conversations that people inform, amuse, update, gossip, review, reassess, reason, instruct, revise, argue, debate, contest, and actually constitute the moments, myths and, through time, the very structuring of the organisation.
>
> *Boden, 1994*

Good interpersonal communication is an essential skill for any healthcare worker, and as we saw in Chapter 4, effective communication is central to the smooth running of the healthcare system as a whole. The care of patients now involves many different individuals, in part because of increasing specialization within the professions. Increased patient mobility means that many individuals do not live in the same area for long. Clinical encounters are also supported by many other players who never see a patient, including laboratory and radiology staff through to administrators. All these trends and factors increase the need for healthcare workers to share information about patients and to discuss their management.

A recurring theme throughout this book is that the specific needs of a given task must drive the choice of technology to assist with that task. Although the range of technical communication options is rich, our understanding of the specific roles they can play in healthcare lags behind.

In this chapter, the basic components of a technologically mediated communication system are explained. The fundamental concepts of a communication channel, service, device and interaction mode are followed by an exploration of the basic communication service types and examples of their application in healthcare. Chapter 19 turns to information and communication networks, which underpin these different communication services, and explains their technical operation and identifies their benefits and limitations. The final two chapters in this section (Chapters 20 and 21) examine the specific types of communication problems that arise in healthcare and critically analyze the ways in which communication technology can sometimes improve health service delivery, first by using social media in Chapter 20, and in Chapter 21, through telemedicine and mobile healthcare.

attention immediately, such as the ringing tone of a telephone. A service that is inherently not interruptive, such as e-mail, can still become interruptive if an alert is triggered when a new message arrives.

- *Communication policies* – A communication system can be bound by formal procedure rather than by technology. Policies can shape communication system performance, independent of the specific technologies used. For example, access control policies dictate who is allowed to see information and describe the steps needed to authenticate identity before access is granted (see Chapter 19).

The utility of any communication system bundle is determined by its components and how they interact with the context of use. If even one element of the system bundle is inappropriate to the setting, the communication system may underperform. For example, sending an x-ray to a small device such as a smart phone is unlikely to be useful, both because the size of the screen will limit viewing the image and because the size of the image may exceed the capacity of the wireless channel used. Sociotechnical variables also have a large impact on the benefit of a communication system. For example, failure to train staff adequately to recognize the importance of good communication will no doubt result in a poor outcome, independent of the amount of money spent on new technology.

18.3 Shared time or space defines the modes of communication system use

The simplest way to model the different modes in which communication can occur is to recognize that individuals can be separated either in time or in space. The nature of the separation changes the characteristics of the interaction and the type of channel and service that are needed (Table 18.1).

Same time, same place – A face-to-face conversation is the most obvious example of communication benefiting from shared location and time. The participants in the dialogue are able to both hear and see each other and to share whatever materials they have to hand. Because they can see and hear so much of each other, the opportunity for exchanging complex and subtle cues is high. In whatever other situations communication occurs, one often seeks to replicate the effectiveness of face-to-face communication. Despite the richness of face-to-face conversation, devices are often still used to augment the interaction. Everything from slide projectors in an auditorium to shared computer screens or surfaces can provide additional channels to enhance communication.

Same time, different place – Separated by distance, conversations can nevertheless occur in the same time. When two parties exchange messages across a communication channel at the

Table 18.1 Communication needs can be characterized by the separation of participants in time or space

	Same time (synchronous)	Different time (asynchronous)
Same place	Face-to-face meeting	Local message
Different place	Remote conversation	Remote message

same time, this is known as *synchronous communication*. Voice telephony is an example of a two-way synchronous channel. Broadcast television is a one-way synchronous channel. It is the nature of synchronous communication that it is interruptive, and as we saw earlier in the book, interruptions may have a negative impact (e.g. on individuals who have high cognitive loads).

Different time, same place – When individuals are separated by time, they require *asynchronous* channels to support their interaction. Because there can be no simultaneous discussion, conversations occur through a series of delayed message exchanges. These exchanges can use anything from sticky notes left on a colleague's desk to electronic messaging systems for clinicians who work on different shifts in the same hospital ward. Asynchronous communication is not inherently interruptive, and if a communication is not urgent, asynchronous channels may be a preferred way of communicating with otherwise busy individuals.

Different time, different place – In many ways, this is the most challenging of the four quadrants because neither location nor time is shared by the communicating parties. Asynchronous messaging is clearly needed. For example, a radiology image stored in a radiology department reporting system can be forwarded along with a report to a requesting physician, who reads it at a later, more convenient time.

Communication systems vary in the media they employ

Communication systems can also be understood in terms of the different *media* they employ. A medium is literally something put 'in the middle', and *communication medium* is a term reserved for the form of a message between two agents (voice, video) (Table 18.2). Sometimes the term is used as a collective noun for information services, such as newspapers or television channels.

Unsurprisingly, the value of one medium over another depends on the context (Caldwell *et al.,* 1995). The nature of a particular task, the setting in which it occurs and the amount of information that a medium can bear all seem to have effects on human performance on a communication task (Rice, 1992). Relatively information-lean media such as electronic mail and voicemail can be used for routine, simple communications. In contrast, for non-routine and difficult communications, a rich medium such as video, and preferably face-to-face conversation, may need to be used. This may be because in routine situations, individuals share a common model of the task (see Figure 4.4), and so they need to communicate less during an exchange. In contrast, in novel situations a significant portion of the communication may need to be devoted to establishing common ground (Clark and Brennan, 1991). Almost paradoxically, rich media decrease our ability to process information because they bring so much of it, but by their very nature they are highly engaging and so encourage interaction (Robert and Dennis, 2005).

Table 18.2   Communication services can be classified according to the media they support and by whether they are asynchronous message–based systems or operate synchronously in real time

	Voice	Image	Data
Synchronous	Telephony	Video-conferencing	Shared electronic white boards, shared documents
Asynchronous	Voicemail	Web access to photographs and videos	Text messages, e-mail

Conclusions

Taking a broad view that communication systems include people, messages, technologies and organizational structures helps in deciding which communication services are most appropriate for a particular task, user group or setting. It can also help identify which social, cultural and organizational changes may be needed along with the technology. In Chapter 19, we delve into the specifics of information and communication networks, which are the substrate for information exchange in healthcare, as elsewhere.

Discussion points

1. Choose a simple episode of care, for example, a patient visiting their GP. Determine all the possible individuals who may be involved in that episode, and sketch out all the conversations that could take place. Describe the different channels and services that could be used in support of the different conversations.

2. Now take the diagram from the previous question and add to it all the information systems that could also be involved in information transactions, starting with the medical record.

3. A colleague drops a letter on your desk and tells you that you have mail. Was receiving the letter a synchronous or an asynchronous event? Break down what happened into its components, including your colleague, and determine which components were synchronous.

4. A pager or bleeper is designed to have an interruptive interaction mode. Can you conceive of ways in which the paging service could behave asynchronously? In what circumstances would such a service be useful, and in which circumstances would it be dangerous?

5. Select a social networking site you are familiar with and describe all the components and attributes of this communication service, using the concepts described in this chapter.

Chapter summary

1. The communication space is the largest part of the health system's information space and contains a substantial proportion of the health system's information 'pathology'.

2. The number of possible conversations that could take place at any one time increases in combination with the number of individuals who need to communicate. Even simple communication systems on analysis involve many different individuals and possible exchanges.

3. A communication system involves people, the messages they wish to convey, the technologies that mediate conversations and the organizational structures that define and constrain the conversations that are allowed to occur. System components include channel, message, policies, agents, social networks, services, device and interaction mode.

4. Communication systems can support communication among individuals separated either by time or by distance.

5. Channels that support communication in real time are known as synchronous channels. Channels that support communication over different times are known as asynchronous channels.

6. When messages are sent from one individual to only one other, this is called *peer-to-peer* communication. Sending a message to a select group of individuals is called *narrowcasting*, in contrast to widespread distribution, which we know as *broadcasting*.

7. Voice services can support rich interactions and have nearly universal application in healthcare. Automated conversations between computer and patient can have a significant impact on health behaviours.

8. Text messaging and e-mail find a wide variety of uses from peer-to-peer interactions for personal messages to narrowcast and broadcast messages. They appear to enable rich interactions between patients and clinicians.

9. Video services can offer some benefits over voice, but they may have their biggest role in sharing objects to create a common physical context for conversation.

10. Social media comprise a diverse collection of information and communication services that facilitate group interaction and vary significantly in design, purpose and target audience.

Interlude – the Internet and the World Wide Web

From a relatively humble beginning, the Internet has transformed through four relatively distinct stages, each one shaped by its predecessors.

1. It began in the United States in the late 1960s as a Cold War military research project, designed to ensure that communication lines remained open after nuclear strikes. This system slowly evolved in size and complexity until, in the mid-1980s, the Internet had become a global computer network.
2. At that time, it was used by many academic institutions and a few commercial companies. During this second phase, its main use was for electronic messaging and the transfer of computer files. What followed next was a period of steady growth, as the population of users slowly expanded beyond industry and academia.
3. It was not really until the third phase, with the introduction of the World Wide Web (WWW), that the massive growth now associated with the Internet occurred. The Web provided a simple and standard way to find and view documents on the Internet. Its ease of use, along with an ever-growing storehouse of publicly accessible information, combined to transform the Internet into a tool that the public at large was able to appreciate and wanted to use.
4. The fourth phase followed soon after the third. It was characterized by the commercial and institutional exploitation of the Internet and its technologies. A constant stream of innovation in the way the Internet is being used, as well as in its underlying technologies, guarantees that such change will be a feature for quite some time.

The Internet as a technological phenomenon

Essentially a network of networks, the Internet permits computers across the globe to communicate with each other. It evolved out of the Advanced Research Projects Network (ARPAnet) developed by the United States Department of Defense in the late 1960s (Lowe et al., 1996). ARPAnet was built with the intention of developing computer networks that would be capable of surviving nuclear war. The challenges at that time were to develop methods for sharing information across diverse sites and to keep these connections operational even if a disruption occurred at individual sites.

The Internet as a commercial phenomenon

The growth of the public's interest in the Internet initially caught most computer and telecommunications companies by surprise. Communication had traditionally been the preserve of the telecommunications industry, rather than the information technology sector. What initially made this particular market so ripe for exploitation was that it was fought over by so many separate industries, each giant in its own right. Telecommunications carriers, cable television companies and computer companies all believed that the Internet had the potential to either transform or wipe out their existing businesses, and so they engaged aggressively in the commercialization of the Internet.

The wealth and competitive aggression of such companies led to significant overinvestment in Internet businesses and fuelled the public equities bubble that resulted in the 'dot com' boom and subsequent bust. It should be remembered that the Internet share market boom had little to do with the technologies being exploited or their true potential. Rather, it was fuelled by greed and panic. So, despite the boom and bust, the use of the Internet and Web continues to grow and is a commonplace element of everyday life for many people.

There are four basic Internet 'businesses' – transport, connection, services and content. *Transport* refers to the industries that provide the physical networks upon which the Internet is built and across which the basic bits of information are moved. This 'bit shipping' is the domain of telecommunication companies and the cable and wireless network operators, and it is fiercely competitive. As it becomes increasingly inexpensive to ship bits, these industries look to diversify into other, more profitable Internet businesses.

Providing *connection* into the Internet is also a business. Service providers offer network connections to the Internet for individuals or groups who do not have the need, or cannot afford to build, their own networks. Along with connection to a network comes *data storage,* and network providers increasingly offer to store user data, for example, through 'cloud' services.

Most Internet businesses provide *services* through applications that are accessed by the Web, often optimized for mobile devices ('apps'). Internet search is a service, as is the provision of a social media space. More fundamentally, the Internet provides traditional 'bricks and mortar' businesses with new ways to interact with the public. Many such businesses are able to transact some or all of their offline services online. Those that are able to move completely online have often seen the rapid decline of the offline businesses, such as book and record stores.

As more of our lives are represented online, our personal information can be aggregated, often without our knowledge or provision. The construction of individual profiles of our interests and activities can be used to market goods to us. Our shopping records become fodder for data analysts who aim to predict the next services or products we want. Even our medical records can be used to predict which pharmaceuticals or health services we may need next.

Further reading

Lowe, H. J., E. C. Lomax and S. E. Polonkey (1996). The World Wide Web: a review of an emerging Internet-based technology for the distribution of biomedical information. *Journal of the American Medical Informatics Association* **3**(1): 1–14.

Negroponte, N. (1996). *Being Digital.* New York, Random House.

CHAPTER 19

Information and communication networks

The simple contrivance of tin tubes for speaking through, communicating between different apartments, by which the directions of the superintendant are instantly conveyed to the remotest parts of an establishment, produces a considerable economy of time. It is employed in the shops and manufactories in London, and might with advantage be used in domestic establishments, particularly in large houses, in conveying orders from the nursery to the kitchen, or from the house to the stable…The distance to which such a mode of communication can be extended, does not appear to have been ascertained, and would be an interesting subject for inquiry. Admitting it to be possible between London and Liverpool, about seventeen minutes would elapse before the words spoken at one end would reach the other extremity of the pipe.

Babbage, 1833

Never underestimate the bandwidth of a station wagon full of tapes hurtling down the highway.

Tanenbaum, 2003

Standards are like toothbrushes. Everybody wants one but nobody wants to use anybody else's.

Morella, 2006

Information sharing in technological systems occurs across a network of connections that both provide the conduits along which data are shipped and which also often dictate message structure. The different communication channels and services introduced in Chapter 18 are all built on top of such networks. Indeed, networks underpin all the information systems that we find in healthcare and provide the connections that allow patient information to move among locations.

A recurrent and still unsolved problem in health informatics is *semantic interoperability* – the desire that when clinical information systems share information, there is a shared understanding not just of the structure or syntax of messages, but also of the semantics or meaning of what is exchanged. We saw in Part 2 of this book that achieving semantic interoperability among people is challenging enough (Pirnejad *et al.*, 2008), and probably it will never be entirely achievable. The challenges for machine interoperability are, in a very different way, just as challenging.

In this chapter, we explore this rich space of machine, as opposed to human, interoperability. We begin by summarizing at a general level some of the basic principles of information and communication networks – not because they are core informatics issues, but because without them it is much more difficult to understand why current approaches to message exchange exist and take the form that they do.

Some of the important health message exchange standards in common use are then introduced. This, too, is a deep and rich topic, and the material in this chapter should be seen as a high-level overview of a very technical area. There are two other technically important issues that need to be addressed when health information is exchanged – how consent to access information is managed and how security measures can help prevent unauthorized network access. The chapter concludes by bringing together these issues to help explain some of the different network architectures that are used for information exchange in healthcare systems, especially on a regional and national scale.

19.1 Communication is governed by a set of layered protocols

For communication to be effective, both conversing parties need to understand the same language. As we saw in Chapter 4, well-behaved agents communicate according to a basic set of rules such as Grice's maxims to ensure that conversations are effective and that each agent understands what is going on in the conversation. The rules governing how a conversation should proceed are called a *communication protocol,* and the design of such protocols is central to understanding the operation of communication networks. When two machines communicate with each other, the communication protocol defines, among other things, how a message is to be constructed, how its receipt is to be acknowledged, how turn taking should occur in the exchange and how misunderstandings or errors may be repaired.

To simplify the design of communication protocols, they are typically decomposed into a number of different layers, each of which accomplishes a different task. Protocol layers are organized hierarchically, with the bottom layers carrying out tasks that then can be forwarded up the hierarchy to be processed by higher layers (Figure 19.1). One advantage of such decomposition is that individual layers do not need to understand how the others work, but need to know only how to interact with them. Thus, each layer has a defined interface with the layers below and above it in a stack, which defines the input and output that will occur between layers. Together the layers form a *protocol stack,* and at the bottom of the stack sits the physical medium that is the channel that transports the data among machines. We notionally consider that any layer n on one machine communicates directly with its counterpart layer n on the other machine at the other end of the network connection.

The International Organization for Standardization (ISO) has developed the Open System Interconnection (OSI) model that is used almost universally as a template to define the protocol layers for communicating among computers. The OSI model consists of seven layers, and the different real world protocols we encounter operate at one or more of the OSI layers (Table 19.1). The OSI layers commence at layer 1, which is directly concerned with translating digital data into a signal that can travel across a channel. Level 1 is therefore interested in

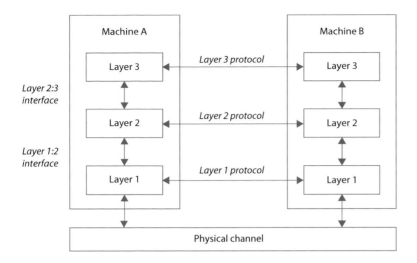

Figure 19.1
When two machines communicate, the conversation is regulated by a series of layered protocols, with defined interfaces insulating one protocol layer from the others. Although all data are in reality transferred across the same channel, notionally it is the individual layers on different machines that talk to each other. (After Tanenbaum, 2003.)

Table 19.1 Summary of the seven Open System Interconnection protocol layers

OSI layer	Function	Example
Application (layer 7)	Supports applications that run over the network, such as file transfer and e-mail.	FTP, e-mail, HL7.
Presentation (layer 6)	Sometimes called the *syntax layer*, translates from application to network format. Encrypts data.	HTTP/HTML
Session (layer 5)	Establishes, manages and terminates connections among applications.	NetBIOS, RPC
Transport (layer 4)	Responsible for end-to-end error recovery and flow control. It ensures complete data transfer.	TCP/IP, NetBIOS/NetBEUI
Network (layer 3)	Responsible for establishing, maintaining and terminating connections. Provides switching and routing by creating logical paths or virtual circuits.	IP
Data link (layer 2)	Encodes and decodes data packets or frames into bits. Is divided into two sub-layers, the media access control (MAC) layer and the logical link control (LLC) layer.	ATM
Physical (layer 1)	Concerned with transmission of unstructured bit stream over a physical link, e.g. electrical, photon or radio signals. Defines cables, cards and physical aspects.	ISDN; Wireless protocols; Fast Ethernet, RS232, and ATM protocols have physical layer components.

ATM, asynchronous transfer mode; FTP, file transfer protocol; HL7, Health Level 7; HTML, HyperText Markup Language; HTTP, HyperText Transfer Protocol; IP, Internet protocol; ISDN, Integrated Service Digital Network; NetBEUI, NetBIOS Extended User Interface; NetBIOS, Network Basic Input/Output System; RPC, remote procedure call; TCP, transmission control protocol.

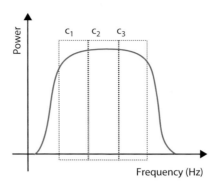

Figure 19.4
Channels can
combine multiple
calls by allocating
each call a different
slot from the
frequencies available
on the common
channel.

channel. It is possible to relate a channel's bandwidth to its data rate. For example, a normal telephone line can carry up to 64 Kbytes per second, based upon a 3.4-kHz voice requirement for the transmission of intelligible speech (Lawton, 1993). In contrast, a common trunk on a telephone network may handle between 1.5 and 2 Mbits per second.

19.3 Broadband systems are designed to carry rich media such as video

Modern networks must both handle traditional high-throughput data traffic (e.g. file transfers) and support real-time, low-latency media such as voice and video. The first globally agreed standard for broadband was the *Integrated Service Digital Network* (ISDN), which was designed to ship both voice and data across traditional telephone networks. ISDN provides two independent data channels to a subscriber. One channel can be used to carry voice, and data are transmitted across the second. A third signalling channel allows the user's equipment to communicate with the network, allowing for rapid call set-up and exchange of other information. For example, caller identification information can be transmitted and read before deciding to accept a voice call. Although ISDN is widely available, it can manage only very low data rates of 64 kbits per second compared with modern computer networks, which can work at rates higher than 10 Mbits per second.

Broadband ISDN (B-ISDN) was developed to fill this gap and bring telephone and computer networks together. One of the main criteria that shaped the design of B-ISDN was the highly variable demand for data capacity expected from different customers. Recall that in normal telephony, a channel is created by assigning a specified time-slot in a sequence of packets that are transmitted down a common channel. This is an example of a *synchronous transfer mode*. For largely voice-based systems, because there is a fixed demand on capacity for each given channel, synchronous communication works well.

If a network is used for other forms of data such as video, then another approach is required. The irregularity with which a user may need to transmit large volumes of video data means that a synchronous method is inefficient. The dedicated packets needed to accommodate video could remain relatively underused if they were used for voice. So, rather than assigning fixed-capacity communication slots, an asynchronous system based on the transmission of data packets (or cells) is used. This method for transmitting data packets is called *asynchronous transfer mode* (or ATM).

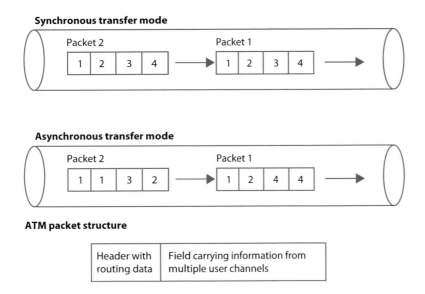

Figure 19.5

Asynchronous transfer mode (ATM) transmission uses a packet transmission system by variably assigning different channels to a given packet, based upon the requirements of individual channels at any given time. Each ATM packet (or cell) carries information in a header segment that describes its particular contents, which are located in the main body of the cell.

In ATM, each packet is filled with information that may come from different channels in an irregular fashion, depending upon the demand at any given time. Because each packet contains information about the channels for which it is carrying data, the channels can be reassembled upon arrival. In other words, ATM allows a communication system to be divided into a number of arbitrarily sized channels, depending upon demand and the needs of individual channels (Figure 19.5). The upper transmission rate for ATM varies depending upon the network interface standard chosen, but typically it is discussed at 1.5 Mbits, with upper limits of 2.4 Gbits per second cited.

ATM is an example of an *isochronous* system because, although packets are sent irregularly, there is a service guarantee of a minimum data rate so that packets will arrive within a certain time frame (Table 19.2). Isochronous transport is required for time-dependent services such as the transmission of live video and audio data. ATM is well suited for applications in which a steady data stream is more important than accuracy. A good example is video-conferencing, in which irregular small 'blips' in the data stream are tolerable, but long pauses are not. Other computer network protocols such as the Internet protocol (IP), Ethernet and Token Ring are truly asynchronous protocols because their packets are transported over the network on a demand or first-come, first-served basis. If the network is busy, packets are delayed until

Table 19.2   Communication protocols can be defined according to the method used to co-ordinate messages between sending and receiving parties

Synchronous – Events that are co-ordinated in time. Technically, a synchronous process depends on other processes and runs only as a result of another process being completed or handed over, e.g. communication that requires each party to respond in turn without initiating a new communication.

Asynchronous – Events that are not co-ordinated in time. Technically, an asynchronous process operates independently of other processes, e.g. sending a communication that does not require a party to respond.

Isochronous – Events that occur regularly in time. Technically, an isochronous process operates at a regular interval to provide a certain minimum data rate, e.g. sending a communication with a guaranteed regularity.

traffic subsides. An isochronous service is thus not as rigid in its timing requirements as a synchronous service, but not as lenient as asynchronous service.

The deployment of ATM depends on the rate with which high-capacity fibre-optic cabling is laid in the community because it cannot run across smaller-capacity circuitry.

19.4 Wireless communication systems support mobility and are implemented at the physical network layer

Wireless communication systems use mainly radiofrequency to transmit data across a network. They are implemented at the physical layer (layer 1) in the OSI stack. For example, wireless ATM is essentially the same as ATM, with the same data packet structure shared between physical and wireless networks; the only differences are the protocol and hardware used to create the wireless link.

The goal of a wireless system is to provide access to voice and data channels, irrespective of location or mobility. Wireless systems are used to create channels for mobile telephones, paging systems and wireless links for computer terminals. Technical requirements vary according to the required data rate and reliability, as well as the expected location and mobility patterns of those using the system. For example, a cordless telephone system that will be used only within a home can be built to far less demanding specifications than a mobile or satellite telephone system designed to be used across a continent, in a moving car or to support simultaneous calls.

Wireless systems vary in the part of the radiofrequency spectrum they use and the way data are encoded when transmitted. Microwaves are used, for example, to create terrestrial line of sight communication systems, as well as communicate with satellites. Wireless local area computer networks ('Wi-Fi') use a spread spectrum approach covering low and high radiofrequencies to allow devices to move within a local area and still remain connected. When a combination of personal devices such as computers and phones needs to share data, ultrahigh-radiofrequency protocols such as Bluetooth can be used to create a *personal area network* (PAN). Infrared links can also be used for very close distance communication within a room between devices such as a computer and printer.

Cellular or mobile telephony has been a major source of growth in the use of wireless technology, and for nations with a poor physical telephone network, wireless systems have allowed rapid and wide penetration of telephone usage without major investments in physical cabling. A cellular network is created by dividing up a geographical area into a number of 'cells'. Each cell has its own radio transmitter to receive signals from handsets and to transmit these to the network's control centre. As a user moves from one cell, the call is handed over to the nearest cell with the strongest reception of the handset. Thus, coverage is limited by the size of the local networks. If radio base stations have not been installed to create cells in a given region, then no network coverage is possible in that area. When coverage is an issue, as it is in regions without dense cellular networks, then satellite-based mobile telephone systems provide a useful alternative. Use of cellular systems can also be limited indoors when the geometry of walls and ceilings impairs radio signal reception. In such circumstances, local computer networks using Wi-Fi base stations can step in to allow continuing access to asynchronous systems such as Internet access using IP.

Mobile telecommunication or cellular systems have undergone rapid change with a new 'generation' of technology appearing roughly every decade. The widely used Global System for Mobile Communications (GSM) is also known as the second-generation (2G) and has been succeeded by 3G and 4G technologies, with 5G in development.

4G systems are an all-IP packet switched network and do not support traditional circuit-switched telephony. They provide mobile ultra-broadband Internet access for smartphones, as well as other mobile computer devices. The applications that can run on 4G include mobile Internet access, as well as IP telephony, video-conferencing and video streaming. Peak data rates when devices are highly mobile are expected to be 100 Mbit per second and increase to approximately 1 Gbit per second when mobility requirements are less extreme. Numerous innovations at the physical transmission layer have been needed to achieve these data rates, including the use of multi-antenna or smart antenna arrays at base stations as well as individual devices, permitting what is known as multiple-input multiple-output (MIMO) communication.

19.5 The electronic exchange of clinical messages is defined by healthcare-specific standards

When information is exchanged along a network, it is not likely that the sending and receiving systems will be built by the same companies or organizations. For exchange of data to occur, each different system must therefore implement its own version of a protocol stack that conforms to the standard of the communication protocol used (e.g. ATM). Such standardization is essential in healthcare if the information sent by one system is to be interpretable by the receiver.

Health level 7 standards define message and document structures

HL7 is an evolving set of standards that are released by the HL7 organization. Health Level Seven Inc. was founded in 1987 and is a not-for-profit standards development organization. HL7 standards are the *de facto* global standard for exchange of clinical and administrative data in healthcare, and together these standards define the format and content of the messages that pass between medical applications (Blobel *et al.*, 2006).

For example, the HL7 messaging standard defines the protocol underpinning the exchange of messages between an electronic health record (EHR) and a laboratory system. This ensures that a test can be ordered for a patient through the EHR and then be sent to and be understood by a different laboratory system, and that a laboratory result can then be transmitted back and be understood by the EHR. HL7 is an abbreviation of Health Level 7, indicating that the messaging standard defines a protocol within OSI layer 7 (see Table 19.1). Thus, HL7 does not specify how messages will be delivered between applications. Other computer network protocols that define operations further down in the stack have that job, and they include IP, transmission control protocol/IP (TCP/IP) and file transfer protocol (FTP). Equally, HL7 does not describe what is done to a message after it has been received because this is the domain of the individual applications.

The HL7 messaging standard covers messages for patient admissions and registration, discharge or transfer, queries, orders, results, clinical observations, billing and master file update information. There are a number of different versions of the HL7 messaging standard

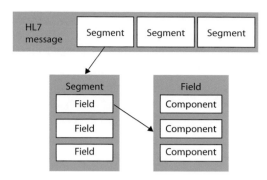

Figure 19.6
HL7 messages have a hierarchically decomposed structure and are assembled from a set or pre-defined components.

in common use, including Version 2 (V2.x) and Version 3. We focus on V2.x in the following description, given its continued widespread use. The messaging standard defines:

- *Message-triggering events,* which initiate message exchanges between systems, e.g. the act of admitting a patient in a hospital EHR.
- *Message structures,* which define a limited form of message semantics using a restricted terminology of recognized data types, i.e. how different types of data are to be labelled and arranged so that their meaning is understood.
- *Encoding rules,* which define message syntax or grammar, i.e. how data structure is to be actually presented, for example the use of different special ASCII characters to delimit the data types defined in the message structure.

The HL7 message structure is simple and hierarchical, built up from *segments, fields* and *components* (Figure 19.6). Each message is first broken down into a sequence of defined segments, each carrying a different piece of data (Table 19.3). For example, the *PID* segment of a message is defined always to carry patient identification data. Version 2.3 of HL7 contains 120 different possible segment definitions that could be used in any given message, but the use of many is optional because they are not relevant in all circumstances. Message length itself is not limited, but the maximum field length suggested is 64k.

Segments are further structured to contain a number of pre-defined fields, which define the contents of the data segment more precisely. Individual fields may repeat within a

Table 19.3   HL7 defines several different types of messages and the segments that each different message must contain*

Message type – ADT (admission, discharge and transfer)
Event – Admit a patient.
1. MSH – Message header (R).
2. EVN – Event type (R).
3. PID – Patient identification (R).
4. NK1 – Next of kin (R).
5. PV1 – Patient visit (R).
6. DG1 – Diagnosis information.

*This ADT message has six separate segments describing the admission of a patient. Required segments are labelled R.

Table 19.4   HL7 message segments may contain a number of pre-defined fields

ST	String	XPN	Person name
TX	Text	XAD	Address
FT	Formatted text	XTN	Telephone number
NM	Numeric	ID	Coded value (HL7 table)
DT	Date	IS	Coded value (user defined)
TM	Time	CM	Composite
TS	Time stamp	CN	Identification and name
PL	Person location	CQ	Quantity and units

segment, for example, to carry a sequence of different values from a laboratory test. For example, the PID segment in HL7 version 2.3 consists of 2 mandatory fields, person name and person identification, as well as 28 others that are not mandatory (Table 19.4).

Fields may have their own internal structure, and these are known as composite data types. For example, XPN is one of the fields in the PID segment, and it stands for extended person name. XPN is composed of seven data elements (Table 19.5).

The HL7 encoding rules translate the message structure into a string of characters that can be transmitted between applications. For example, encoding rules state that fields are delimited by '|', and that components are separated by ^ characters. For example, we could encode the name 'Mr. John M. Brown' into the XPN field as follows:

`|Brown^John^M^Mr|`

and a whole PID segment could be encoded as

```
PID||05975^^^2^ID|54721||Brown^John^M^Mr|Brown^John^M^Mr|19591203|M||B|
54HIGHST^^KENSINGTON^NSW^2055^AUSTRALIA||(02)731-
359|||M|NON|8000034~29086|999|
```

In some ways we can liken the HL7 message structure to a compositional or post–co-ordinated terminology (see Chapter 22), in that we build up messages from pre-defined

Table 19.5   The extended person name (XPN) field within the patient identification (PID) segment of a HL7 V2.x message has a number of pre-defined components

#	Name
1	Family name
2	Given name
3	Middle initial or name
4	Suffix
5	Prefix
6	Degree
7	Name type code

components, according to encoding rules that in a limited way control that composition. However, since HL7 does no more than define data types, it is neutral to the meaning of any message's contents. There are no mechanisms in HL7, for example, to make sure the contents of a message are clinically meaningful or correct. Such details may be addressed in implementation guides, as message semantics are considered to be in the domain of the applications that send or receive HL7 messages.

The HL7 standard family has broadened from messaging standards and now includes a number of other significant standards:

- The HL7 Reference Information Model (RIM) is HL7's overarching ontological model of the healthcare domain. The RIM describes the data content needed in a specific clinical or administrative context and defines semantic and lexical connections between information carried in HL7 message fields.
- The HL7 Clinical Document Architecture (CDA) is a standard representation for the syntax of clinical documents such as discharge summaries, consultation notes, imaging and pathology reports (Dolin *et al.*, 2001). CDA documents are encoded in Extensible Markup Language (XML) and use RIM data types.

19.6 Semantic level standards are required to ensure meaning is unchanged when a message is sent between two dissimilar systems

Ensuring that documents are syntactically interoperable is a significant achievement. It means that when a system receives a message, it has a sense of how to read it, in the same way that an understanding of grammar allows us to interpret the likely role that a word plays in a sentence, e.g. acting as a noun. It does not, however, guarantee semantic interoperability, which would see the meaning of what is contained in a message also being agreed on by both sending and receiving systems. As we will see in Part 6, for such meaning to be shared, systems also need to share an understanding of all the concepts that may be discussed, as well as the ontology, or set of relationships, that can exist between such concepts.

HL7's RIM was designed as a framework for such ontological structuring, but it has its critics, who see inconsistency in its structure and in its ontological content (Schadow and Mead, 2006; Smith and Ceusters, 2006). If systems today want to ensure that they understand the same concepts, they typically subscribe to the same terminological standard, such as the International Classification of Diseases (ICD). Agreeing on terminology is essential, when we move from information systems that passively record data to those that try to act on what they receive. For example, a decision support system may trigger clinical alerts based on its belief that a particular clinical measurement is outside an acceptable range.

The Semantic Web seeks to make Web content semantically interoperable and actionable

The desire to see machine-shared data behave in a semantically interoperable way is not limited to healthcare. Most of the Web's content today is designed for humans to read, not for computer programs to manipulate meaningfully (Berners-Lee *et al.*, 2001; Feigenbaum *et al.*, 2007;

Shadbolt *et al.*, 2006). One page of text is as meaningful as another to an application such as a Web browser, which is interested only in how to display the content, not act upon it.

Much effort is now devoted to creating Web documents that are machine interpretable. This would allow intelligent programs to make decisions based upon the information they find as they traverse the Web. For example, an intelligent agent could 'read' a Web page, understand that it describes the results of a trial testing a treatment for a disease and then seek out other documents that provide alternate treatment options. For this to happen, the document's content must be sufficiently standardized that machine interpretation is possible. The task for the developers of this *Semantic Web* (sometimes called Web 3.0) is to provide a common framework that allows data to be shared, interpreted and re-used across software applications, within organizations and across the global World Wide Web (WWW). To achieve this, methods and languages need to be agreed on that allow software to make inferences based upon the information contained in Web sites.

We saw earlier that the OSI protocol stack is designed to establish a connection among computers on a network from the physical transport layer up to the application layer, which is where we expect semantic interoperability to be achieved. A number of individual elements are needed to achieve this type of functionality, and so a new Semantic Web stack has emerged to define the relationships between items such as terminological taxonomies, ontologies, rules and establishment of trust relationships (Figure 19.7). As with OSI, each layer higher up in the stack can exploit capabilities of layers below it. The bottom two layers are the foundation of the pre-semantic Web, and they define the operation of traditional hypertext documents (Figure 19.8). The middle layers are devoted to standardized Semantic Web components and include the following:

- *Resource Description Framework* (RDF) – The Web is built on the basic notion of a resource, which originally was a document that could be found by its address or Universal Resource Locator (URL). In the Semantic Web, resources are generalized to

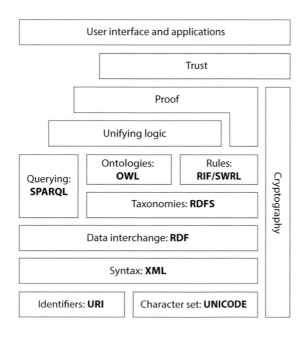

Figure 19.7
The Semantic Web stack is an architecture that explains the relationships between the different languages and standards needed to allow Web content to be interpreted by machine, and it can be considered mainly to occupy the topmost Open System Interconnection (OSI) stack layer. (From Obitko, 2007.)

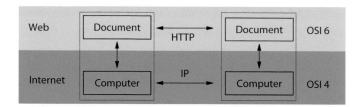

Figure 19.8 World Wide Web protocols such as HyperText Transfer Protocol (HTTP) sit higher up in in the Open System Interconnection (OSI) stack than basic Internet protocols such as Internet protocol (IP) and provide a standard way for creating, finding and accessing documents. Semantic Web Protocols sit above HTTP and reside largely within OSI stack layer 7.

any information object or entity that can be given a name, an address and accesses. RDF provides a way of describing resources or capturing their metadata. RDF describes a resource using a set of triples of the form (resource, property, data/other resource) and is written in XML.

- *RDF Schema* (RDFS) provides the basic vocabulary for RDF and permits the creation of hierarchies of resource classes and definition of their properties.
- *Web Ontology Language* (OWL) provides a means to define the legal relationships among concepts such as a resource or its properties, and it is based on description logic that allows computers to make inferences about the content they find.

Part 6 of this book is devoted to terminology and ontology, where we explore the many different healthcare-specific approaches to defining concepts and their ontological relationships. Part 7 describes different approaches to machine reasoning, which can take such knowledge and use it to make automated decisions.

FHIR is a next-generation approach to messaging standards

To combat what is perceived as unnecessary structural complexity in HL7 standards such as RIM (which, for example, makes it difficult to update a standard as well as implement it in a given system), more modern, lightweight standards are emerging. The FHIR (Fast Healthcare Interoperability Resources) specification (pronounced 'fire') is a next-generation standards framework developed in accordance with principles that are emerging out of the Semantic Web program. It is created under the HL7 umbrella to be consistent with other HL7 standards, but it is designed so that messages that contain data are able to support automated clinical decision support and other applications requiring semantic processing (HL7, 2014).

FHIR takes a compositional or post–co-ordinated approach to constructing messages out of resources. Resources can be any clinical content that needs to be exchanged, just as they are in the WWW. Each unique resource type defines the structure for the data elements they will contain, and it may also define how they can relate to other resources. The philosophy behind FHIR is to build a basic set of resources that, either by themselves or when combined, will satisfy the majority of common user cases.

OpenEHR allows clinicians to specify document models independently of software design

The OpenEHR program takes an open source approach to standardizing clinical documentation (Kalra *et al.*, 2005). OpenEHR allows clinicians to define the semantic structure of a clinical document by creating a specific document model called an *archetype*. Archetypes are external to any clinical software that may use them, thus cleanly separating clinical modelling from software implementation.

An archetype may be created for a low-level item such as a specific investigation, measure or examination and the possible results that could be recorded for it, e.g. blood pressure, examination of the middle ear. Archetypes exist for all the typical concepts that would be found in a record, and clinician authors can construct a specific model for their system's needs from a library of archetypes and add new models when they do not exist. Archetypes are published as shareable XML schemas, and the archetype specification itself is an ISO standard (ISO 13606-2). The OpenEHR community extends well beyond support for archetypes. Tools and definitions exist for a wide variety of document types, user interfaces, application programming interfaces (APIs) and use Semantic Web technologies such as OWL and RDF. OpenEHR has been used for several large international systems such as national summary care records.

Substitutable Medical Apps Reusable Technologies (SMART)

Interoperability standards typically define either the syntax (structure) of a message or the semantics (allowed intended meanings) of a message, but make no assumption about how a message is to be used. Standards can however operate at a higher level, specifically defining the purpose for which a message is to be applied.

Such *task-interoperability*, or *substitutabilty*, allows different pieces of software to be functionally interoperable, meaning that one is able to substitute for the other to accomplish the same task (Mandl and Kohane, 2009). A program may for example take as input data from an EHR, and then calculate a patient's cardiac risk. If the program is designed to conform to a functional standard, then we could directly replace it with an alternate cardiac risk calculator without needing to modify any other parts of our software environment. The advantage of functional interoperability is that it provides a modular and controlled way in which clinical information systems can be updated or modified to accomplish new tasks.

The Substitutable Medical Apps, Reusable Technologies (SMART) platform was initially developed at Harvard Medical School and Boston Children's Hospital to provide such a way for clinical 'apps' to be developed and be substitutable (Mandl *et al.*, 2012). Data sources such as an EHR are conceptually placed into 'containers' that conform to the SMART application programming interface (API). Any SMART conformant application will then be able to see the data source in a consistent way that allows substitutability.

To allow substitutability, SMART takes the stance that a task has a predefined set of data that need to be presented, and that these data need to conform to a format best suited to the task requirement – in other words each task description is a kind of task-oriented template (see Chapter 4). When it is queried, a container must thus search within itself for the data associated with a task request, and then reshape the data to transform it to meet the needs of the task, before sending it out.

SMART is built to conform with the HL7 FHIR standard, which ensures that it is integrated into a major international messaging standards family.

19.7 Message exchanges containing sensitive data must be encrypted

When data are shipped across a network, individuals who are not the intended recipients of the data may intentionally intercept them. Such interceptions occur without our knowledge and may be made by national security organizations or criminal enterprises. As a result, when sending sensitive information such as a health record or financial data, basic security measures are essential to minimize the risks of unauthorized access, as well as taking measures that make any intercepted data unreadable as an additional line of defence.

There are thus two complementary ways that a degree of security can be ensured for data placed in a network. The first involves setting up barriers to accessing data files. For example, an institution such as a hospital may set up an internal network or intranet. Access to the intranet depends on users' knowing passwords to authenticate that they are privileged to use the system. By controlling which computers can access the network and which users have accounts, and by the complexity of the password system, intranets can be relatively closed and secure systems. If a network is more open, for example, by using the Internet to allow access to documents, then the gateway between the Internet and the local system needs to be controlled. *Firewalls* are thus placed at the gateway to limit, as much as is possible, access to appropriately authenticated users.

The second component of security is to prevent eavesdroppers outside a secure network from intercepting information traffic. To prevent access to confidential information, these data need to be encrypted. *Encryption* basically scrambles data according to a pre-defined method. The scrambling of data is done by an algorithm that transposes each original letter or number in a message with another one. To read the message as intended, the receiver of the message must take the scrambled message and apply the algorithm in reverse. To prevent an intercepting party from also having the algorithm, both sender and receiver can share a specific encryption code or *key* (typically a long string of numbers). The key is used by the algorithm to decide how to transpose characters, and every key produces a different result. Without the key a message can be very difficult to decode, and messages encrypted with longer keys are increasingly difficult to unscramble. In information model terms, only those in possession of the model or key are able to interpret the data (Figure 19.9).

One standard way to encrypt messages that does not require sender and receiver to share the key ahead of time uses what is known as *public key infrastructure* (PKI). All users of the system have a public and a private key created for them by a third-party certificate authority. They keep their private key to themselves, and the public key is published. When a message is sent to a receiver, the sender first retrieves the receiver's public key and uses it to encrypt

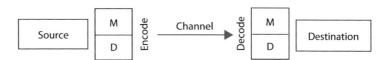

Figure 19.9   Once data (D) have been encrypted according to a code, they can be securely transported across a communication channel like the Internet. To be able to decode the data, one must possess a key or code that is the model (M) used to encrypt the data.

the message. When the receiver receives a message, it is decrypted using the private key. The system works because the public and private keys are created at the same time and are mathematically related to each other.

Encrypted data are secure as long as the encryption code is itself secure. As powerful encryption schemes are created, others try to develop methods to crack these codes. As a consequence, when it is absolutely essential that data remain secure, there is a constant pressure to adopt ever more powerful encryption mechanisms. For situations in which total security is not necessary, such as healthcare, it is still reasonable to use codes that could in principle be decodable by those with access to advanced technology while accepting that it is unlikely that most people would have the capability or desire to do so.

19.8 Electronic consent mechanisms allow patients to control access to their data

Although encryption mechanisms are used to protect data as the information is sent along insecure networks, other methods are needed to control access within defined organizational boundaries, such as a health service. As we saw earlier, one level of control is to create access accounts for individuals and issue them with unique passwords. When it comes to patient data, password control is insufficient. When a patient agrees to be cared for by a clinician or a health service, that patient implicitly give consent for their data to be accessed for that purpose alone. This consent typically extends only to healthcare professionals directly involved in the patient's care or who have been given permission to see the data, and it is deeply influenced by the privacy laws in place in any specific region or nation.

Yet in an electronic environment, many more clinical workers can access such patient information, sometimes from many different locations. A clinician working in a hospital thus may not be directly involved in a patient's care, but may be tempted to look at the EHR for any number of reasons. The clinician may be curious because the patient is known to them, is a relative, a celebrity or because the clinician could personally benefit from what is in the record. Electronic consent (e-consent) systems create a mechanism that controls who has access to a patient record and indeed may limit access to only some portions of a record.

There are four broad types of consent that can be given (Coiera and Clarke, 2004):

- *General consent* – Blanket consent is given by a patient for any healthcare professional working within a specified health context to access any and all of their health information for any purpose relating to their care. It corresponds to what is known as *opt-in consent* and persists into the future, unless specifically revoked. One benefit of opt-in consent is that for any future episode of care, additional consent is not required.
- *General consent with specific denial(s)* – Here a patient provides a general consent, but partially withholds consent. The patient may choose to limit disclosure of a particular portion of the information in the record or prevent disclosure to a particular named individual or category of clinical or administrative role. Patients may wish, for example, to put tight restrictions on psychiatric history, infectious status such as human immunodeficiency virus exposure or their history of pregnancy and contraception. Patients may also limit the purposes for which their data can be accessed, e.g. limit its

Figure 19.10 (a) to (d) Four different possible architectures of a health information exchange. CDR, clinical data repository; EHR, electronic health record; PHR, patient health record; RDR, research data repository; SCR, summary care record.

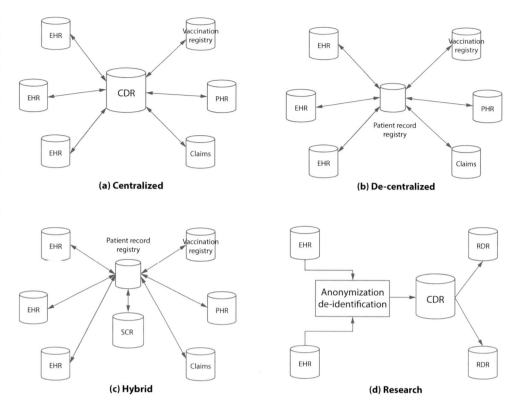

(a) Centralized

(b) De-centralized

(c) Hybrid

(d) Research

et al., 2011). The creation of a centralized HIE can be expensive because it requires the creation of the CDR, which can require a substantial and ongoing investment. However, it allows for fast access to data when needed.

- *Federated or de-centralized* – Patient-level data stay with the organizations that create and use them in this HIE model. A patient registry is created centrally that lists the names of all patients for whom there is a record in the region covered by the HIE, and this registry is updated by local organizations as they see new patients. A provider can query the registry to find out whether a certain patient has more records stored at other institutions. If the provider finds that these records exist, the provider can request them from that institution, which may send the records by a number of means including secure e-mail, dedicated private networks or secure Web services. For the central patient registry to work effectively, it is ideal if the region uses a single and unique patient identifier for every individual, to make it easy to identify the records of a specific individual. In the absence of unique identifiers, statistical matching algorithms can be employed that use multiple attributes of a patient such as name, age, address and so forth to decide whether two records are both likely to belong to the same patient.

- *Hybrid* – HIEs can combine various elements of these two approaches to extend the functionality offered. In one variant, regional CDRs are created under a centralized model, and then a supra-regional or national patient registry is created from these CDRs. This approach allows regions to create and manage their own CDRs and for these

CDRs to all come together in support of a larger national HIE. An alternate hybrid design stores only summary record data centrally along with a patient registry (see Figure 10.4). This approach allows some patient data to be easily accessed by other institutions, for example, in an emergency situation, and requests for additional, more detailed information are made only if required.

- *Research network* – Clinical data are captured by health services as part of the care process. Research organizations have an interest in the secondary use of the same clinical data, typically at a population level. HIEs can be built to support such re-use when research and clinical organizations join the same HIE (Safran *et al.*, 2007). A research organization cannot directly access clinical records but must make the request through some intermediating systems, and a formal information governance process tightly controls how data are passed to any research organization. First, on the clinical side, some form of consent certificate store is likely to be needed, so that it can be determined whether a record is available for research use. Next, any patient records that are made available will need to be *anonymized,* meaning that the patient identifier is stripped so that the record is not linked to an individual. Records also need to be *de-identified,* meaning that any data elements that could result in the identity of the patient being discovered are removed (e.g. occurrences of the patient's name, medical record number, Social Security number and other data fields that directly link a patient to their data) (Kushida *et al.*, 2012). One may also try to assess whether the record can be willfully *re-identified,* for example, by combining it with other information sources (El Emam *et al.*, 2011). As health records start to incorporate genetic data in particular, it becomes possible to use such information in the process or re-identification (e.g. identifying gender, racial background and disease state) (Knoppers *et al.*, 2012). The patient data accessed by research organizations are not likely to be stored in live clinical systems, but rather warehoused in a data bank that is regularly updated from clinical systems (Ford *et al.*, 2009). The specific HIE architecture chosen to support research use of clinical data depends on whether it is a local system designed to suit the needs of a particular partnership between research organizations and clinical services or is intended to be a scalable system with regional or national coverage (Harris *et al.*, 2009; Mandl *et al.*, 2014; McMurry *et al.*, 2007).

Any debate over which is the best architecture for a region or nation is not one that can be decided in the abstract. The decision to create an HIE and the architecture chosen are shaped by the goals of the HIE, the maturity of the existing clinical information systems that store the primary health data, the governance of the organizations (whether they are public or private entities), the available resource and expertise to build the HIE and the financial model that will support HIE operations. Moreover, the use cases for which the HIE is designed are critical. If the use cases emphasize rapid retrieval of data, then a decentralized model is unlikely to work because of the potential for lags involved in requesting and receiving information among organizations.

Independent of the architecture of the technology in an HIE, there is a larger question of the overall approach to managing the implementation of such a project. Centrally co-ordinated approaches to building an HIE (e.g. by a government) create a single point of failure vulnerability, and such projects can suffer large cost and time overruns and be hostage to political fortune (Greenhalgh *et al.*, 2010). HIE implementations that are locally co-ordinated but have weak central leadership are also likely to experience difficulties. This suggests that rather than a top-down centralized approach to HIE development, or a bottom-up distributed approach, the best strategy is to go 'middle-out', with central agreement of roles and responsibilities, but local ownership (Coiera, 2009).

Discussion points

1. IP is the asynchronous networking protocol used on the Internet. How suited is IP to real-time services such as voice telephony (sometimes known as voice over IP) compared with ATM?

2. There are usually several competing standards or technological systems in the marketplace for any given application. What do you think determines whether a technology, protocol or standard is ultimately dominant?

3. Is an HL7 messaging standard sufficient to support exchanging messages between an EHR and a clinical decision support system?

4. The finer details of different technologies are probably not relevant or even of interest to most healthcare workers. They want to drive the car, not know what goes on under the hood. Do you agree with this sentiment?

5. What are the major barriers to achieving semantic interoperability in healthcare?

6. Can opt-out consent ever guarantee that every patient whose data are stored in a record has truly given informed consent?

7. What is the most cost-effective health information exchange architecture?

8. Explain how a patient's record could be re-identified despite removing all personal details from the document.

9. Is opt-in or opt-out the best approach to handling consent for health information exchanges or national record systems?

10. Compare HL7 V2 messages with OpenEHR archetypes and SMART task descriptions in terms both of how restrictive they are on what data can be placed in a message, as well as the kind of interoperability they support.

Chapter summary

1. Rules that govern how a message exchange may proceed over a network are called a communication protocol, and this defines how a message is to be constructed, how its receipt is to be acknowledged, how turn taking should occur and how errors may be repaired.

2. The International Organization for Standardization (ISO) has developed the Open System Interconnection (OSI) seven-layer model that is used almost universally to define the protocol layers for communicating among heterogeneous computers.

3. A communications channel can be either a dedicated circuit or a shared resource. Circuit-switched networks provide a complete circuit among the communicating parties. Packet-switched systems transport separate packets of data that can come from a number of different sources on a common channel.

4. A channel's capacity to carry data is called its bandwidth, usually measured in bits per second.

5. The type of data transfer protocol used over a communications network contributes to the eventual bandwidth. The Integrated Service Digital Network (ISDN) and asynchronous transfer mode (ATM) systems are currently the most important standard protocols for communicating with multimedia such as video.

6. Wireless communication systems use mainly radiofrequency to transmit data across a network. They are implemented at the physical layer (layer 1) in the OSI stack.

7. HL7 (Health Level 7) is a set of international standards for electronic data exchange in healthcare, and the standards can be used to define the format and content of the messages and documents that pass between medical applications.

8. Semantic level standards are required to ensure meaning is unchanged when a message is sent between two dissimilar systems. The Semantic Web is a set of standards that seek to make Web content semantically interoperable and actionable.

9. Message exchanges containing sensitive data must be encrypted, and public key encryption is a robust method based upon certified individuals' sharing a public key and retaining a private key.

10. Electronic consent mechanisms allow patients to control access to their data, and they can range from opt-in models to selective consent and opt-out models.

11. Health information exchanges are networks designed to allow multiple clinical information systems to share patient data, as well as permit clinical data to be used for research purposes.

CHAPTER 20

Social networks and social media interventions

Social processes underpin everything from our lifestyle choices, our health decisions, to the way healthcare is conceived and delivered. Social media, a class of information tools that support group interactions, find many applications across healthcare from disease management through to supporting biomedical research. They provide channels for consumers to interact with each other and for health services to provide online services to the community or to supplement existing services online. Social processes also underlie the causation of many diseases, whether through direct transmission of infectious diseases or by sharing of behaviours that are associated with health risks. There is thus also a therapeutic role for social media in the treatment of socially shaped conditions such obesity, depression, diabetes, and heart disease.

This chapter introduces the concept of social networks and the basic properties that dictate how networks form and function. The pivotal role that social processes play in the genesis of many diseases is described, followed by an exploration of the way social media can be used in healthcare both to support health services and to manage health conditions. The important concept of a network intervention (NI), in which the target of the intervention is to change the network around an individual, rather than necessarily the individual himself or herself, is explained, and a set of design requirements for social media interventions to manage health conditions effectively is outlined.

20.1 Social networks are a means of representing the relationships and interactions among a group of individuals

Social networks are a way of representing the ties that bind us as individuals into families, groups, organizations and societies (Tichy *et al.*, 1979). Social networks help explain many aspects of human interaction. They provide evidence for how information or messages spread in a community along the connections among individuals. They help explain why some individuals in a community are more effective in spreading information or having that information influence others. Initially, social network studies focussed on family and friendship networks because these relationships were thought to be most influential in our lives. However, it soon became clear that even weak social ties have the power to influence our behaviour (Granovetter, 1973). We do not have to have a direct relationship with an individual for that person to influence the way we behave. If there is a pathway of interme-diating individuals, then their influence can reach us indirectly through these connections.

Sociograms illustrate connections between individuals and can be used to calculate measures of role in a network

Social networks are typically represented graphically in a *sociogram*. The basic elements of a sociogram are network nodes, which represent individuals, and the connections between those nodes, which represent the existence of a social tie between two individuals. Sociograms allow us to calculate some basic properties of individuals, their paired (dyadic) relationships and indeed the network as a whole:

- *Network size* is usually estimated from the number of individuals connected in the network. *Isolates* are those individuals who are not connected to a group.
- If a tie has a direction to it, then the *in-degree* is the count of the number of incoming connections to a node. Socially, this may correspond to the notion of 'popularity'. *Out-degree* counts the number of connections from a node to others. This can be thought of as a measure of an individual's gregariousness.
- *Tie strength* is a measure of the importance of the interactions between two individuals. Strong ties exist, for example, between close family members. Weak ties are also very important, however, because they are the connectors between tightly tied groups. They are likely to be major conduits of novel information, such as information about a new job opportunity, because tight groups already tend to know the same thing (Granovetter, 1973). One measure of tie strength is the frequency of interactions over it. Weak ties support very infrequent interactions, and strong ties see regular interaction. Other measures of tie strength include the amount of time spent interacting, as well as the emotional intensity, intimacy, mutuality and reciprocity of interactions.
- *Density* counts how many of the members are connected to each other within a group. A simple measure of density is the number of actual connections between individuals divided by the number of possible connections. *Reciprocity* is a related measure that looks at how many network connections are bi-directional.
- A *path* describes the route one can take to go from one individual in a network to another, and path metrics provide us with an indication of the distance between any two individuals, or indeed they can be used to compute average paths between group members for a given network. Average path length is behind the *small world* or 'six degrees of separation' idea in which for certain networks, most individuals can find a path to another only using a relatively small number of connections through other intermediate individuals.
- *Degree centrality* is a measure based on a count of connections and is used to compare the in-degrees and out-degrees of all nodes in a network. It can be thought of as a measure of having the most 'friends' and can help locate those individuals who are most central and thus may be more essential for the distribution of information within a group or who may be more influential in a group. There are many other related measures of centrality (Figure 20.1).

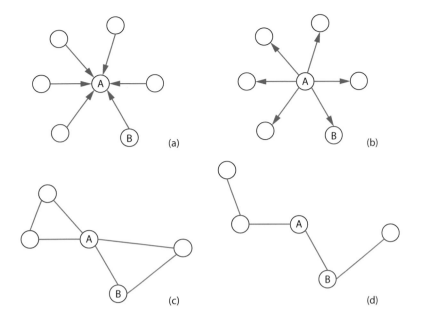

Figure 20.1
Centrality is a measure of where a node sits within a network. Node A has a greater centrality than node B when measured by (a) the number of in-degrees, (b) out-degrees, (c) betweenness centrality and (d) closeness centrality.

- *Betweenness centrality* is a related measure used to help identify those individuals who are boundary spanners. These are individuals who can broker between different parts of a network because they are among the few individuals who are common to both parts. It measures the number of pairs of individuals that would need to be involved in connecting two individuals. Because betweenness emphasizes position in a network, rather than how many 'friends' you have, someone who is an important connector between groups with high betweenness centrality can have low degree centrality.
- *Closeness centrality* counts the length of the shortest path between a node and others and so emphasizes how much an individual is 'in the middle' of things. It does not emphasize how many 'friends' you have or how important you are in sitting between groups.

Social network structure is a function of network size, the individuals in the network and the purpose of the network

Natural networks are not uniform or random constructs, but they have a topological structure. The way different subsets of nodes are densely connected, or some nodes act as connectors or boundary spanners to joining these subgroups, can be highly informative. This *modularity,* or denser subgroupings, can occur for a number of natural reasons, such as shared purpose or interest in the subgroup compared with other subgroups (Newman, 2006).

Identifying *community structure* in a network assists in interpreting the role that the network plays (Figures 20.2, 20.3 and 20.4). A *community* is any group of nodes that has a relatively higher degree of connection to each other than to other nodes. For any given node, its *neighborhood* is all the nodes that directly connect to it. Communities can overlap, with some members belonging to both, and can be hierarchical in larger networks, with smaller communities appearing within larger ones (Ahn *et al.,* 2010; Palla *et al.,* 2005).

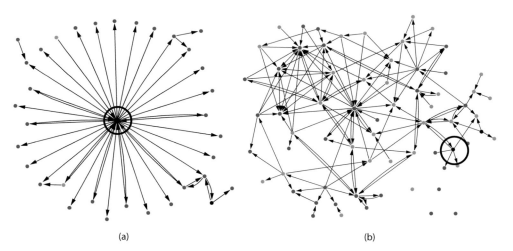

(a) (b)

Figure 20.2   Network structures for online health forums vary with the nature of forum interaction. In (a), a primary care practitioner dominates (circled) at the center of a question and answer forum that forms a star network, with consumers scarcely interacting with each other at all. In (b), a similar forum is focussed on women's health issues, and the doctor's role is peripheral to the active engagement of forum members in discussing each others' issues. In (a), the doctor has the highest degree and betweenness centrality measures of anyone in the forum, but these measures drop significantly and they move to the periphery of the network in (b). (Adapted from Lau *et al.*, 2013a.)

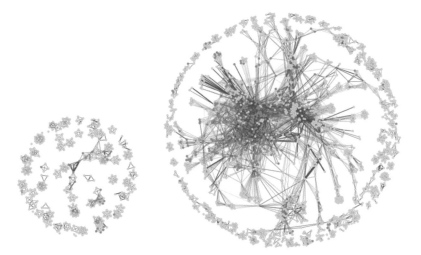

Figure 20.3   Networks of individuals who collaborate on research, as measured by their shared co-authorship on research papers about the drugs mirtazapine (left) and olanzapine (right). The mirtazapine network is smaller and sparser than the olanzapine network, which has a large and dense core. Researchers who are directly affiliated with the company marketing the drugs are represented by the dark nodes, and non-industry researchers are represented by light nodes. The olanzapine network features a high proportion of industry authors who are predominantly in the core and therefore are more influential in the production of evidence about this drug. (From Dunn *et al.*, 2012b.)

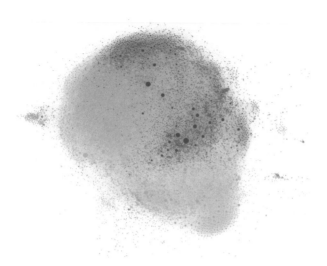

Figure 20.4   A network of Twitter users that posted tweets about human papillomavirus vaccines in a 6-month period in 2013 and 2014, connected by follower relationships and coloured by community affiliation. The community structure reveals a separation between users predominantly posting negative opinions (purple, bottom right) and other communities of public health, media and scientific groups. (Copyright Adam Dunn.)

Small networks of up to 100 nodes tend to have a number of tightly connected communities with limited connections to the rest of the network. Larger networks appear to become less like a community, with nodes blending more into the core of the network (Leskovec *et al.*, 2009). Thus, cohesive communities appear to have a network size in the order of 100 nodes. This correlates with evidence from anthropology, which suggests that human social groups, such as tribes, reach a natural limit at a size of approximately 150 individuals (known as *Dunbar's number*), after which there is a tendency to split (Dunbar, 1996).

Community structure can be very helpful in understanding the way a network behaves. For example, a social contact network can be used to trace the spread of an infectious disease such as influenza (Figure 20.5), gastroenteritis, or human immunodeficiency virus (HIV). Two outbreak clusters could end up being connected by one individual who interacts with both communities, but is not a close member of either (demonstrating the importance of weak ties in spread across networks).

Social networks underpin many aspects of health service delivery

There is often a formal process description of the way a particular health service is delivered that captures the individuals that are meant to be involved and how they interact to execute a workflow. Social network analyses reveal that these idealized representations of work have little to do with what really happens, which is often deeply shaped by social connections.

Social networks, for example, underpin the way hospital clinicians seek advice from each other on medication questions. Social network analysis shows that nursing and medical staff members tend to seek advice on medications from within their own professional group (Figure 20.6). It is left to a few individuals, such as senior nurses or the pharmacist, to play

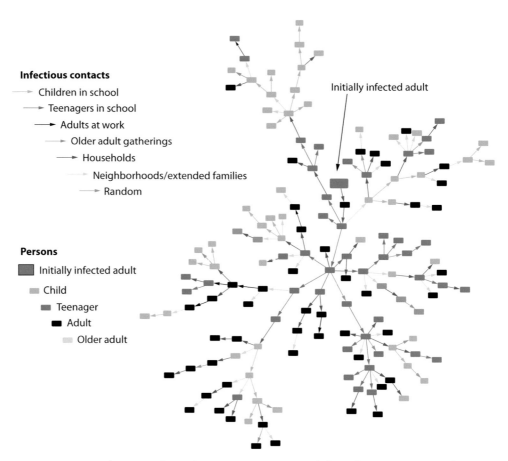

Figure 20.5   Initial stages of an infectious contact network for influenza spread. Colored rectangles represent individuals in a community, and colored arrows represent infectious transmission. An adult is the first to be infected in the community (large purple rectangle) and through two household contacts (light purple arrows) brings influenza to school (dark purple arrows), where it spreads among other teenagers. Teenagers then spread influenza to children in households, who spread it to other children in the elementary schools. Children and teenagers form the backbone of the infectious contact network and are critical to its spread. The infectious transmissions in this network occur mostly in the household, neighborhood and schools. (From Glass *et al.*, 2006.)

the role of boundary spanner linking these two groups (Creswick and Westbrook, 2010; Patterson *et al.*, 2013). The rate of adoption of new drugs similarly appears influenced by social network structures, with adoption times becoming shorter in group practices in primary care (Williamson, 1975).

The degree to which clinical groups are tightly bound may impede the rate at which evidence-based practices are adopted (Mascia and Cicchetti, 2011). Similarly, the diffusion of safety and quality practices within clinical groups is shaped by social network structures. Cohesive and collaborative health professional networks appear to facilitate care co-ordination to contribute to improving quality and safety of care. The presence of cliques, professional and gender homogeneity and over-reliance on central agencies or individuals appear to impede the spread of good practices (Cunningham *et al.*, 2012a).

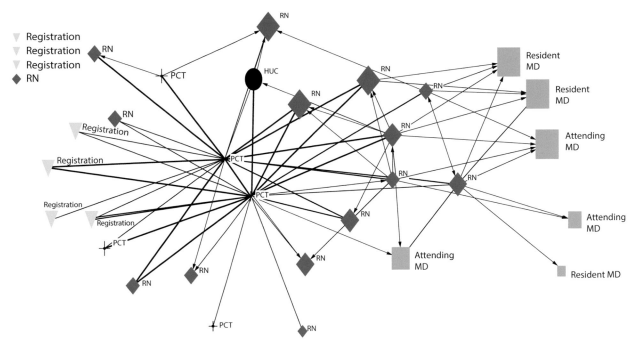

Figure 20.6   A medication advice-seeking network representing the communication interactions among doctors, nurses and administrative staff in a hospital emergency department during a day shift. The size of each node corresponds to its degree centrality, and the width of a connection represents the amount of interaction that occurs between two individuals. Community structure shows that interaction between professional groups follows defined patterns. Just a few individual nurses connect the medical group to the rest of the network, and some groups have no interaction at all with doctors. Doctors are designated by squares, nurses by diamonds and registration clerks by triangles. Four individuals with no connections in the network are collected at the top left. HUC,Health Unit Co-ordinator; PCT, Patient Care Technician; RN, Registered Nurse. (From Patterson *et al.*, 2013).

20.2 Members of social networks become more like each other with time

It is well known that people tend to have friends that are similar to themselves – in interests, beliefs and behaviour (Aiello *et al.*, 2012). Individuals who cluster together can also share attributes such as weight or exercise patterns. It is easy to come to the immediate conclusion that social network membership somehow causes this similarity to evolve over time. The underlying causes of similarity are more complex, however, and there are at least three alternate explanations for why attributes such as weight cluster in social networks (Cohen-Cole and Fletcher, 2008; de La Haye *et al.*, 2011a):

● *Social contagion* – Social networks may 'transmit' behaviours and beliefs from contact to contact, in a manner analogous to the transmission of an infective organism through physical contact networks. Individuals do, in some circumstances, alter their behaviours so that they match those of their peers – a very common phenomenon in adolescent groups, for example.

- *Social selection* – People tend to associate with others who share similar interests, beliefs, and behaviours, a phenomenon known as *homophily* (Rogers, 1995). This selection process can often explain the correlation found between belonging to a network and having a belief, behaviour or physical attribute without any individual causally affecting others through contagion. Social selection may also have more basic biological drivers. Friends appear to share significant genetic similarities such as gene sets associated with smell, as well as genetically determined immunological differences that would enhance group survival (Fowler *et al.*, 2011; Christakis and Fowler, 2014).
- *Demographic confounders* – Race, culture, ethnicity and socioeconomic status can determine the locality in which an individual resides and the social networks that they develop. Shared exposure to events at a location can thus often explain apparent associations between network membership and individual attributes. For example, we know that individuals in a social network tend to be similar to each other in weight. Different neighborhoods vary in the availability and cost of foods through stores and fast food restaurants, as well as gyms, parklands and sporting venues, all of which are able to affect the weight of individuals in a location (Cohen-Cole and Fletcher, 2008). Hence any association between networks and weight may simply reflect the underlying confounding influence of demography (Ellen, 2009).

Many social network studies confound homophily, contagion and structural effects such as demography (Shalizi and Thomas, 2011), but carefully designed studies can tease apart their separate contributions (Aral and Walker, 2012; Centola, 2011; Iyengar *et al.*, 2011). When testing for the influence of social networks on a process or outcome, we therefore require study designs that control for homophily, adjust for demographic confounders and test for contagion effects over a sufficient time for such behaviours to move across a network.

Behaviour change models can explain the mechanisms underlying social contagion

Many 'middle'-level theories compete to explain how social networks may influence health behaviours. Social networks are a source of interpersonal support, as well as resources to cope with stressors (Heaney and Israel, 2002). *Behavioural imitation* or social modelling theories suggest that our peers provide us with exemplar behaviours that we can then imitate (Salvy *et al.*, 2012). In contrast, *social norm* theories suggest that our mental models of what is or is not an acceptable state or behaviour are shaped by the norms implicit in the behaviours of our peers. In norm theory, a personal behaviour or attribute becomes more acceptable the more frequently our peers exhibit it. For example, after becoming aware that a friend has gained weight, an individual may relax his or her exercise programme or diet, in part because the standards and social norms for weight have been altered (Salvy *et al.*, 2012). The fact that geographical distance does not seem to attenuate social contagion effects provides some support for norms over imitation, which may require direct observation (Christakis and Fowler, 2007).

Experimental psychology provides us with evidence of a number of more basic processes in human decision-making, which may explain phenomena such as the effect of social norms or imitation on behaviour, and are of direct relevance to understanding social contagion. In *decision by sampling* theory (see Chapter 8), our personal judgements are shaped by our personal sample of the available evidence, drawn from memory or the environment (Brown and Matthews, 2011). Because our personal sample of events is typically small and unrepresentative of the total distribution, our decisions appear equally skewed. Such distortions are common in human assessments of health risks, in which individuals play down risks associated with behaviours such as smoking, drinking or exposure to HIV. It seems likely that most of the observed difference in personal risk estimates does come down to how well the likelihoods of risk are modelled by our experience.

The *relative rank hypothesis* posits that people's judgements about their own state are driven by where they rank within our personal information sample (Brown and Matthews, 2011). This has been confirmed in numerous experimental studies. An individual's perceptions of the health benefits of his or her own current exercise is influenced by how it ranks in comparison with others, and this can be manipulated by experimentally changing the ranked position (Maltby *et al.*, 2012). Similar effects have been found with judgements of depression and anxiety, which are mainly predicted not by the objective severity of symptoms, but rather by where individuals ranked the severity of their symptoms in comparison with others (Melrose *et al.*, 2013).

20.3 Many diseases appear to spread along social networks

Although it has long been known that infectious disease can be socially transmitted, more recent work has shown that the spread of disease along social lines is much more widespread. Many observational studies have identified a clear association between various disease states and the composition of an individual's social network. Obesity, smoking, alcohol consumption and depression have all been shown to 'spread' along social networks (Christakis and Fowler, 2007; Christakis and Fowler, 2008; Fowler and Christakis, 2008), as do patterns of health screening, sleep and drug use (Christakis and Fowler, 2012). It appears that many major 'non-communicable' conditions may be nothing of the sort.

Association is not causation, however, and as we saw earlier, individuals in a network may share attributes such as health behaviours or disease states for a number of reasons, only one of which is social contagion. These observational studies have thus generated controversy when they move from identifying the association between social network and disease to imputing direct cause. Some observational studies have used the temporal sequencing of events in social network data to show that changes in network structure preceded changes in rates of a health state, thereby implying that network structure drove changes in disease state (Christakis and Fowler, 2007). It is thus crucial for studies that explore network and disease association to identify the different contributions made by contagion, homophily and demography.

Obesity rates appear to be influenced by contacts across social networks

Obesity rates provide a good example of the complexity involved in unpacking causation of disease states across social networks. Several reviews have examined the evidence base for the association between social networks and obesity and all find a significant, although variable, relationship between the two (Badaly, 2013; Cunningham *et al.*, 2012b; Fletcher *et al.*, 2011; Salvy *et al.*, 2012). It is estimated that the rate of becoming obese increases by 0.5 percentage points for each obese social contact we have (Christakis and Fowler, 2007).

Although obesity has complex determination, including biological factors, it is clear that changing diet and exercise patterns are major contributors to the growth in obesity rates and also that such patterns are heavily shaped by social factors (Wellman and Friedberg, 2002). It is not that obesity literally spreads by social contact, but rather that the norms and behaviours that lead to them may do through social contagion. Our individual lifestyle choices appear shaped by the behaviours of those with whom we have close social ties, and these behaviours propagate along the networks created by these ties. For example, friends can be weight referents, by shaping weight norms and hence behaviours associated with weight management (Burke and Heiland, 2007). Friends can also share weight-related behaviours that cause their body mass index (BMI) to become increasingly alike over time (de La Haye *et al.*, 2011b), and eating habits appear socially contagious (Pachucki *et al.*, 2011).

In adolescents, both BMI and obesity-related behaviours such as energy-dense food intake, physical activity and inactivity cluster in friendship groups and larger peer networks (de La Haye *et al.*, 2010). It is estimated that for every 1-unit increase in a friend's BMI, an adolescent's weight increased by 0.3 BMI units (Trogdon *et al.*, 2008).

Some studies have moved from observation to experimentation in an attempt to understand the relative contribution of contagion, homophily and demography on the association between networks and obesity, diet and exercise. There appears to be a divergence of views on the relative contribution of contagion and selection on weight similarity. The Framingham Study data suggest that in adult populations, contagion is the main driver. In contrast, among adolescent social networks, strongly influenced by school and shared experience, friendship selection appears the stronger driver of weight similarity (de La Haye *et al.*, 2011b).

A controlled experiment that studied the diffusion of a diet diary along networks showed the strongest contagion effects occurred in more homophilous networks (Centola, 2011). This suggests that contagion effects are enhanced by homophily (friends who are more similar have more influence on each other), and that both processes are likely to be in operation in varying extent, depending on context. Network size also appears to be an important variable in the effect of networks on weight, cholesterol and triglyceride levels, as well as compliance with weight reduction strategies such as diary keeping or attending weight loss sessions (Kaplan and Hartwell, 1987).

20.4 Social media are software systems designed to support interactions among groups of individuals

Social media is a general term used to describe a diverse set of information and communication system elements that, when assembled, facilitate group interaction (Grajales *et al.*, 2014). Social media create online communal spaces where groups of people can choose to interact, discuss, co-ordinate or co-produce. Social media have the characteristic that in one way or another they make visible a group's activity to its members and thus support interactive collaboration. A social media application may, for example, allow users to narrowcast to their friends, sharing messages, images, video or music and may foster collaborative engagement about the value and meaning of such content. Such applications differ from more traditional broadcast media because they directly support or create social networks (Kaplan and Haenlein, 2010).

Crowdsourcing refers to the practice of seeking contributions from a group to solve particular problems or elicit particular information (Brabham, 2008). For example, Wikipedia, the online encyclopedia, is entirely created and maintained by the community. Although such crowdsourced information can be remarkably useful, it can be inaccurate (Rector, 2008), for example, about drug information (Clauson *et al.*, 2008).

The social networks created in online communities are as diverse as other human social structures and can be anything from loose, open and opportunistic through to closed, tight and secretive. It is this capacity for social media to create loosely aggregated coalitions of individuals who share short-term common purpose that often captures attention.

Social media play many different roles in health service delivery

Social media are used in many different ways across the health sector, by allowing old things to be done in new ways and creating entirely new models of care delivery (Eysenbach, 2008a; Indes *et al.*, 2013; Lau *et al.*, 2011; Maher *et al.*, 2014; The Change Foundation, 2011a; The Change Foundation, 2011b). Clinicians, especially younger ones, can be active users of social media (Butcher, 2010), but the ways in which health professionals use social media in daily practice are poorly defined (von Muhlen and Ohno-Machado, 2012). One study of US physician Twitter accounts found that although clinicians shared medical information with the public in a potentially beneficial way, privacy and ethical breaches and unprofessional content were also observed (Chretien *et al.*, 2011). Indeed, public social media services may not conform to the security and privacy rules that govern transmission of health information. Such concerns have led professional organizations to formulate policies on the appropriate use of social media because clinicians may be unaware of how public their comments may be (Australian Medical Association, 2012).

Social media applications in healthcare include:

1. *Measuring the quality and safety of clinical services* – Patients and their families are a potent source of 'signal' about healthcare quality (Iedema *et al.*, 2012), and social media can tap into this information (Greaves *et al.*, 2013). Crowdsourced public ratings of health service safety and quality found on the Internet correlate with more traditional quality measures (Bardach *et al.*, 2013), as well as hospital mortality and infection rates (Greaves *et al.*, 2012). Social media are also an important conduit for the reporting of patient safety events, including potential drug interactions to assist in pharmacovigilance (Banerjee *et al.*, 2013).

2. *Emergency services* – Social media are being used both as an emergency broadcast channel and a mechanism to track first-hand accounts of citizens, enriched with video, audio and global positioning system (GPS) location data (Merchant *et al.*, 2011). Sites such as Facebook can help establish emergency communication cascades and buddy networks or communicate emergency room locations and current waiting times. The Red Cross has developed smartphone apps that help people create an emergency plan and share it with others (Dunbar, 1996; Verizon, 2013). After the 2010 Haiti earthquake, social media facilitated interactions among the multiple agencies and nations that responded. Wikis and collaborative workspaces facilitated knowledge sharing, bypassing traditional formal liaison structures that previously blocked such interaction (Yates and Paquette, 2011).

3. *Public health messaging and health promotion* – Social media provide a channel for broadcasting of public messages. They have the potential to reach a broader and more diverse audience than broadcast media, and they provide mechanisms to foster engagement and partnerships with consumers around health promotion (Neiger *et al.*, 2012). Online communities are also of value where behaviour change is important, such as smoking cessation (van Mierlo *et al.*, 2012).

4. *Infectious disease surveillance:* Digital disease surveillance can assist in the early detection of disease outbreaks, as well as continuously monitoring disease levels, and it can track population sentiments to disease control measures (see Chapter 29) (Salathé *et al.*, 2013). Large-scale and popular social media sites such as Facebook and Twitter have a role in crowdsourcing patient-level data that can contribute to disease surveillance and epidemiology (Eysenbach, 2009). Communities can share messages online during a disease outbreak such as influenza and can both report their own infectious state and discuss protective measures (Collier *et al.*, 2010). As a result, social media provide an important source of data for public health officials trying to track the spread of epidemics (Signorini *et al.*, 2011). Tweets are a valuable channel for disseminating health messages during a pandemic, and analysis of their content can track a pandemic in real time (Chew and Eysenbach, 2010). Similarly, analyses of the terms used in public search engines can predict influenza outbreaks, although the models used to make such predictions require recalibration over time as public search behaviours change. For example, increased awareness of a disease can trigger higher than expected Web searches and an overshoot in the prediction of the number of likely influenza cases (Butler, 2013).

5. *Disease management* – Social media can directly support disease management by creating online spaces where patients can interact with clinicians and share experiences with other patients. Patients with cancer use Twitter to discuss treatments and provide psychological support (Sugawara *et al.*, 2012), and online engagement appears to correlate with lower levels of self-reported stress and depression (Beaudoin and Tao, 2008). Personally controlled health management systems (PCHMSs) integrate personal health records with consumer care pathways, booking and scheduling services, communication channels such as e-mail that link consumer with provider and social forums where consumers can ask questions and share experiences. Social media thus comprise one component of a complex bundle of online services brought together to support consumers (Lau *et al.*, 2013b). PCHMSs have been applied in diverse settings such as *in vitro* fertilization (Aarts, 2012; Lau *et al.*, 2012b) and mental health and well-being support (Lau *et al.*, 2013b). PCHMSs can influence consumer behaviours. For example, influenza vaccination rates and visits to primary care providers are significantly increased when consumers are provided both with the information and social feedback needed to decide to act and with tools such as online booking to translate that intention into an action (Lau *et al.*, 2012c).

The use of social media is associated with some health risks

Any new technology brings potential new risks. One analysis of online social networks in diabetes found wide variation in the quality and scientific validity of discussions and in auditing, moderation of discussions and governance (Weitzman *et al.,* 2011). The health risks associated with online content and discussions for consumers include the following (Lau *et al.,* 2012a):

- Marketing material prompting potentially harmful or risky products targeted at consumers (e.g. pro-tobacco videos or direct-to-consumer drug advertising) may be posted on social media.
- Public displays of unhealthy behaviour (e.g. people displaying self-injury behaviours, harming others or injecting or otherwise consuming drugs) may be shown. Pro-anorexia videos in one study represented only a small amount of the total number of anorexia-related content, but they were disproportionately accessed, suggesting a higher degree of visibility and engagement with them (Syed-Abdul *et al.,* 2013).
- Public health messages can be tainted over social media, which are frequent outlets for controversial views. For example, social media can give space to negative voices that disagree with public health messages, such as the need for vaccination. One study of YouTube videos found that the majority of content about human papillomavirus (HPV) vaccination was negative in tone (Briones *et al.,* 2012).
- Individuals may suffer a negative psychological impact after accessing disturbing, inappropriate, offensive or biased social media content. They may also be stigmatized by viewing videos that portray their illness or symptoms negatively (e.g. epilepsy or obesity).
- Social media may be used intentionally to distort public policy or research funding agendas. Controversial treatments that have yet to be fully scrutinized in clinical trials may be still promoted in social media, perhaps with patient testimonials. This may lead to increased demand by patients for access to potentially harmful therapies, some of which may be obtainable over the Internet. It may also lead patients to discontinue proven therapies in favor of those treatments with weaker or no evidence to support them.

Social media contribute to the conduct of research as well as sharing and analysis of trial data

Social media have a variety of applications in the execution and translation of health research (Shneiderman, 2008). They can be used to identify people interested in participating in a clinical trial (West and Camidge, 2012), or they can bring these people in as research collaborators (Swan, 2012). Patients have a vested interest in the outcomes of research, and many have an appetite to share their medical records and personal data with the research community. Web sites that provide personal health records often provide social mechanisms for community members to discuss their conditions and exchange information. Such sites can support the collection, aggregation and analysis of such patient interaction and outcome data in the service both of treatment decisions and of more basic research.

Traditionally, researchers have gathered their own data, analyzed the data and then published results, but the data have remained behind academic or commercial walls (see Chapter 14). Clinical trial data are now required to be made publicly available in many circumstances (Rathi *et al.,* 2012). Online social collaborative systems allow researchers to engage with each other as they explore such public data sets. In the social collaborative model, research data sets are placed in open, perhaps publicly funded, databases where others can access and re-analyze a data set or can pool data sets to answer new questions (Dunn *et al.,* 2012a). A community can formulate research questions, suggest analyses and interpret findings. In one example, the task of aligning multiple gene sequences was turned into a computer game that ordinary Web users could engage in with minimal knowledge of the biological context. The 'gamification' of this scientific task reportedly led to a 70 per cent improvement in the accuracy of sequence alignment (Kawrykow *et al.,* 2012).

20.5 Network interventions harness social media to change the behaviour of individuals within a social group

Network interventions (NIs) are the purposeful use of a social network to influence behaviour. NIs shift the treatment target from the individual to those around them in their social network. They seek to harness network effects such as social contagion to target individuals, organizations, communities or indeed whole populations. Targeting a social group rather than just an individual is sometimes called *network medicine* (Barabási, 2007). The design of an NI varies with its goals. During an epidemic, the design of an NI to increase infection control behaviours across a whole population would be very different from an NI that is targeted at identifying and isolating infected individuals in a contact network. Social networks can thus be manipulated in a number of ways, depending on the state of the existing network and the goal of the NI (Valente, 2012):

- *Individuals* – Depending on the goal of a NI, different individuals within a network can be targeted. By influencing the 'champions' who are central to a network, one can increase the diffusion of evidence-based practices (Mascia and Cicchetti, 2011). When the desired change requires diffusion of a behaviour across separate network communities, then the NI may be targeted at those individuals who are bridges or boundary spanners, with membership of multiple communities.
- *Groups* – Some behaviours result from group norms, as we saw earlier, and the only way to change the behaviour of individuals is to target the behaviour of the whole group, e.g. communities of practice are defined by shared professional norms (Ranmuthugala *et al.,* 2011).
- *Network induction* – Networks can be used as a conduit for information distribution. Word of mouth, snowballing and 'viral' interventions are mechanisms that propagate information widely by stimulating communication among social network members. HIV prevention messages, for example, appear to be more effectively distributed when a peer network is used to disseminate information compared with traditional public health messaging methods (Broadhead *et al.,* 1998).
- *Network alteration* – When existing networks are unable to support a desired change, they can be manipulated by adding or removing individuals or by changing the nature of connections. Changing the social network of alcohol-dependent patients from one supportive of drinking to one supportive of abstinence appears to be both effective and sustainable over the long term (Litt *et al.,* 2009). Changes in our circumstance may

trigger the need for different support structures, and individuals sometimes substitute one social network for another to compensate. The death of a spouse, for example, may trigger the formation of new social ties, the rekindling of dormant ties or the intensification of existing ties, all attempts at engineering social networks to repair losses or meet new needs (Simons, 1983; Zettel and Rook, 2004).

Network therapy has long been used to help manage alcohol and substance misuse, for example, by using members of a network to provide social support (Copello *et al.*, 2002). It also appears to be useful in the management of a number of chronic illnesses including type 2 diabetes, asthma, heart disease and epilepsy (Gallant, 2003). NIs are the basis of the Weight Watchers programme. Peer support is associated with statistically significant improvements in glycaemic control, blood pressure, cholesterol, BMI, physical activity, self-efficacy, depression and perceived social support (Dale *et al.*, 2012).

Social media can be used as a mechanism for network interventions if they satisfy certain conditions

For diseases such as depression or obesity that are socially shaped, social media provide a mechanism to support the design of NIs. Such social media interventions have the potential to directly affect the primary pathological pathway by targeting individual and community behaviours that lead to disease. The *strong social media hypothesis* proposes that where a disease is socially mediated, then social media are a channel for its cure (Coiera, 2013).

Engagement in weight-loss communities online, for example, appears to play a prominent role in weight loss (Hwang *et al.*, 2010). Many studies have explored the impact of online social intervention on weight loss (e.g. Funk *et al.*, 2010; Gold *et al.*, 2007; Harvey-Berino *et al.*, 2004; Napolitano *et al.*, 2013; Pullen *et al.*, 2008; Webber *et al.*, 2008; Womble *et al.*, 2004). Interventions in this group include the use of online peer support from text messaging, bulletin boards and chat rooms through to Facebook. Some studies show moderate to large effect sizes on weight, but unfortunately they do not account for any impact of homophily and often suffer from small sample size, lack of clarity about the nature of the intervention (often blending a bundle of online and offline components) and short duration of follow-up (Li *et al.*, 2013; Williams *et al.*, 2014).

For an online NI to satisfy the strong social media hypothesis, we first need evidence that the NI is treating a socially mediated health condition and then need to assemble evidence that the NI is altering social ties in a way that is causally associated with an improvement. Specifically, several conditions must be satisfied:

1. The pathogenesis or spread of the disease being treated by an NI must be mediated by a social network.
2. The social networks should be susceptible to manipulation to treat the disease.
3. If the 'pathological' network is offline, then an online social network must be able to *substitute* for the offline one.
4. The online social network should itself be susceptible to manipulation to treat the disease.

We have already seen that the first two requirements hold for many disease conditions. When designing an NI to treat such diseases, we thus need to design the social media intervention in such a way that it creates genuine social relationships that can substitute for the 'pathological' relationships causing the health issue and that can then be manipulated online to manage the problem.

It is clear that online relationships can substitute for offline relationships in many cases. When computer networks link people, they become social networks (Wellman, 2001). Just as in offline relationships, those close to each other in online networks are more homophilous, sharing common interests (Aiello *et al.*, 2012). Although the choice of social media used differs by tie strength (different groups have their preferred ways of interacting online), what is communicated between them seems not to vary with the medium chosen, e.g. work-only pairs talk about work (Haythornthwaite, 2005). It is also clear that social media allow new relationships to develop by facilitating previously unavailable interactions. Experiments with 'matched health buddies' show that participation in online health forums is more likely when individuals receive social reinforcement from multiple buddies in their social network (Centola, 2010).

Young adult cancer survivors appear to use social media to fulfill needs that are not being met in their offline lives (McLaughlin *et al.*, 2012). Use of social media in this group of patients appears to be higher among those whose pre-existing social support was low and who have little social support from friends and family, lower family interaction and weaker social bonds. Similarly, Facebook provides a mechanism for maintaining existing ties as individuals move on from social settings such as college, thereby creating a proxy network to build or maintain 'social capital' in the group (Ellison *et al.*, 2007). Indeed, there is good evidence that network substitutability goes both ways. When relationships formed online reach a certain strength, they often translate into offline relationships (Parks and Floyd, 1996; Bargh and McKenna, 2004).

There is now also clear evidence that some online networks can change offline behaviour. Engagement with online communities has the potential to influence cancer outcomes directly by increasing social interaction among patients and reducing anxiety and depression (Beaudoin and Tao, 2008; Eysenbach, 2008). We also know that consumers' opinions about the meaning of health information they read on the Web can be shaped by the views of others on the Web (Lau and Coiera, 2008). A randomized controlled trial involving 61 million Facebook users during the 2010 US congressional elections showed that online political mobilization messages directly influenced voting behaviour. Messages shared through social media were significantly more effective than traditional targeted messages, and most transmission occurred between 'close friends' with a face-to-face relationship (Bond *et al.*, 2012).

Conclusions

Social shaping of human behaviours exploits a human need to conform and model those in our close social group. Social networks are both a way of looking at human relationships and a way of understanding how particular groups and communities aggregate, interact and shape each other's beliefs and behaviours. Such an understanding puts us in the position to intervene through social networks to achieve different goals. Online social media provide a powerful vehicle to redefine social ties and reshape individual views of conformity and normality. If one's social group is obese, it is difficult to avoid sharing common behaviours that lead to obesity. If a virtual social group can be harnessed to redefine diet and exercise norms, then that disease destiny may also be redefined.

McLuhan famously contended that the way a medium restructures human interactions is at least as important as the things we say over it (McLuhan, 1964), Technical systems have social consequences, just as social systems have technical consequences (Coiera, 2004). When it comes to online social media, the technical and the social become one. By harnessing social media to change behaviours that lead to disease, the medium is not just the message. The medium is the medicine (Coiera, 2013).

Discussion points

1. Is a social network a real thing or is it just a model?

2. Draw a sociogram that describes the ties between you and your friends or between you and your work colleagues. Can you see any groupings or community structures in the network? If so, what do you think has driven the creation of these groupings?

3. Look up methods to calculate degree, closeness and degree centrality, and then calculate these for your position in the network you created in the previous question. Can you see any differences in the centrality values, and what could be the causes of such differences? Which measure of network centrality do you think is most important for you?

4. What aspects of social interaction do you think are missing from a typical sociogram?

5. Why do drug companies send sales representatives to visit doctors in their practice when they could just as easily send new drug information to them in an e-mail or through the post?

6. Consider a clinical workflow or process you are familiar with (e.g. the referral of a patient by a primary care physician to a specialist or seeking advice on how to manage the care of a patient in a hospital ward). Contrast what the 'official' description of the process could be, compared with the way it is socially enacted.

7. Do you think doctors are more influenced by the latest research evidence or by what they are told about new treatments by their colleagues?

8. Do you think researchers who work for a pharmaceutical company are more central in research collaboration networks by accident or design?

9. Do you think it is safe for a community member to crowdsource a diagnosis and treatment?

10. Describe the different categories of social media you are familiar with (e.g. blogs, social networking sites, wikis). Compare and contrast the content types of these services and the mechanisms they provide for sharing, interacting or co-producing.

11. What rules are used to govern who can write or edit a public document by using a wiki? Why are any rules necessary at all?

12. Explain how obesity is socially transmitted.

13. Design an online NI that you think will lead network members to reduce weight to a healthy range.

14. Why do some social media interventions work in changing behaviour and others do not?

Smaller hospitals often lack the patient volume or financial resources to justify hiring dedicated intensivists and running specialized intensive care units (ICUs). Telemedicine ICU (tele-ICU) may partially compensate by assisting in managing locally patients who would otherwise need to be transferred or who would otherwise have received less expert care. Tele-ICU is a bundle of services, combining video, patient telemetry and access to some elements of the electronic health record. It can be demand driven, with requests for assistance, or provide comprehensive and continuous remote monitoring by a team of dedicated physicians and critical care nurses who may order laboratory and radiographic studies, initiate preventive treatments and aid in diagnosis and treatment planning.

Tele-ICU coverage is associated with a significant reduction in ICU mortality and length of stay, but not in-hospital mortality or length of stay (Young *et al.*, 2011). This may be explained in part by the bundled nature of the intervention, which includes technological as well as process improvements that may reduce mortality while patients are in the ICU but not once they are transferred to normal wards that have no special provisions. It is also the case that any implementation of tele-ICU is shaped by local models of care, local staff skills, whether remote expertise is available from a dedicated team and whether a dedicated ICU facility is available at the local hospital.

Teleradiology

It is now standard for radiological practices to be largely if not entirely digitized, with radiological information systems (RIS) supporting day-to-day radiological practice, and picture archiving and communication systems (PACS) supporting the storing and sharing of images. It should therefore no longer matter where a set of images is read, as long as the information infrastructure allows images to be uploaded in a reasonable time frame. This allows after-hours cover for facilities where there is no radiologist on site. It also allows a general radiologist to consult with a remote specialist, sharing difficult images, and can lead to improved diagnostic accuracy for the general radiologist (Franken and Berbaum, 1996).

Teleradiology appears to work best when it fits the workflow of the task. Emergency teleradiology generally works well because there are limited indications for it and less need to review prior examination results and clinical information. For example, accessing remote electronic radiological images appears to result in comparable diagnoses and treatment plans for the management of upper extremity orthopaedic conditions (Abboud *et al.*, 2005). In contrast, an examination of a patient with a complex medical condition typically requires comparison of new images with the prior studies and a review of information such as pathology and laboratory reports. In this non-urgent setting, teleradiology can be more difficult if the supporting technology makes it cumbersome for the remote radiologist to gather such additional information (Thrall, 2007). This 'missing information' may explain why, in some studies, diagnostic performance is lower for remote radiologists when compared with a patient presenting at their service, where record access should be better.

Telepathology and dermatology

Sharing of images of pathology skin samples can be of use when a local reader of the image is not expert in the task, and the diagnostic performance is similar, if not equal, to that of expert diagnosis alone (Piccolo *et al.,* 2002). Teledermatology, which involves sharing of skin images to either make a diagnosis or decide on the need for referral, appears to achieve a somewhat lower diagnostic accuracy than attendance at a standard dermatology clinic (Warshaw *et al.,* 2011). However, overall rates of patient management decisions appear to be equivalent, and it is difficult to measure clinical outcome differences between clinic and remote diagnosis.

Multimedia Messaging Services (MMS) on a mobile phone can also be used to send teledermatology referrals to a dermatologist. Digital photographs of skin conditions can be sent to dermatologists along with clinical information. In one study, dermatologists were able to make a correct diagnosis in 78 per cent of cases based solely on the MMS referral and provided adequate management recommendations for 98 per cent of patients (Börve *et al.,* 2012).

Real-time telepathology for light microscopic diagnosis can aid intra-departmental consultation between duty staff and senior or expert staff with frozen-section diagnosis. The result appears to be quicker and better diagnostic rates compared with routine intra-departmental consultation (Liang *et al.,* 2008). Internet-based telepathology also appears of value across nations, by allowing developing countries to access subspecialty expertise that is not locally available (Wamala *et al.,* 2011).

Mobile communications can help clinical teams interact but may contribute to the overall level of work interruptions

Hospitals are complex organizations, and good communication processes are fundamental to their operation. Hospital workers are highly mobile, with medical staff often moving widely across a hospital campus or even having to move off campus to attend other hospitals or clinics. Nevertheless, it is important that teams remain within reach of each other to deal with emergent inpatient issues or to make admission and discharge decisions.

Various different mobile wireless technologies and devices have been used to help keep teams in contact with each other, as well as enhancing contactability for urgent requests (Wu *et al.,* 2012). Alphanumeric pagers are ubiquitous, and some clinical staff may carry several of these. Pagers are issued not just to named individuals but also for specified roles such as members of medical emergency teams. One-way pagers have several drawbacks, including 'telephone tag', which results when multiple pages and calls are needed to connect the person making the page with the person being paged.

Mobile telephones avoid many of these problems. They enable synchronous voice interaction but also offer asynchronous channels such as text messaging. Text messages can be generated by *clinical decision support systems* (see Chapter 25), for example, notifying a clinician that a test result is available, that a particular test value is significantly abnormal (Rind *et al.,* 1994) or is at 'panic' levels (Kuperman *et al.,* 1999).

Hands-free communication devices (HCDs) are an alternate mechanism for contacting individuals in hospital. They are typically lightweight devices that are either worn around the neck or clipped to a lapel and use Voice over Internet Protocol (VoIP) through a hospital's Wi-Fi network. HCD systems allow users to make outgoing calls, pick up incoming calls or dictate call-handling instructions using verbal commands (Richardson and Ash, 2010). For

Language, coding and classification

CHAPTER 22

Terms, codes and classification

> By an almost instinctive impulse, similar to that which leads to the use of language, we are induced to collate or group together the things which we observe – which is to say, to classify them … to imagine them combined or grouped in a certain order… Accordingly, every science and art has endeavoured to classify as completely as possible the things belonging to it; hence, in our field of enquiry, the objects classified are the phenomena and processes of the living body, diseases, remedies, the hundred influences and agencies of external nature, etc.
>
> *F. Oesterlen, Medical Logic, 1855*

Both conceptually and practically, the study of clinical language is central to informatics. Clinical languages are the building blocks from which we construct models of health and disease, and thus they exert their influence at the very foundations of clinical reasoning. Practically, language is important because so much of the clinical record is expressed in text or narrative. If one wishes to monitor population-level disease for public health surveillance, or simply audit clinical practice, there needs to be some way of condensing the content of clinical text into core concepts such as specific diseases, treatments and outcomes.

This chapter introduces foundational concepts underpinning clinical terminologies, coding and classification. Chapter 23 reviews some of the more important real-world terminological systems and their uses and limitations. The concluding chapter in this part, Chapter 24, critically examines the differences between formal terminological systems and natural language. Chapter 24 also demonstrates the way in which computer approaches to natural language processing must accommodate the inherent messiness of written and spoken language as they try to interpret the meaning of clinical texts.

22.1 Language establishes a common ground

Human beings are designed to detect differences in the world. We distinguish different objects, name them and then categorize them. This process of discovering and then naming the difference between two things is basic to the way in which we learn about the world, develop language and proceed to interact with the world (Wisniewski and Medin, 1994). Language evolves as we interact with the world, discover new things about it and do different things within it. However, this growth in language is tempered by the need to communicate with others and share experiences. When members of different cultures meet, they must establish a linguistic common ground. To do this, there must be some shared language with agreed meaning. There is little value in each of us developing a complicated set of words if no one else understands what they represent.

The story in healthcare is similar, with a long history of discovery and the creation of new ideas. As a result, the words used in clinical practice change both their meaning and form over time (Feinstein, 1988). A clinician today has a very different understanding of the word asthma from a clinician of 100 years ago. Further, different societies have different concepts of illness. Even among similar Western cultures, there can be quite different notions of what constitutes a disease and what is normal. Hypotension, or low blood pressure, has been a routinely treated disease in some European countries, but it is regarded as normal in others.

Even among the different clinical 'cultures', there are differences. Different groups of health professionals – nurses, the medical specialities, health economists and administrators – all evolve slightly different words or jargon.

22.2 Common terms are needed to permit assessment of clinical activities

Much effort has been devoted to formal clinical language development for the purpose of epidemiology, resource management and clinical audit. Audit is the process of assessing the outcomes associated with different diseases and their treatments. To make all such assessments, it is first necessary to make measurements by pooling patient data. Although it is possible to compare patient outcomes based upon measurements, for example serum biochemistry, these are rarely sufficient to describe a patient's state. In healthcare, language is often the basis of measurement. Words describe observed findings such as 'pitting oedema', 'unconscious' and the diagnoses that cause these findings.

Yet the words used by people to describe conditions vary, as do the meanings attached to words (see Box 22.1). With an agreed-on set of terms to describe clinical disease and the process of care, data analysis can be much simplified (Board of Directors of the American Medical Informatics Association, 1994). Once created, controlled clinical terminologies can be used not just for audit, but also to enable computerized decision support. Clinical notes, for example, can be interpreted using a terminology, and the appearance of specified words in a patient record can trigger computer alerts.

22.3 Terms, codes, groups and hierarchies

Clinical terminologies (or nomenclatures), like all languages, start with a basic set of words or *terms* (Box 22.1). A term, like any normal word, has a specific meaning. In this case, a term stands for some defined clinical *concept* such as 'diabetes', 'tibia' or 'penicillin'. Most languages permit words that have the same or similar meanings, and this is usually the case in healthcare,

Box 22.1
The basic level

When people are asked to name objects, they instinctively pick words that describe them at a level that is most economical, but still adequately describes their functionality. For example, people usually use the word 'chair' in preference to the more general word 'furniture', which loses much sense of function, or the more specific description 'dining chair', which adds little.

This cognitively economical level of description has been called the *basic level* by Eleanor Rosch, who developed her classification theory to describe this feature of human cognition (Rosch, 1988). Rosch proposed that objects in the basic level have the quality that they are statistical prototypes of their class. Such prototypical objects contain most of the attributes that represent objects inside their category and the least number of attributes of those outside the category. Thus, if people were asked to describe 'a chair', they would list a set of attributes that could be used to describe most, but not all, kinds of chair. A stool may be a special kind of chair, even though it does not have a back support that could be considered part of the features of a prototypical chair.

The basic level is thus formed around a natural word hierarchy based upon the level of detail of description, coupled with the utility of description. The basic level therefore is not absolute, but it varies with the context within which a word is used. Sometimes 'dining chair' actually is the most appropriate description to use. Similarly, in some circumstances, it is sufficient to classify a patient as having 'acidosis'. Clinically however, it is probably more useful to use a description such as 'metabolic acidosis', which becomes basic in this context because it is at this level that treatment is determined.

too. To permit some flexibility, most clinical languages allow the same concept to be named in several different ways. However, because several terms may be used for the same concept, it is usual to define a single alphanumeric *code* for every distinct concept in the language (Figure 22.1). This gives rise to the process of *coding*, in which a set of words describing some clinical concept is translated into a code for later analysis.

The terms and codes in different terminologies vary, depending upon the reasons for which they are created. For example, if a coding system exists for epidemiological analysis, the concepts of interest are at the level of public health, rather than at the level of a particular medical specialization. The level of detail captured in the codes would be much finer in the latter case, and the concepts would be different. When determining the cost of providing care, more aggregate-level data are needed. A *group* is used to collect into a single category a number of different codes that together are considered to be similar for the purpose of reimbursement (see Figure 22.1).

Classification hierarchies

Once a set of terms and codes is collected together, they can quickly become so large that it is difficult to find individual terms. They consequently need to be organized in a way that the

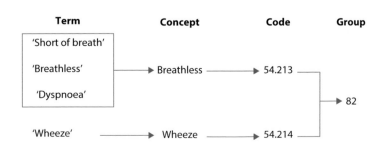

Figure 22.1
Multiple terms may map onto a single concept, which has its own unique numeric code in clinical languages. Groups collect similar codes together for more coarse-grained analysis.

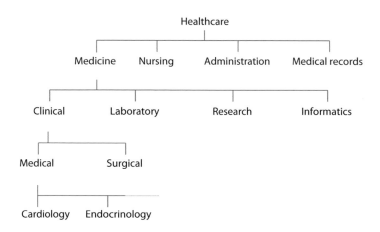

Figure 22.2 Classification hierarchies organize terms in some conceptual structure that gives meaning to terms through their relationship with other terms in the hierarchy.

terms can be easily searched. A straightforward alphabetical listing of terms is of limited value, and so clinical terminologies need to be organized in a way that permits concept-driven exploration. For example, it should be easy to locate the word 'pericarditis' by knowing that one is seeking a word describing inflammation of the pericardium. From a user's point of view, a terminology needs to be more like a thesaurus than a dictionary, by organizing terms into conceptually similar groupings.

As we saw in Chapter 7, one of the most common ways to organize ideas is to produce a classification hierarchy. The essence of a hierarchy is that it provides a structured grouping of ideas, organized around some set of *attributes* or *axes*. The hierarchy provides some meaning to terms through the way they relate to others. For example, in Figure 22.2, it is clear without knowing anything more about the term 'endocrinology' that it is a branch of clinical medicine and not a part of healthcare administration.

Just as a hierarchy may serve as a map to help locate unknown terms, it can also help uncover new relationships among concepts. A researcher, for example, may try to arrange concepts in such a way that a deeper set of relationships becomes apparent. If this has explanatory power, then the classification system can be used to direct further research, explain or teach. The periodic table of elements, developed by Mendeleev, was used in this way. Atomic weights of the elements, along with some of their chemical properties, were the attributes used to construct the initial classification system. Where no elements were known to exist, gaps were left that were later filled as new elements were discovered. The regularity of the table also led to a deeper understanding of the underlying atomic structure of the elements.

The meaning of terms in a classification hierarchy is determined by the type of link used

There are many ways in which terms can relate to one another in a hierarchy, depending upon which attributes of the concept are of interest. In each case, the meaning of the linkage between terms is different (Figure 22.3):

- A *part–whole* link connects related anatomic structures, organizations or the components of a device.

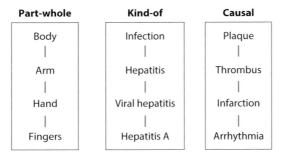

Part-whole	Kind-of	Causal
Body	Infection	Plaque
|	|	|
Arm	Hepatitis	Thrombus
|	|	|
Hand	Viral hepatitis	Infarction
|	|	|
Fingers	Hepatitis A	Arrhythmia

Figure 22.3
Depending on the type of attribute used to classify concepts, many different types of hierarchical structure are possible. Each type of link implies a different relationship among the terms in the hierarchy.

- In a *kind-of* (or *is-a*) hierarchy, elements are assembled because of some underlying similarity. For example, a drug such as penicillin is a kind-of antibiotic.
- *Causal* structures are used to explain how a chain of events may unfold over time.

Each of these different types of link allows one term to inherit properties from other terms higher up in the hierarchy. What is inherited depends on the type of link. In a part-whole hierarchy, terms inherit their location from parent terms higher in the tree. In kind-of hierarchies, many different properties of parent terms can be inherited by child terms. Thus, there are many chemical and pharmacological properties that amoxicillin inherits from the parent class of penicillins and that the penicillins inherit from their parent class antibiotics. In contrast, in a causal structure one would not expect a concept such as 'thrombosis' to be a kind of 'coronary plaque', but only that it takes its temporal ordering in a chain of events from it.

This leads to an obvious but critical point about classification hierarchies. For the meaning of terms in a classification system to be as explicit as possible, the links between terms should be clearly defined, so there is no confusion about which properties a term can inherit from its parents. Confusion is easy, and it is common to see classifications mixing part-whole and kind-of relations. Ideally, a hierarchy should use only one kind-of link.

Some complex clinical terminologies permit multiple axes of classification. These *multi-axial classification systems* allow a term to exist in several different classification hierarchies, and this minimizes duplication of terms and enhances the conceptual power of the system. In a multi-axial system, a term such as 'hepatitis' could exist both as a *kind-of* infection and as a *cause of* jaundice.

22.4 Compositional terminologies create complicated concepts from simple terms

Many coding systems are *enumerative,* listing out all the possible terms that could be used in advance. Terminology builders strive to make such systems as complete as possible and to contain as few errors or duplications as possible. As the numbers of terms grow, this task becomes increasingly difficult. When many people contribute to a terminology, the natural

CHAPTER 23

Healthcare terminologies and classification systems

The terms disease and remedy were formerly understood and therefore defined quite differently to what they are now; so, likewise, are the meanings and definitions of inflammation, pneumonia, typhus, gout, lithiasis … different from those which were attached to them thirty years ago… great mischief will in most cases ensue if, in such attempts at definition and explanation, greater importance is attached to a clear and determinate, than to a complete and comprehensive understanding of the objects and questions before us. In a field like ours, clearness can in general be purchased only at the expense of completeness and therefore truth.

Oesterlen, Medical Logic, *1855*

Coding and classification systems have a long history in medicine. Current systems can trace their origins back to epidemiological lists of the causes of death from the early part of the eighteenth century. François Bossier de Lacroix (1706–77) is commonly credited with the first attempt to classify diseases systematically. Better known as Sauvages, he published the work under the title *Nosologia Methodica*.

Linnaeus (1707–78), who was a contemporary of Sauvages, also published his *Genera Morborum* in that period. By the beginning of the nineteenth century, the *Synopsis Nosologiae Methodicae*, published in 1785 by William Cullen of Edinburgh (1710–90), was the classification in most common use.

It was John Graunt who, working about a hundred years earlier, is credited with the first practical attempts to classify disease for statistical purposes. Working on his *London Bills of Mortality*, he was able to estimate the proportion of deaths in different age groups. For example, he estimated a 36 per cent mortality rate for liveborn children before the age of 6 years. He did this by taking all the deaths classified as convulsions, rickets, teeth and worms, thrush, abortives, chrysomes, infants and livergrown. To these he added half of the deaths classed as smallpox, swinepox, measles and worms without convulsions. By all accounts his estimate was good (World Health Organization, 2011).

It has only been in the last few decades that these terminological systems have started to attract wider attention and resources. The ever-growing need to amass and analyze clinical data, no longer just for epidemiological purposes, has provided considerable incentive and published in 1979 by the College of American Pathologists. SNOMED intellectual property rights transferred in 2007 to the International Health Terminology Standards Development Organization (IHTSDO), a not-for-profit organization.

Level of acceptance and use

SNOMED is reportedly used in more than 40 countries, presumably largely in laboratories for the coding of reports to generate statistics and facilitate data retrieval (Cornet and de Keizer, 2008).

Classification structure

SNOMED is a hierarchical, multi-axial classification system. Terms are assigned to 1 of 11 independent systematized modules, corresponding to different axes of classification (Table 23.3). Each term is placed into a hierarchy within one of these modules and is assigned a 5- or 6-digit alphanumeric code. Each code carries with it a packet of information about the terms it designates that gives some notion of the clinical context of that code (Figure 23.2). Terms can also be cross referenced to multiple modules (Table 23.4).

SNOMED also allows the composition of complex terms from simpler terms and is thus partially compositional. SNOMED International incorporates virtually all the ICD-9-CM terms and codes and thus allows reports to be generated in this format if necessary.

SNOMED RT (Reference Terminology) was released in 2000 to support the electronic storage, retrieval and analysis of clinical data (Spackman *et al.*, 1997). A reference terminology provides a common reference point for comparison and aggregation of data about the entire healthcare process, recorded by multiple different individuals, systems or institutions. Previous versions of SNOMED expressed terms in a hierarchy that was optimized for human use. In SNOMED RT, the relationships between terms and concepts are contained in a

Table 23.3   The SNOMED International modules (or axes)

Module designator
Topography (T)
Morphology (M)
Function (F)
Diseases/Diagnoses (D)
Procedures (P)
Occupations (J)
Living Organisms (L)
Chemicals, Drugs and Biological Products (C)
Physical Agents, Forces and Activities (A)
Social Context (S)
General Linkage-Modifiers (G)

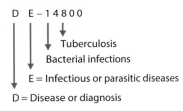

Figure 23.2
SNOMED codes are
hierarchically
structured. Implicit in
the code,
tuberculosis is an
infectious bacterial
disease.

Table 23.4   An example of SNOMED's nomenclature and classification

Axis		Nomenclature			Classification
Axis	T	+ M	+ L	+ F	= D
Term	Lung	+ Granuloma	+ M. tuberculosis	+ Fever	= Tuberculosis
Code	T-28000	+ M-44000	+ L-21801	+ F-03003	= DE-14800

Some terms (e.g. tuberculosis) can be cross-referenced to others, to give the term a richer clinical context.

machine-optimized hierarchy table. Each individual concept is expressed using a description logic, which makes explicit the information that was implicit in earlier codes (Table 23.5).

Limitations

It is possible, given the richness of the SNOMED International structure, to express the same concept in many ways. For example, acute appendicitis has a single code D5-46210. However, there are also terms and codes for 'acute', 'acute inflammation' and 'in'. Thus, this concept could be expressed as Appendicitis, acute; or Acute inflammation, in, Appendix; and Acute, inflammation NOS (not otherwise specified), in, Appendix (Rothwell, 1995). This makes it

Table 23.5   Comparison between implicitly coded information about 'postoperative esophagitis' in SNOMED III codes and the explicit coding in SNOMED RT

SNOMED III code and English nomenclature:	D5-30150 Postoperative esophagitis
SNOMED III components of the concept:	T-56000 Esophagus
	M-40000 Inflammation
	F-06030 Postoperative state
Cross-reference field in SNOMED III:	(T-56000)(M-40000)(F-06030)
Parent term in the SNOMED III hierarchy:	D5-30100 Esophagitis, NOS
Essential characteristics, in SNOMED RT syntax:	D5-30150:
	D5-30100 &
	(assoc-topography T-56000) &
	(assoc-morphology M-40000) &
	(assoc-etiology F-06030)

From Spackman et al., 1997.

difficult, for example, to compare similar concepts that have been indexed in different ways or to search for a term that exists in different forms within a patient record. The use of a description logic in SNOMED RT was designed to solve this problem. Further, although SNOMED permits single terms to be combined to create complex terms, rules for the combination of terms have not been developed. Consequently, such compositions may not be clinically valid.

23.5 SNOMED Clinical Terms

Purpose

SNOMED Clinical Terms (SNOMED CT) is designed for use in software applications such as the electronic patient record and decision support systems and to support the electronic communication of information among different clinical applications. Its designers' ambitious goal is that SNOMED CT should become the accepted international terminological resource for healthcare, by supporting multilingual terminological renderings of common concepts.

History

In 1999, the College of American Pathologists and the UK NHS announced their intention to unite SNOMED RT and Clinical Terms Version 3 (Stearns *et al.*, 2001). The intentions in creating the common terminology were to decrease duplication of effort and to create a unified international terminology that supports the integrated electronic medical record. SNOMED CT was first released for testing in 2002.

Level of acceptance and use

SNOMED CT supersedes SNOMED RT and the Clinical Terms Version 3. It will gradually replace CTV3 in the United Kingdom as the terminology of choice used in the NHS, and it is used in many countries around the world.

Classification structure

The SNOMED CT core structure includes concepts, descriptions (terms) and the relationships between them (Figure 23.3). Like SNOMED-RT and CTV3, SNOMED CT is a compositional and hierarchical terminology. It is multi-axial and uses description logic to define the scope of a concept explicitly. There are 15 top-level hierarchies (Table 23.6). The hierarchies go down an average of 10 levels per concept.

SNOMED CT incorporates mappings to classifications such as the ICD-9-CM and ICD-10. It is substantially larger than either SNOMED-RT or CTV3 alone, and it contains more than 300 000 concepts, 400 000 terms and more than 1 000 000 semantic

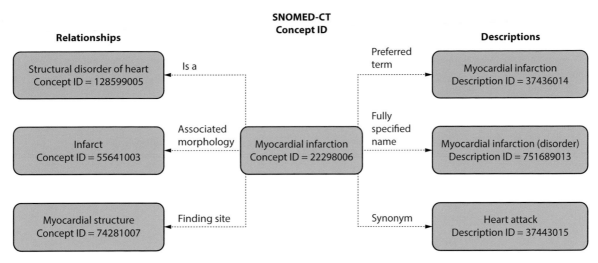

SNOMED-CT Concept ID

Relationships

Structural disorder of heart
Concept ID = 128599005

Is a

Infarct
Concept ID = 55641003

Associated morphology

Myocardial infarction
Concept ID = 22298006

Myocardial structure
Concept ID = 74281007

Finding site

Descriptions

Preferred term

Myocardial infarction
Description ID = 37436014

Fully specified name

Myocardial infarction (disorder)
Description ID = 751689013

Synonym

Heart attack
Description ID = 37443015

Figure 23.3 Outline of the SMOMED CT core structure. (Adapted from the National eHealth Transition Authority [NEHTA] Clinical Terminology Overview, 2012.)

relationships. SNOMED CT also integrates LOINC (Logical Observation Identifier Names and Codes) to enhance its coverage of laboratory test nomenclature. Most of the features of the parent terminologies are incorporated into SNOMED CT. For example, the CTV3 templates, although not explicitly named in the new structure, are essentially preserved in SNOMED CT.

Independent evaluations of the comprehensiveness of SNOMED CT demonstrate that it does a fairly good job of covering most common concepts. One study that examined about 5000 of the most common patient problems found that SNOMED CT could exactly represent about 92 per cent of the terms used in this problem list (Elkin *et al.*, 2006). Coverage of multidisciplinary concepts associated with the management of chronically ill patients was assessed using chart review in another study and was found to be adequate, with about 82 per cent of required concepts covered (Sampalli *et al.*, 2010). All such evaluations represent points in time because a terminology such as SNOMED CT is under constant revision, with new editions produced on a regular basis.

Limitations

Because SNOMED CT is a compositional terminology, there is continuing requirement to prevent illogical compositions from being created as new terms and modifiers are added. Although type checking is implemented, explicit compositional controls were not evident in the early releases. A sample of 1890 descriptions from the initial merging of the 2 parent terminologies found a 43 per cent redundancy in terms (Sable *et al.*, 2001). Some were simply common to both parent systems, but many terms were problematic. Some terms were vague or ambiguous, had flawed hierarchy links or contained knowledge about disease processes that should have been beyond the scope of the terminology. Whereas many

Table 23.6   The top-level hierarchies of SMOMED CT

Procedure/intervention includes all purposeful activities performed in the provision of health care.

Finding/disorder groups together concepts that result from an assessment or judgement.

Measurable/observable entity includes observable functions such as 'vision', as well as things that can be measured such as 'hemoglobin level'.

Social/administrative concept aggregates concepts from the CTV3 'administrative statuses' and 'administrative values' hierarchies, as well as concepts from the SNOMED RT 'social context' hierarchy.

Body structure includes anatomical concepts as well as abnormal body structures, including the 'morphologic abnormality' concepts.

Organism includes all organisms, including micro-organisms and infectious agents (including prions), fungi, plants and animals.

Substance includes chemicals, drugs, proteins and functional categories of substance, as well as structural and state-based categories, such as liquid, solid, gas, etc.

Physical object includes natural and human-made objects, including devices and materials.

Physical force includes motion, friction, gravity, electricity, magnetism, sound, radiation, thermal forces (heat and cold), humidity, air pressure and other categories mainly directed at categorizing mechanisms of injury.

Event is a category that includes occurrences that result in injury (accidents, falls, etc), and excludes procedures and interventions.

Environment/geographical location lists types of environment, as well as named locations such as countries, states and regions.

Specimen lists entities that are obtained for examination or analysis, usually from the body of a patient.

Context-dependent category distinguishes concepts that have pre-coordinated *context*, i.e. information that fundamentally changes the type of thing it is associated with. For example, 'family history of' is *context* because when it modifies 'myocardial infarction', the resulting 'family history of myocardial infarction' is no longer a type of heart disease. Other examples of contextual modifiers include 'absence of', 'at risk of' etc.

Attribute lists the concepts that are used as *defining attributes* or *qualifying attributes,* i.e. the middle element of the object–attribute–value triple that describes all SNOMED CT relationships.

Qualifier value categorizes the remaining concepts (those that have not been listed in the categories above) that are used as the *value* of the object–attribute–value triples.

From Bos, 2006.

problematic terms were identified automatically, some required visual inspection and discussion to be resolved.

23.6 The Unified Medical Language System

Purpose

The Unified Medical Language System (UMLS) is something like the Rosetta Stone of international terminologies. It links the major international terminologies into a common structure and provides a translation mechanism between them. The UMLS is designed to aid in the development of systems that retrieve and integrate electronic biomedical information from a variety of sources and to permit the linkage of disparate information systems, including electronic patient records, bibliographic databases and decision support systems.

History

In 1986, the US National Library of Medicine (NLM) began a long-term research and development project to build a unified medical language system (Humphreys and Lindberg, 1989; Humphreys *et al.,* 1998).

Level of acceptance and use

Broad use of the UMLS is encouraged by distributing it free of charge under a license agreement. The UMLS is widely used in clinical applications, and the NLM itself uses the UMLS in significant applications including PubMed and the Web-based consumer health information initiative at *ClinicalTrials.gov.*

Classification structure

The UMLS is composed of three 'knowledge sources' – a Metathesaurus, a semantic network, and a lexicon. The *UMLS Metathesaurus* is intended for system developers and provides a uniform format for more than 150 different biomedical vocabularies and classifications. Systems integrated within the UMLS include the ICD-9, ICD-10, Medical Subject Headings (MeSH), ICPC, WHO Adverse Drug Reaction Terminology and SNOMED CT. The 2014 edition of the Metathesaurus included 2.9 million concepts and 11.6 million unique concept names.

The Metathesaurus is organized by concept and does not include an over-arching hierarchy. It can be conceptualized as a web rather than as a hierarchical tree, by linking alternative names and views of the same concept together and identifying useful relationships among different concepts. This method of structuring UMLS allows the component terminologies to maintain their original structure within UMLS, as well as linking similar concepts between the component terminologies.

Each concept has attributes that define its meaning, including the semantic types or categories to which it belongs, its position in the source terminology hierarchy and a definition. Major UMLS semantic types include organisms, anatomical structures, biologic function, chemicals, events, physical objects and concepts or ideas.

Numerous relationships between different concepts are represented, including those that are derived from the source vocabularies. Where the parent terminology expresses a full hierarchy, this is fully preserved in UMLS. The Metathesaurus also includes information about usage, including the name of databases in which the concept originally appears.

The UMLS is a controlled vocabulary, and the *UMLS Semantic Network* is used to ensure the integrity of meaning between different concepts. It defines the types or categories to which all Metathesaurus concepts can be assigned and the permissible relationships among these types (e.g., 'virus' causes 'disease or syndrome'). There are more than 133 semantic types that can be linked by 54 different possible relationships. The primary link is the 'isa' link, which establishes the hierarchy of types within the network. A set of non-hierarchical relationships among the types includes 'physically related to', 'spatially related to', 'temporally related to', 'functionally related to', and 'conceptually related to'.

The *SPECIALIST Lexicon* is intended to assist in producing computer applications that need to translate free-form or natural language into coded text. It contains syntactic information for terms and English words, including verbs that do not appear in the Metathesaurus, as well as multi-word expansions of generally used acronyms and abbreviations. It can thus be used to generate natural language or lexical variants of words. For example, the word 'treat' has three variants that all have the same meaning as far as the Metathesaurus is concerned – treats, treated or treating.

Limitations

The very size and complexity of the UMLS may be barriers to its use, by offering a steep learning curve compared with any individual terminology system. Its size also poses great challenges in system maintenance. Every time one of the individual terminologies incorporated into UMLS changes, technically those changes must be reflected in the UMLS. Consequently, regular and frequent updates to the UMLS are issued. As the system grows, the likelihood of errors being introduced naturally increases, as we will see in Chapter 24.

The richness of the linkages between concepts also offers subtle problems at the heart of terminological science. For example, the 'meaning' of a UMLS concept is derived from its relationships with other concepts, and these relationships come from the original source terminologies. However, a precise concept definition from one of the original terminologies such as the ICD or SNOMED may be blurred by the addition of links from another terminology that contains a similar concept (Campbell *et al.*, 1998). For example, 'gastrointestinal transit' in the MeSH is used to denote both the physiologic function and the diagnostic measure (Spackman *et al.*, 1997). Because UMLS does not contain an ontology which could aid with conceptual definition, it is difficult to control for such *semantic drift*.

23.7 There are many specialized classification system terminologies in routine use

The classification systems reviewed so far are intended for broad use across the health system, but as we have seen, they often require extensions to allow them to be useful for more clinically related tasks. These systems typically are inadequate for use in specialized settings, and as a result many systems have been developed to cover such gaps. Some of the more important specialist classifications include the following:

- The *Diagnostic and Statistical Manual of Mental Disorders* (DSM) provides a common language and standard criteria for classifying mental disorders. The DSM-5 was released in 2013 (Regier *et al.*, 2009).
- The *Logical Observation Identifier Names and Codes* (LOINC) provides a set of names and identification codes for identifying laboratory and clinical test results (McDonald *et al.*, 2003).
- *RxNORM* is another product from the NLM, and it provides a standard set of drug names and relationships derived from a number of different source vocabularies (Nelson *et al.*, 2011).

- The *International Classification of Primary Care* (ICPC) was introduced in 1987 and is currently in its second edition ICPC-2 (Soler *et al.,* 2008).
- The *Current Procedural Terminology* (CPT) is a US nomenclature developed by the American Medical Association, and it is used to report medical procedures and services for health insurance purposes (American Medical Association, 2007).
- *RadLEX* is a radiology specific terminological system designed for use in a broad range of radiology information systems such as picture archiving and communication systems (Langlotz, 2006).

23.8 Comparing coding systems is not easy

Unsurprisingly, the same clinical concept may look very different when coded using different classification systems (Table 23.7). The different origins of the systems, and the different revision histories each has had, inevitably result in the use of different terms for similar concepts. Although it is beguiling to try to compare different coding systems, such comparisons are often ill considered. This is because it is not always obvious how to compare the ability of different systems to code concepts found in a patient record. Coding requirements vary from setting to setting and from task to task. It is thus not meaningful to compare performance on one task and infer that similar outcomes will result for tests on other tasks.

As critically, term use varies among user populations. The terms used in a primary care setting differ from those used in a clinic allied to a hospital, thus reflecting different practices and patient populations. Differing disease patterns and practices also distinguish different nations. A system such as Read Version 2, designed for UK primary care, may not

Table 23.7 A comparison of coding for four different clinical concepts using some of the major coding systems

Clinical concept	UMLS	ICD-10	ICD-9-CM 4th edition	Read, 1999	SNOMED International, 1998	SNOMED CT, 2002
Chronic ischaemic heart disease	448589 Chronic ischaemic heart disease	I25.9 Chronic ischaemic heart disease	414.9 Chronic ischaemic heart disease	XE0WG Chronic ischaemic heart disease NOS	14020 Chronic ischaemic heart disease	84537008 Chronic ischaemic heart disease
Epidural haematoma	'453700 Hematoma, epidural'	S06.4 Epidural haemorrhage	432.0 Nontraumatic extradural haemorrhage	Xa0AC Extradural haematoma	89124 Extradural haemorrhage	68752002 Nontraumatic extradural haemorrhage
Lymphosarcoma	'1095849 Lymphoma, diffuse'	C85.0 Lymphosarcoma	200.1 Lymphosarcoma	B601z Lymphosarcoma	'95923 Lymphosarcoma, diffuse'	'1929004 Malignant lymphoma, non-Hodgkin'
Common cold	1013970 Common cold	J00 Acute nasopharyngitis (common cold)	460 Acute nasopharyngitis (common cold)	XE0X1 Common cold	35210 Common cold	82272006 Common cold

ICD, International Classification of Diseases; UMLS, United Medical Language System.
From the National Centre for Classification in Health, Australia.

perform as well in US clinics as a US-designed system. The reverse may also be true of a US-designed system applied in the United Kingdom.

Coding systems should thus be compared on specified tasks and for given contexts, and the results should only cautiously be generalized to other tasks or contexts. Equally, the poor performance of coding systems on tasks outside the scope of their design should not necessarily reflect negatively on their intended performance.

Conclusions

Clinical languages are created for a variety of different purposes, and the great differences in their structure and size reflects those origins. Originally designed for use by humans as they label clinical records to help with codifying and analyzing population level events, they are now being used in an entirely different way. With clinical texts now computerized, clinical languages are used to identify specific events or elements within individual patient records. To do this requires a sometimes nuanced understanding of what is written in the text. Where humans are fairly adept at interpreting natural language, doing the same task automatically remains challenging – and it is the subject of Chapter 24.

Discussion points

1. How likely is it that a single terminology system will emerge as the international standard for all clinical activities?

2. Take the two terminologies created from the discussion in Chapter 22, and now merge the two into one common terminology. As you go, note the issues that arise and the methods you used to settle any differences. Explain the rational (or otherwise) basis for the merger decisions.

3. Are there any clinically significant differences that could arise out of the different codings in Table 23.7? What impact could such differences make on epidemiological surveys of population health?

4. You have been asked to oversee the transition from ICD-9-CM to ICD-10-CM at your institution. What social and technical challenges do you expect to face? How will you plan to deal with them?

5. Why was the Rosetta Stone important, and what lessons does it have for modern terminology building?

6. Many countries take a major terminology such as ICD and customize it to suit their local needs. Discuss the costs and benefits of this approach from an individual country's point of view. What could the impact of localization be on the collection of international statistics?

Chapter summary

1. The International Classification of Diseases (ICD) is published by the World Health Organization. Currently in its tenth revision (ICD-10), its goal is to allow morbidity and mortality data from different countries around the world to be systematically collected and statistically analyzed.

2. Diagnosis-related groups (DRGs) relate a patient's diagnosis to the cost of treatment. Each DRG takes the principal diagnosis or procedure responsible for a patient's admission and is given a

corresponding cost weighting. This weight is applied according to a formula to determine the amount that should be paid to an institution for a patient with a particular DRG. DRGs are also used to determine an institution's overall case-mix.

3. The Systematized Nomenclature of Medicine (SNOMED) is intended to be a general-purpose, comprehensive and computer-processable terminology. Derived from the 1968 edition of the *Manual of Tumour Nomenclature and Coding*, the second edition of SNOMED International is reportedly being translated into 12 languages.

4. The Read codes are produced for clinicians, initially in primary care, who wish to audit the process of care. Version 3 is intended, like SNOMED International, to code events in the electronic patient record.

5. SNOMED CT merges SNOMED RT and Read CT3 into an international terminology suitable for use in clinical information systems.

6. The Unified Medical Language System (UMLS) links the major international terminologies into a common structure and provides a translation mechanism among them.

7. Specialist terminologies are created to meet the need for fine-grained detail in specific professions or applications and are needed when one of the main general terminologies is inadequate to the task.

8. Coding systems should be compared on specified tasks, and results should only cautiously be generalized to other tasks and populations. Equally, the poor performance of coding systems on tasks outside their design should not reflect negatively on their intended performance.

CHAPTER 24

Natural language and formal terminology

> The problem was that every system of classification I had ever known in biology or in physical science was designed for mutually exclusive categories. A particular chemical element was sodium, potassium or strontium, but not two of those, or all three. An animal might be a fish or fowl, not both. But a patient might have many different clinical properties simultaneously. I wanted to find mutually exclusive categories for classifying patients, but I could not get the different categories separated. They all seemed to overlap, and I could find no consistent way to separate the overlap.
>
> *Feinstein, 1967, p 10*

Terminological systems are usually created with a specific purpose in mind. The International Classification of Diseases (ICD) was initially created to collect morbidity and mortality statistics. The Read codes were developed for primary care physicians, and SNOMED (Systematized Nomenclature of Medicine) was developed to code pathological concepts. As these systems grow, their use extends beyond their initial domain, and some systems are redeveloped as general purpose systems. It is often a declared intention that such general systems are complete and universal healthcare languages.

In this chapter, we first explore how the nature of human language limits the ability of terminologies ever to truly be complete or universal. Terminologies are just one kind of information model, and are subject to the same limitations inherent in all models, a foundational and recurring theme of this book. We also explore the pragmatic challenges faced in building and maintaining a terminology in an ever-changing world. The second part of this chapter examines the process of terminology assignment from a computational point of view. The basic steps involved in computer detection of data stored in clinical texts such as the patient record and the methods by which the assignment of a term or code is made to that text are summarized. The chapter concludes with an exploration of different natural language processing methods and their broader application in health and biomedicine.

24.1 The accuracy of coding health records is variable and never perfect

Coding is a process of data compression or summarization. The data captured in a record are scrutinized to decide which of a limited number of labels should be assigned to the entire record, for a specific purpose. It has been known for a long time that this process is imperfect and is associated with its own systematic biases (Romano and Mark, 1994). The 'view' of a patient created by the terminology likely varies among different terminological systems, each of which has a slightly different representation of similar concepts, reflecting partly the purpose of the terminology and partly the natural variations introduced in the development of the terminology.

Like any other measurement instrument, the coding process incorrectly labels some records by assigning a label to patients who do not warrant the label (false-positives) or failing to assign a label to patients who should have it (false-negatives). It thus becomes important to benchmark the accuracy of coded data before these data are used, for example, to support population health decisions. One large review of the accuracy of routinely collected data sets in the United Kingdom found an overall median accuracy of about 83 per cent, with considerable variation in accuracy rates among studies (50 to 98 per cent) (Burns *et al.,* 2012) These overall results are reflected in analyses of coding accuracy in other countries (e.g. Austin *et al.,* 2002; Henderson *et al.,* 2006; Lorence and Ibrahim, 2002).

Coding errors can arise for a number of reasons:

- There may be *errors in the patient record,* perhaps introduced by the clinician writing the record or because test results and reports from one patient end up in the record of another.
- Crucial *data may not be available* at the time of coding. Some laboratory tests, for example, may require weeks before a report is issued because the testing laboratory receives only a few requests and waits until it has accumulated a sufficient number to run the test in a single batch.
- Coding sometimes differs in the selection of a primary reason for an episode of care. However, *the notion of 'primary' is likely to be subjective.* Patients with multi-morbidity have more than one trigger for needing care. Is the hospital admission because the patient has lung cancer or because the patient has pneumonia associated with the cancer?
- Assignment of a code requires some understanding of the care process, and *coding quality varies with the coder's expertise* and with the coder's understanding of disease and the care process.
- *Data entry errors* add their own distortion to the data. A coder may intend to use the correct code but inadvertently enter the wrong one because of mistakes made when using a coding system (see Chapter 13 for a discussion of how such human factors are a cause of errors when using information technology).

24.2 Universal terminological systems are impossible to build

Although some of the inaccuracy in coding of patient records is related to errors in the process of code or term assignment, more foundational issues also bedevil the process. The terms and related concepts themselves are sometimes the problem. The ideal terminological system would be a complete, formal and universal language that allowed all healthcare concepts to be described, reasoned with and communicated. In the past, some researchers explicitly asserted that building such a singular and 'correct' language was their goal (Cimino, 1994; Evans *et al.*, 1994).

This task has two clear requirements – the ability for the terminological language to cover all the concepts that need to be reasoned about and the independence of the terminology from any particular reasoning task. Where alternative terminologies exist, they must be logically related so that one can be translated into the other. For example, if a set of clinical codes is extracted from a patient record, those codes should then be translatable into ICD codes or diagnosis-related groups (DRGs).

There are two fundamental obstacles to devising such a universal terminology. The first is the *model construction* problem. Terminologies are simply a way of modelling the world, and as we saw in Chapter 1, the world is always richer and more complex than any model that humans can devise. The second related issue is the *symbol grounding* problem (Norman, 1993). Words are labels, and as individuals we develop some cognitive match (or grounding) between a label and events we perceive in the world. Some labels are abstractions built out of other labels and may never be experienced at all – any theoretical construct falls into this category. So, it is no surprise that not everyone will match a label to exactly the same phenomena. If there is no way of guaranteeing a universal definition of a concept, then we resort to consensus processes in which most people agree on a label and its real world match.

Concepts are probabilistic but terminologies are not

It is perhaps intuitive to think that the words we use correspond to objective and clearly definable parts of the world. Words should clearly correspond to observable objects. However, cognitive studies of the way people form word categories have shifted us from the view that categories exist objectively. Research suggests that all concepts are relative and are structured around probabilistic prototypes.

These concept prototypes at the *basic level* are the product of pooling many examples observed from the world (see Box 22.1). They capture aspects common to all the examples and exclude aspects that are not universally shared. Thus, the qualities of prototypical categories are generally true only of the examples they classify (Figure 24.1). For example, most people would say that flight was a property of birds and cope with the fact that some birds are flightless. The category 'bird' has no pure definition. The same is true of the words used in healthcare. The term 'angina' corresponds to a wide variety of different presentations of pain. Students are taught the classical presentations of angina, but they quickly learn that there are many variations to the general case.

Concept creation is thus a learning process of generalization from example. The creation of concept prototypes is an ongoing part of human activity because language development tracks changes in our view of the world (Goldberg, 2006). We also saw in Chapter 22 that different hierarchies can be created, depending on the attributes used to link terms. One could categorize a bird by attributes such as size, colour, whether it can fly, wingspan and so

6. On balance, should the electronic health record be mainly structured or unstructured text? Perhaps consider the balance between the loss of narrative and the workflow impact of asking clinicians to enter structured text and the challenges of automatically assigning labels to narrative text afterward.

7. Take a segment of text from a clinical record. Define a set of Markov models you think would be sufficient to interpret the lexical roles of all the words in that paragraph correctly. Compare your model set with those of others, and try to understand why any differences exist.

8. Apply the Markov model you built in question 7 to another paragraph that you have not seen previously. How well do the models perform now?

9. Your organization is moving from ICD-9 to 1CD-10. Discuss the challenges of the move from a technical and then from a socio-technical perspective.

Chapter summary

1. The process of coding introduces systematic biases and is associated with errors. Errors may be associated with gaps in the patient record or with the expertise or subjective view of the individuals doing the coding, or they may be associated with human factors problems associated with the coding system.

2. There is no pure set of codes or terms that can be universally applied in healthcare. There is consequently no universal way in which one healthcare language can be mapped onto another. Terms are subjective, probabilistic, context-dependent and purposive, and they evolve over time.

3. There are two fundamental and related obstacles to devising a universal terminological system. The first is the model construction problem – terminologies are just models of the world, and the world is always richer and more complex than any model. The second is the symbol grounding problem. The words we use to label objects or events do not necessarily reflect the way we think about objects, nor do they accurately map to defined objects or events.

4. The process of terminology growth and alteration introduces huge problems of maintenance and the very real possibility that the system will start to incorporate errors, duplications and contradictions. Introducing changes into a mature terminological system becomes increasingly expensive over time, and as a consequence maintaining a terminological system will become increasingly expensive over time.

5. Compositional terminological systems are intended to be easier and less expensive to maintain and update than enumerative systems. Early in construction, the cost of building a compositional system is higher than the cost of an enumerative system, but over time the cost is lower because maintenance costs are comparatively lower.

6. Labelling clinical texts with concepts requires natural language methods, which approach a text at multiple levels, starting with individual words, then looking at text structures and finally interpreting text against external knowledge such as an ontology.

7. Natural language methods have widespread application in health, by assisting with search engine design, text mining and text summarization and generation, as well as question answering.

PART 7

Clinical decision support and analytics

CHAPTER 25

CHAPTER 25

Clinical decision support systems

As we have seen throughout this book, clinicians face many substantial challenges when making decisions. They must contend with the ceaseless change in clinical evidence and the resulting challenge to keep knowledge up-to-date. Decision-making is best when there is pre-existing experience with a specific circumstance, but it is challenging when conditions are new to the reasoner. Finally, our decisions are distorted by inherent biases both in the way we estimate probabilities and in the way we assign utilities to outcomes.

We can assist human decision-making and improve the decision outcome in many circumstances by using a *clinical decision support system* (CDSS). These computer programs range from systems that simply present data to aid a human make a decision, some generating prompts or alerts when a clinician's decision appears problematic, through to systems with the capability of making decisions entirely on their own.

In this chapter, the focus is on the different applications for CDSSs in clinical practice, particularly with regard to where clear successes can be identified. Chapter 26 takes a more technological focus and looks at the computational reasoning processes that can underpin a CDSS and the main computational approaches used to encode and apply knowledge. Chapter 27 focusses on how such knowledge is created, through machine learning, data analytic and computational discovery methods.

25.1 Decision support systems can assist with a wide variety of clinical tasks

Knowledge-based systems are the most common type of CDSS in routine clinical use. Sometimes known as *expert systems,* they contain clinical knowledge, usually about a very specifically defined decision task or problem, and apply this knowledge to patient-specific data to generate reasoned conclusions. Clinical knowledge is typically encoded as a set of decision rules, e.g. 'if the patient data equal x then do y'.

CDSSs can be applied to any well-structured decision problem. The extent to which theses systems are actually used depends on the mix of tasks and patients seen, the

Box 25.1
Common limitations
of clinical decision
support system
evaluation studies

- A focus only on post-system implementation evaluation of users' perceptions of systems rather than outcomes.
- Reliance upon retrospective designs that are limited in their ability to determine the extent to which improvements in outcome and process indicators are causally linked to the CDSS.
- Failure to adopt a comprehensive approach to evaluation using a multi-method design to capture the impact of CDSSs across multiple dimensions.
- Ignoring sociotechnical issues and instead concentrating on assessment of technical and functionality issues, which may explain only a small proportion of information technology failures.
- Expectations that improvements will be immediate. In the short term, there may even be a decrease in productivity. Long-term evaluations are often required to show improvements both materialize and be sustained.

Nevertheless, the growing pool of evidence on the impact of CDSSs in delivering improvements in the quality, safety and efficiency of health is promising, mainly in relation to alerts, reminders and PSSs. The following sections demonstrate the value of CDSSs in clinical practice, but also the complexity of the evaluation task, the gaps in our knowledge about their effectiveness and the richness and variety in form of decision support.

Improvement in patient safety

There is now a clear body of research that provides evidence of the effectiveness of CDSSs in increasing the safety of patients by reducing errors and adverse events and by increasing the proportion of appropriate and safe prescribing decisions.

Reduction in medication errors and adverse drug events

The interest in electronic prescribing systems is based upon the evidence that medication errors are among the most significant causes of iatrogenic injury, death and costs in hospitals (Kohn et al., 2001; Thomas et al., 1999). In the United States, it is estimated that more than 770 000 people are injured or die each year in hospitals as a result of adverse drug events (ADEs) (Kaushal and Bates, 2001). The greatest proportion (56 per cent) of preventable ADEs occurs at the drug ordering stage, and only 4 per cent of ADEs occur during dispensing (Bates et al., 1995). Errors occurring at the earlier stages are more likely to be intercepted (48 per cent) compared with those occurring at the administration stage, which are usually missed.

CPOE systems help automate the process of prescription by assisting in the generating and communicating of computerized scripts. CPOE systems typically include a prescribing decision support module to check the prescription produced. Electronic prescribing does reduce the risk of medication errors and ADEs. Multiple studies of the effects of CPOE on medication error rates show a 13 to 99 per cent relative risk reduction, a 35 to 98 per cent reduction for potential ADEs (i.e. errors which did not result in injury but had the potential to do so) and a 30 to 84 per cent reduction for actual ADEs (Ammenwerth et al., 2008).

Computer-assisted prescriptions were shown in one study to contain more than three times fewer errors than handwritten prescriptions and to be five times less likely to require pharmacist clarification (Bizovi et al., 2002). The first convincing evidence that such performance translates into a clinically significant reduction in medication errors and ADEs comes from two seminal studies undertaken at the Brigham and Women's Hospital in Boston, Massachusetts (Bates *et al.,* 1998; Bates *et al.,* 1999). The CDSS was developed specifically by the hospital and offered clinical decision support such as allergy alerts and suggested drug doses.

The first study demonstrated a 55 per cent reduction in potential ADEs following system implementation (Bates *et al.,* 1998). The rate of ADEs fell from 10.7 per 1000 patient days to 4.9 per 1000 patient days. The second study (Bates *et al.,* 1999) demonstrated an 86 per cent reduction in potential ADEs 4 years after implementation. Unexpectedly, the number of life-threatening potential ADEs increased from 11 per cent before implementation to 95 per cent after 5 months. The majority of these related to orders regarding potassium chloride because the CDSS system made it easy to order large doses of intravenous potassium without specifying that it be given in divided doses. Once changes were made to the order screen for this drug, the number of life-threatening intercepted potential adverse events fell to zero. If these systems were implemented nationwide in the United States, the study authors calculated that they would prevent approximately 522 000 ADEs each year, and if only 0.1 per cent of such errors was fatal, more than 500 deaths would be avoided (Birkmeyer *et al.,* 2000).

This mixed benefits picture – one of overall benefit but of also smaller but unanticipated risks and harms – is most likely the rule and not the exception with CDSSs and probably most clinical information systems. Electronic prescribing systems, either through their design or functionality, have now been shown to introduce new error classes at the same time that they minimize existing ones. The particular system errors introduced do depend on the specific design of a system and workflow, and as such different systems manifest different error profiles (Westbrook *et al.,* 2012). In one study, about 40 per cent of the residual error rates after implementation of electronic prescribing were system rather than prescriber related (Westbrook *et al.,* 2013).

Clinicians themselves are often unaware of the mistakes made when they prescribe. In one study, doctors stated that they were unaware of the potential clinical situation leading to 44 per cent of clinically significant ADEs identified by an alert system (Raschke *et al.,* 1998). However, alerting a clinician to an ADE may not result in changes to clinical behaviour, possibly because in many cases no change is necessary. A US ambulatory setting study of 2.3 million people's prescriptions identified 43 000 alerts for 23 697 people. In 15 per cent of instances when the physician was contacted, the alerts resulted in an immediate change in drug management, and in a further 9 per cent, there was agreement to review management at the next patient visit (Monane *et al.,* 1998).

Enhancing prescribing behaviour

CPOE systems functions that have the potential to change prescribing patterns and result in more cost-effective drug selection include:

1. Prompts to use a less expensive generic drug when a more expensive drug was initially ordered.
2. Presenting a list of suggested drug doses for each medication ordered.
3. Highlighting recommended frequency of dose for specific intravenous drugs.
4. Prompts to suggest recommended orders for specific patient groups (e.g. order an anticoagulant for patients prescribed bed rest).

Box IC2.1
The Turing test

How will we know when a computer program has achieved an intelligence equivalent to that of a human? Is there some set of objective measures that can be assembled against which a computer program can be tested? Alan Turing was one of the founders of modern computer science and artificial intelligence, and to this day his intellectual achievements remain astonishing in their breadth and importance (Figure IC2.1). When he came to ponder this question, Turing brilliantly side-stepped the problem almost entirely (Turing, 1950).

In his opinion, there were no ultimately useful measures of intelligence. It was sufficient that an objective observer could not tell the difference in conversation between a human and a computer for us to conclude that the computer was intelligent. To cancel out any potential observer biases, Turing's test put the observer in a room, equipped with a computer keyboard and screen, and made the observer talk to the test subjects only using these tools. The observer would engage in a discussion with the test subjects by using the printed word, much as one would today by exchanging e-mail with a remote colleague. If a set of observers could not distinguish the computer from another human in more than 50 per cent of cases, then Turing believed that one had to accept that the computer was intelligent.

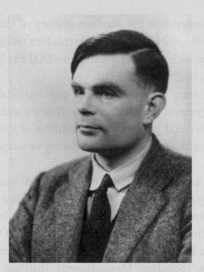

Figure IC2.1
Alan Turing.

Another consequence of the Turing test is that it says nothing about how one builds an intelligent artefact, thus neatly avoiding discussions about whether the artefact needed to in any way mimic the structure of the human brain or our cognitive processes. In Turing's mind, it really did not matter how the system was built. Its intelligence should be assessed based only upon its overt behaviour.

There have been attempts to build systems that can pass Turing's test. Many have managed to convince at least some humans in a panel of judges that they, too, are human. A version of the Turing test in which only 30 per cent of judges had to be convinced was first passed on 7 June 2014 by a 'chatbot' at the University of Reading in the United Kingdom, albeit in controversial circumstances – the program that won cleverly impersonated a Ukrainian teenager who did not speak English as a first language.

Further reading
Muggleton, S. (2014). Alan Turing and the development of Artificial Intelligence. *AI communications* **27**(1): 3–10.
Turing, A. M. (1950). Computing machinery and intelligence. *Mind* **59**(236): 433–460.

one extreme, we find a camp that believes that intelligence emerges from the interaction of simple reasoning agents and their environment. These workers in the field of robotics and 'artificial life' are inspired by biology and cite, for example, the way a colony of ants can exhibit intelligent behaviour even though each ant is a relatively simple creature. As a consequence, they see little need to fill AI systems with detailed knowledge about the world (Steels and Brooks, 1995).

At the other extreme sit those researchers who believe that an AI system needs to have its intelligence pre-programmed (e.g. Genesereth and Nilsson, 1987). These researchers believe that an AI system should contain large amounts of knowledge about the world. This knowledge could need to cover everything from what most of us would call common sense through to complex technical knowledge that could come from a textbook.

In reviewing the emerging field of AI in medicine in 1984, Clancey and Shortliffe provided the following definition:

Medical artificial intelligence is primarily concerned with the construction of AI programs that perform diagnosis and make therapy recommendations. Unlike medical applications based on other programming methods, such as purely statistical and probabilistic methods, medical AI programs are based on symbolic models of disease entities and their relationship to patient factors and clinical manifestations.

Much has changed since then. Today, the use of statistical methods sits side by side with symbolic approaches to disease representation, and the decision to use one or the other is pragmatic, and not philosophical. The importance of diagnosis as a task requiring computer support in routine clinical situations also now receives much less emphasis (Durinck *et al.*, 1994). The strict focus on the medical setting has broadened across the healthcare spectrum, and instead of AIM systems, it is more typical to describe them as *clinical decision support systems* (CDSSs). Intelligent systems today are thus found supporting medication prescribing, in clinical laboratories and educational settings, for clinical surveillance or in data-rich areas such as the intensive care setting.

CDSSs are by and large intended to support healthcare workers in the normal course of their duties, by assisting with tasks that rely on the manipulation of data and knowledge. An AI system could be running within an electronic patient record system, for example, and alert a clinician when it detects a contraindication to a planned treatment. It could also alert the clinician when it detects patterns in clinical data that suggest significant changes in a patient's condition.

Along with tasks that require reasoning with clinical knowledge, AI systems also have a very different role to play in the process of scientific research. In particular, AI systems have the capacity to learn, leading to the discovery of new phenomena and the creation of clinical knowledge. For example, a computer system can be used to analyze large amounts of data and look for complex patterns within the data to suggest previously unexpected associations. Equally, with enough of a model of existing knowledge, an AI system can be used to show how a new set of experimental observations conflicts with the existing theories.

Although there certainly have been ongoing challenges in developing such systems, they actually have proven their reliability and accuracy on repeated occasions (Shortliffe, 1987). Much of the difficulty experienced in introducing them has been associated with the poor way in which they have been incorporated into clinical practice, either solving

In this case, the inference engine would produce a ranked set of conclusions, based upon statistical likelihood, with asystole being most likely explanation of a zero heart rate. One of the most common probabilistic inference rules used in expert systems is Bayes' theorem (see Chapter 8).

Belief networks provide a structure to modelling statistical associations

For many clinical decisions, we can do better than write multiple rules and instead can structure the decision process, in effect creating a set of linked rules that can guide reasoning. One example of a more structured approach to machine representation of statistical knowledge is the *decision tree* (see Chapter 8).

More often, probabilities in a CDSS are expressed using a *belief network,* which is a more generalized way of representing probability relationships among different events than a decision tree and is similar to a finite state machine. Belief networks are also often called Bayesian networks, influence diagrams or causal probabilistic networks. They find great use in temporal reasoning tasks, in which the state of a system evolves over a period of time.

Finite state machines were introduced in Chapter 15 as a way of connecting related clinical events. A finite state machine represents processes as a series of different states and connects them together with links that specify a *state transition* (see Figure 15.3). In a probabilistic network, the states represent clinical events such as the presence of a symptom or diseases, and the links represent conditional probabilities among the events (Figure 26.1). Typically, each node is assigned a probability that represents its likelihood in the population in question. Next, connections between nodes record the conditional probability that if a parent node is true, then the child node will also be true.

Bayes' rule is typically the inference procedure used on belief networks. So, for example, if we are told that certain clinical findings are true, then based upon the conditional probabilities recorded in the belief network, Bayes' rule is used to calculate the likelihood of different diseases. Often networks are many layers deep, and the inference procedure essentially percolates through the network and calculates probabilities for events. Intermediate nodes

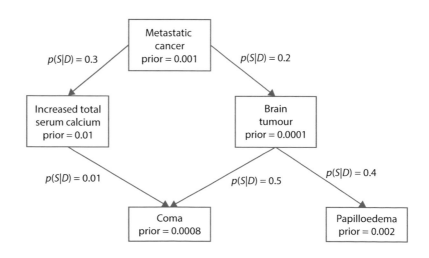

Figure 26.1
A simple Bayesian belief network for metastatic cancer. The prior probability of each event is recorded at the node representing it, and the conditional probability of one event giving rise to another is encoded in the links between the nodes. (After Cooper, 1988.)

between clinical findings and diseases may include intermediate pathophysiological states such as right-sided heart failure.

Several potential restrictions with belief networks may limit their usefulness in some clinical situations. First, Bayes' rule in its traditional form works only for independent events, as we saw in Chapter 8. Belief networks, however, may need to record dependent states, and alternative formulations to Bayes' rule, designed for such dependencies, must be used in such situations. Second, probability values may not always be available to build the network.

Interestingly, decision trees and most belief networks record two different types of knowledge. Each branch in a tree or link in a network expresses a probability, but the structure of the tree or network is *declarative*. In other words, we create a logical structure of events and then add probabilities to guide the navigation of the structure. Thus, although the formal statistical basis of Bayesian inference is attractive, the actual construction of network structures has a much weaker theoretical base, and it can be very empirical, based on the understanding of the individuals creating the structure alone. This is not a trivial point because the choice of states to include in the network and the way they are or are not connected strongly influence the behaviour of the network.

Markov processes can represent the time evolution of a system

There are a number of related approaches to modelling sequences of states and probabilities that are in one way or another related to belief networks. *Markov chains,* in particular, are a common way to record a directed graph or sequence of states in a process and the probabilities linking them, For a process to be a Markov process, it needs to be memoryless – in other words, only the current state has a role in determining the next state, and the history of where one comes from in a graph does not matter.

Markov models are used to simulate the time varying risks of different states, and the transition probabilities we assign to the models are based upon a given period of time – the Markov cycle. For example, in Figure 26.2, the probability of staying well or having an infarct would be estimated from population data over a defined period such as a month or a year, as would all other transition probabilities in the same model. We then repeatedly calculate the

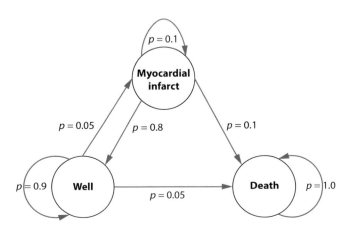

Figure 26.2
A Markov model showing probabilities of moving among three mutually exclusive states. The process is memoryless in that only the current state affects your likelihood of moving to another state. Probabilities leaving a node sum to 1.0, and self-links show the probability of staying in the current state at the next period in time.

Model-based systems are designed to use underlying disease models to allow for such first-principles reasoning (Uckun, 1991). Such models may be constructed from a variety of different representations. A model could be built from a set of mathematical equations describing the physiological relationships between measured variables. In pharmacology, kinetic models of drug distributions in the body, also known as compartmental system models, help work out whether a particular drug dose is therapeutic or toxic. *System dynamics* models treat the world as a set of stocks and flows and allow a wide variety of different processes to be modelled (see Figure 26.5); simulations can then be run under different initial circumstances, to see how the modelled system is likely to behave (Meadows, 2008).

As is often the case in healthcare, complete models of disease phenomena are frequently not available and our knowledge of processes and relationships among variables is incomplete. In such cases, there is evidence that clinicians carry around looser models, expressible in non-numeric or qualitative terms (Kuipers and Kassirer, 1984). Such qualitative representations of knowledge have now been formalized and can be used to capture useful portions of healthcare knowledge (Coiera, 1992). These representations have proved to be useful in diagnosis (e.g. Ironi *et al.*, 1990), for patient monitoring (e.g. Coiera, 1990; Uckun *et al.*, 1993; Widman, 1992) and for modelling relatively unspecified genetic or metabolic processes (see Figure 26.6) (Garrett *et al.*, 2007).

Model-based systems are perceived as being better at explanation than 'shallow' rule-based or probabilistic systems They are, however, more computationally expensive to run. Thus, there is a move among researchers to build CDSSs that combine the two, having both a facility to invoke deep models should they be needed and also being able to rely on efficient rules whenever they are applicable.

Important application areas for model-based systems are drug development, testing of new devices or health service configurations and modelling the likely impacts of a change in

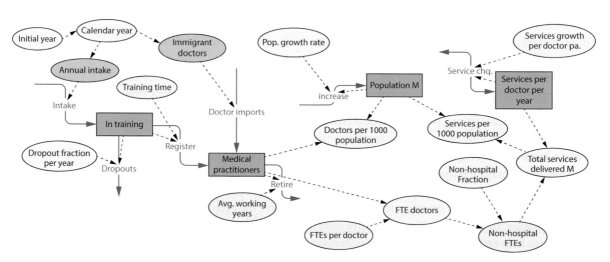

Figure 26.5   A system dynamics model of the processes governing the number of doctors working in a population and the services they provide. Squares represent 'stocks', which are dynamically varying quantities, and arrows are the flows between each stock. Ovals represent either input values to a stock or output values. Mathematical relationships between these entities are captured within the model elements and are not shown here. FTE, full-time equivalent. (Adapted from a model by Mark Heffernan and Geoff McDonnell, with permission.)

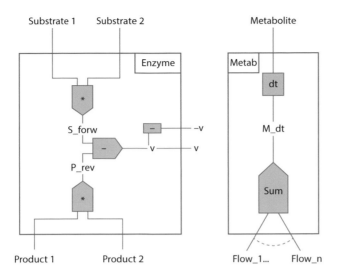

Figure 26.6 Qualitative models of basic metabolic reactions for an Enzyme (left) and Metabolite (right). V+ and V− are used to indicate the amount of consumption or production of the metabolite. Each variable (e.g. Substrate 1) represents the concentration of a different metabolite or substance. Links between these are built from a library of known mathematical relationships (sum, −, *, div) and more complex functions like the time derivative (dt). The model can be read as a consistent set of equations that specifies the general qualitative behaviour of each variable over time (increasing, steady, decreasing) but not specifying its actual quantitative value. forw, forward; M, metabolite; P, product; rev, reverse; S, substrate. (After Garrett et al., 2007.)

policy or governance. Models can become quite large and have layers that correspond to physiological, disease, health service delivery and population health (e.g. Eddy and Schlessinger, 2003). Such *in silico* trials can be conducted fairly inexpensively compared with their *in vitro* or real world counterparts, and they have a valuable role in establishing potential impact and clinical safety and avoiding real world trials that are flawed. In arenas such as policy or health service improvement, clinical trials may be too expensive, impractical or impossible, and *in silico* models provide our best guesses at real world impact, by assisting in intervention design and debugging, before they are implemented in the real world.

26.7 Intelligent decision support systems have their limits

Although CDSSs can perform to clinically acceptable levels, as with humans there are always inherent challenges in the reasoning process. These limitations need to be made explicit and should be borne in mind by clinicians who use automated interpretation systems.

Data

CDSS do not have eyes or ears, and are limited to accessing data provided to them electronically. Although this constitutes a potentially enormous amount of data to work with, it does mean that critical pieces of contextual information may be unavailable. Thus, interpretations need to be judged partly on the data available to the system when it makes its decision. This highlights the importance of designing an explanatory facility into expert systems, so that clinicians can understand the reasoning behind a particular recommendation by tracing the pieces of data that were used in its formulation.

The task of validating data may have to be one of the first tasks that an interpretative system undertakes. Although there are many clues available to suggest whether a datum represents a real measurement or is an error, this cannot always be decided based solely on the electronic evidence. There may be no way for a machine to decide that a transducer is incorrectly positioned or that blood specimens have been mixed up. Clinicians will always need to be wary of the quality of the data upon which interpretations have been made.

Knowledge

Knowledge is often incomplete, and this is an everyday reality in the practice of healthcare. Clinicians deal with physiological systems they only incompletely understand and have evolved techniques for dealing with this uncertainty. Although clinicians are able to acknowledge that they are performing at the edge of their expertise and adjust their methods of handling a problem accordingly, it is much more difficult to incorporate such a facility in a computer system.

Computers typically treat all knowledge equally. Although they are able to weigh probabilities that a set of findings represents a particular condition, they do not take into account the likelihood that some pieces of knowledge are less reliable than others. Further, most current systems are forced to use a static knowledge base. There are many techniques to update knowledge bases, but it will not necessarily be the case that a system incorporates the latest knowledge on a subject.

26.8 Conclusion

The technical problems associated with the process of knowledge acquisition mean that there are always potential mistakes in the system. Just as a normal computer program can contain 'bugs', so a knowledge base can contain errors because it is simply another form of program. Wherever possible, the explanation offered by a system should be examined to ensure that the logical flow of argument reflects current clinical understanding. As we saw in Chapter 8, the use of intelligent systems is also limited, not because of technical flaws, but because of the cognitive limitations of their human users. The next chapter explores the challenge of creating and updating the knowledge-bases destined for use within a CDSS, as well as for assisting in the more basic knowledge discovery task – the domain of health analytics.

Discussion points

1. Can machines think?

2. Which representational formalism is best suited to clinical decision support problems?

3. Which is the best reasoning method – a neural network, a Bayesian network, or a rule-based expert system?

4. If a CDSS needs to provide explanations in support of its recommendations, which technology approach would you take and why?

5. Think of five related logical statements of the form $A \Rightarrow B$, that together summarize knowledge about a particular task such as diagnosing a given disease. Now assume that one or two of the variables in the

statements are known to be true, and work out what else you can now demonstrate to be true, using both *modus ponens* and *modus tollens* as your inference procedures.

6. Using the Markov model in Figure 26.2, calculate the likelihood of each state over a sequence of four cycles.

7. Build either a system dynamics model (Figure 26.5) or a qualitative model (Figure 26.6) of the impact of antibiotic prescribing on the rate of antibiotic resistance in bacteria and hence on infection rates.

8. What negative consequence do you imagine could arise from using a CDSS?

9. If you were treating a patient, in which circumstances would you rely on information from a clinical trial to guide a decision, and when would you prefer to make a prognostic assessment based upon finding out what happened to past patients who are similar to the current patient?

Chapter summary

1. Once a task has been identified, the designer of a clinical decision support system (CDSS) needs to consider which reasoning method and which knowledge representation will be used. For example, the different reasoning methods one could use in arriving at a diagnosis may be the rules of logic or statistics, rules of thumb, neural networks and comparison with past cases. The knowledge representation chosen is closely related to the reasoning method.

2. An expert system is a program that captures elements of human expertise and performs reasoning tasks that normally rely on specialist knowledge. Expert systems perform best in straightforward tasks, which have a pre-defined and relatively narrow scope and perform poorly on ill-defined tasks that rely on general or common sense knowledge.

3. An expert system consists of three basic components.

    a. A knowledge base, which contains the rules necessary for the completion of its task.

    b. A working memory in which data and conclusions can be stored.

    c. An inference engine, which matches rules to data to derive its conclusions.

4. Although probabilities can be expressed in rules, it is more common for them to be captured in a belief network, which is a graphical way of representing probability relationships among different events, typically by using Bayes' rule to draw inferences.

5. Markov models are related to Bayesian networks and can simulate the probability of events over a number of time cycles, under the assumption that networks are memory free. Monte Carlo simulations help determine the statistical properties of such simulations over multiple cycles.

6. Neural networks are computer programs whose internal function is based upon a simple model of the neurone. Networks are composed of layers of neurones (or nodes) with interconnections between the nodes in each layer.

7. Model-based systems are designed to use process and system models to solve problems from first principles. These models may be constructed from a variety of different representations including mathematical models of physiological relationships, compartmental system models, system dynamics models, qualitative models or statistical models. *In silico* trials can simulate the impact of changing the initial conditions under which a model operates.

8. Clinical decision support systems are limited by the data they have access to and by the quality of the knowledge captured within their knowledge base.

Literature-based discovery

Discovery methods can be applied directly to the research literature, to uncover previously unsuspected associations. The Arrowsmith system is a classic literature-based discovery system, allowing a user to ask questions such as, 'Are there any things that are shared by patients with disease A as well as disease C?' Such questions allow insights about the management of one condition to be re-applied to the associated condition. In 1986, Don Swanson used Arrowsmith to connect papers about dietary fish oil with papers about Raynaud's syndrome. Some papers described how dietary fish oil reduced blood lipids, platelet aggregability, blood viscosity and vascular reactivity. Papers about Raynaud's syndrome noted that it was a peripheral circulatory disorder associated with and exacerbated by high platelet aggregability, high blood viscosity and vasoconstriction (Swanson, 1986). Swanson hypothesized that fish oil would thus be beneficial in the prevention and treatment of Raynaud's syndrome, a hypothesis that has since been tested and validated.

Biological model discovery

Beyond such associational discoveries, it is possible to use patient data to construct pathophysiological models that describe the functional relationships between various measurements. For example, a learning system can take real-time patient data obtained during cardiac bypass surgery and then create models of normal and abnormal cardiac physiology (Hau and Coiera, 1997). These models may be used to look for changes in a patient's condition if they are applied at the time they are created. Alternatively, if used in a research setting, these models can serve as initial hypotheses that can drive further experimentation. Model discovery finds great use in hypothesizing new genetic regulatory mechanisms, metabolic pathways and disease processes.

Drug discovery

One particularly exciting application of learning systems is to discover new drugs. The learning system is given examples of one or more drugs that weakly exhibit a particular activity, and based upon a description of the chemical structure of those compounds, the learning system suggests which of the chemical attributes are necessary for that pharmacological activity. Based upon the new characterization of chemical structure produced by the learning system, drug designers can try to design a new compound that has these characteristics. Traditionally, drug designers synthesized a number of analogues of the drug they wished to improve upon and experimented with these analogues to determine which exhibited the desired activity. By using discovery tools, the development of new drugs can be speeded up and the costs significantly reduced. Statistical analyses of drug activity have been used to assist with drug analogue development (exploring different molecular variations of a drug), and computational discovery techniques have been shown at least to equal if not outperform chemists, as well as having the benefit of generating knowledge in a form that is easily understood by them (King *et al.,* 1992).

27.3 Manual knowledge acquisition methods can guide interactions with human experts to reveal the basis for their judgements

The first CDSSs used manually developed knowledge bases, typically obtained by describing the reasoning used in the heuristic judgements of experts. These rules described the features associated with different diagnoses and were used to generate a differential diagnoses or suggest the most appropriate therapy for a clinical case. The methods used to craft these rules ranged from the highly informal to the systematic use of robust processes designed to elicit the rationale underpinning human judgements. Despite their often qualitative nature, these 'manual' methods remain an important model building tool, both used alone and to help guide automated processes. In the latter situation, although we may have huge data sets with very many data types, the process of automated model building often needs direction from those who understand the problem domain – for example, identifying which patterns are interesting or which data types are most likely to be significant in shaping an outcome.

There are several classic approaches to *knowledge acquisition* or *knowledge engineering,* and these are very similar to qualitative methods widely used by researchers when they seek to answer a variety of other questions (Cooke, 1999; Olson and Rueter, 1987; Welbank, 1990):

Interviews

Especially early in the process of understanding a decision task, interviews can be very illuminating. Both unstructured (free flowing) and structured (following a question script or describing a typical scenario) interview methods can be used. Structuring interviews is more appropriate when there are clear questions to be answered, and unstructured approaches are more useful in the very early sense-making stages of the process. Interview data can be collected on anything from note form through to full video recording.

Observation

By observing humans as they make judgements, either in real world settings or, for difficult situations, in response to artificial cases, we can develop an understanding of the types of decision tasks they face and how they resolve them. Observers can take on active, non-participatory or highly passive roles and capture what they observe through notes, audio, images or video. Many of the methods used to analyze data are borrowed from anthropology and ethnography. These include *grounded theory* (Strauss and Corbin, 1994), in which researchers gather data in as neutral a way as possible and then seek the concepts implied by the data by constant comparison across data types, supported by additional data gathering. Researchers take note of how frequently new concepts emerge from the data analysis and seek the point of *saturation* (when no further new concepts are evoked) to indicate that the knowledge acquisition task is likely complete. Advantages of observation are the richness of the data that can be captured and their reflection of reality, as opposed to recollection. Disadvantages include the difficulty in capturing rare events or understanding complex processes by observation alone.

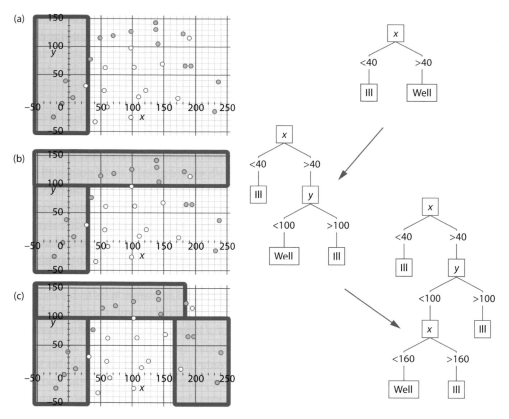

Figure 27.3 (a), (b) and (c) A supervised learning algorithm tries to find a function that partitions positive examples from negative examples. In this illustration, the learner is trying to discriminate between patients who are labelled as ill (purple) from well (white). Using two clinical measurements as the discriminating features (x and y), it builds a decision tree in stages, starting with a branch that best separates out the classes and then adding further branches to improve class separation.

partitions until it has fully separated the two classes, as shown in Figure 27.3 (b) and (c). A decision tree is the result, and it can be used as a CDSS, with the leaf nodes assigning a class to future unseen patients.

27.5 Statistical learning methods try to discover classes in data based on statistical properties of data distributions

Statistical methods find wide application in machine learning and discovery, given their long pedigree and natural fit to the task. Although they were initially created to allow humans to test hypotheses about how data can be separated into classes, statistical methods are equally suitable to be used in an automated setting, in which a learning algorithm tries to find the best discriminant function that can separate classes in a data set. Statistical methods can be used to discover trend lines, regression lines, rules and trees.

Bayesian inference methods use conditional probabilities between features and classes to create a classification model

Bayes' theorem has wide application in medical decision-making and can also be used as a supervised learning method. The frequency with which a feature is associated with a class is estimated from the training data set and is assumed to mimic the distribution in the wider population. The simplest approach is known as a *naïve Bayes classifier,* which makes the strong assumption that each feature is independent of every other feature (an assumption that is often not true and requires use of more complex methods to manage).

In the training stage, the algorithm calculates the probability that a given value for a feature (e.g. gender = female) is associated with the classes that are to be separated. A high probability (close to 1) indicates that examples with this feature value are likely to be in the positive class, and low probabilities (close to 0) predict that the example is likely to be in the negative class. Indeterminate probabilities (close to 0.5) indicate that the feature value is independent of either class and can be ignored.

The resulting feature probabilities for each class can then be used as a decision rule. When a new case is presented to a CDSS with the rule, the system calculates the probability that the case belongs to one class or another, and the class with highest probability is chosen as the most likely one for the case.

Hidden Markov models can be estimated from sequential data sets

Hidden Markov models (HMMs) were introduced in Chapter 26 and are a simple yet powerful method for dealing with sequential data. They can be used to interpret DNA data (e.g. knowing the probability that a guanine nucleic acid is followed by a cytosine in a genetic sequence can help in assembling a long sequence from a number of fragments). HMMs are used for time series analysis of phenotype data and for 'omics' data sets, and they find great application in text and language analysis.

In the learning setting, the task is to take a sequential set of data and to estimate the maximum likelihood or transition probability that one label is followed by another, based upon the frequencies found in the example sequences. The resulting model should approximate the transition probabilities to be found in the wider population of unseen examples. It can thus predict whether an unseen sequence belongs to the same class as the sequences in the training set. Conditional random fields (CRFs) can also be generated from example data, and they are increasingly replacing HMMs in many complex pattern recognition applications such as text interpretation.

Clustering algorithms identify classes in a data set by finding groups of data points that are close to each other in feature space

One common approach to unsupervised learning is to use a clustering algorithm. This family of methods typically calculates a *distance function* between data points and seeks to find arrangements of the data where the distance is minimized. The simplest method is known as *k-means clustering*, where k is the predefined number of clusters we are trying to

Figure 27.4
(a) A clustering algorithm first selects random points from a data space as centroids. (b) It then computes the distance between each and the nearest points. (c) If a point can be identified within each group with a shorter distance between all points, it becomes the new centroid. (d) When no better centroids can be found, the process stops, and we are left with our clusters, which should represent separate classes.

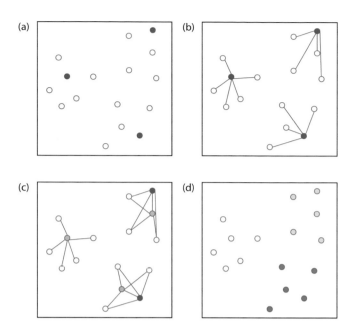

discover. In this approach there are two basic steps, which are repeated until no further improvement in class separation is possible. First, in the assignment step, we identify k points in the data set (initially randomly) and calculate the distance between each such point and its nearest neighbours (Figure 27.4). This distance is usually calculated as *Euclidian distance*, which is the sum of the squared distances between points in a cluster. In the update step, we seek a new centroid from the cluster that has the smallest within-cluster sum of squares compared to the current centroid. The process iterates until no better centroids can be found. The final clusters found depend heavily on the initial choices of centroid, and there is no guarantee with this simple method that an optimal partitioning of the data set has been found. As with many learning algorithms, the process is best repeated a number of times, so that the best performing model can be selected from the multiple learning trials.

27.6 Statistical learning theory has created a new class of algorithms that are better able to discover concepts from data

The motivation behind many of the algorithms described in this and the previous Chapters has been to mimic biological processes (e.g. neural nets), to apply well-understood statistical methods (e.g. Bayes' theory, Markov processes) or the emulation of how humans seem to learn (e.g. rules and decision trees).

Learning a model from data, as we have seen, can be thought of as finding a mathematical function that best separates data points into discrete classes. If we are trying to separate two classes of points in the *xy* plane, that function needs only to be a line. If we move to three dimensions, the function now needs to be a plane surface. With more than three data dimensions, our task is to discover the hyperplane that is best able to discriminate among classes.

Statistical learning theory emerged in the 1990s as a more principled and general approach to discovering such discriminant hyperplanes. These methods were also computationally tractable, meaning not only that the algorithms were capable of learning correct models, but also they were time and computer memory efficient while doing so.

Support-vector machines try to find the hyperplane that provides the maximum separation between classes

Statistical methods (e.g. linear regression, Bayes' theorem) and all the methods reviewed so far use every data point when computing a function to separate classes (e.g. Figure 27.4). In the *support-vector machine* (SVM) approach, we disregard those points that are obviously in one or another class. Instead, we focus only on those examples that are consequential or most difficult to classify – the points that lie closest to the potential line of discrimination among classes. SVMs are an example of a non-probabilistic binary linear classifier, which is capable of discovering hyperplanes that separate data with many dimensions (Cortes and Vapnik, 1995).

SVMs begin by trying to find any line or plane that is capable of separating data into different classes, as shown in Figure 27.5 (a), and there are usually potentially many such candidates. For each candidate, we find the points nearest it, from both the positive and negative examples of a class if it is a two-class task. Those points provide the evidential support of the goodness of the separation achieved, and together the set of points nearest to the plane become its support vector, as shown in Figure 27.5 (b) and (c). The learning task is to find the plane that gives the widest possible separation between the classes in the data set, so the distance between every candidate plane and its support vector is calculated. The plane with the widest separation between the points in its support vector is chosen as the best approximation of the function that separates the classes – the maximum margin hyperplane seen in Figure 27.5 (c).

Figure 27.5
(a), (b) and (c) There are potentially many lines that could separate two classes. For each such hypothesis (h_1, h_2), those points closest to the line constitute its support vector, and the distance (d+, d−) between the line and its support vector is computed. The line with the support vector that has the greatest distance or separation between the positive and negative points in its support vector (h_2) is chosen as the best function separating the classes.

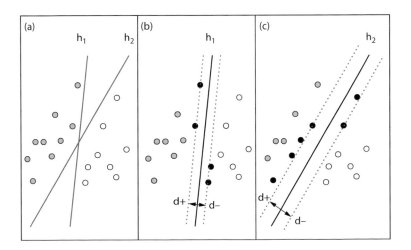

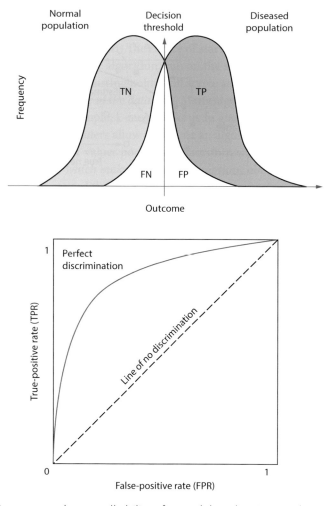

Figure 27.8   To measure the overall ability of a model to discriminate between two populations (e.g. normal and diseased), we measure true- (T) and false- (F) positive (P) and negative (N) rates at a given threshold value of a discriminating variable, e.g. body weight. We do this multiple times by varying this decision threshold value. For each threshold value, we plot the true-positive rate – TP / (TP + FN)– and the false-positive rate – FP / (FP + TN). The resulting curve is called the receiver operating characteristic curve and the area under this curve provides a measure of the goodness of discrimination.

We are thus looking for a model that is the best generalization of the data it was trained on (it is simpler than just a mere description of all the points). This degree of model generalization can be measured in many ways:

- The number of characters of symbols used to write a model down is one metric of model size, and we can simply compare models by counting the length of the string needed to write them down. We prefer the model with the *minimum description length* (or *message length*), which turns out to have a strong relationship with Bayesian model theory (Grünwald, 2007; Wallace, 2005).

- We can measure the Shannon information content of a model, also related to the description length. This can be thought of as a measure of how compressed the model is. A minimal model cannot be compressed any more, and an overly general model has plenty of padding that still can be removed. The *Akaike Information Criterion* (AIC) is a common measure of the goodness of fit or complexity of a model, and it penalizes models that have more parameters than comparable models (but it does not tell us whether the model is a good or bad one – that is the role of measures such as the AUC). A closely related metric is the *Bayesian Information Criterion* (BIC), but it gives a higher penalty to additional model parameters (Burnham and Anderson, 2002).

These measures of model fit to data can also be used to refine any models learned. For example, if the learning algorithm has built a decision tree, we can actively prune the tree by seeing what happens to model performance when particular branches are removed. The result of pruning is a more compact tree that has classification performance equivalent to that of the unpruned version. By definition, such a tree is a better generalization of the data and is therefore more likely to have better performance on unseen data because it is less likely to have been fitted to noise.

Conclusions

As clinical and health service data sets accumulate, we can use machine discovery methods to start to make sense of the many patterns we find there. The process of doing science is now one in which even hypothesis building can be automated to some extent. The process of learning is challenging, not just from a technical perspective (i.e. building the best model given a data set). The greater challenge is to realize that only some of the models that can plausibly be built are useful at any given time. The larger the data set, the more likely it is that something will correlate with something else. Deciding what is meaningful in such patterns requires some understanding of the context from which the data came and the purpose for which the model is needed.

Discussion points

1. When training a learning algorithm, we try to give it an equal number of positive and negative examples of a class. What would happen if one class had significantly more examples than the other (to become the 'majority class')?

2. You have been asked to analyze a hospital's medical records to look for reasons behind an unexplained spike in deaths. Do you use a supervised or unsupervised approach to learning?

3. You have trained a classifier on several hundred examples of patients with and without a disease, and it has an AUC of 0.95. When you use this classifier on patient records from another hospital, you discover that the AUC is now 0.63. How many reasons can you think of to explain this decrease in performance?

4. A binary classifier tries to guess whether a patient has a disease or not, based upon a blood test. As we vary the cut-off value that separates ill from well, using the test, the error rates will change. Here are two confusion matrices with raw number of errors for the classifier at two different blood concentrations of the measured substance. Which value of the blood test is better at discriminating health from disease, and why?

(a)

Cut-off: 1.3 mmol/L	Positive	Negative
True	30	8
False	3	15

(b)

Cut-off: 2.3 mmol/L	Positive	Negative
True	30	8
False	15	3

5. What method is used to train a neural network from examples?

6. What is the best method to choose if you want to train an algorithm that can discriminate between patients who have hypertension and patients with both hypertension and diabetes?

7. What is the curse of dimensionality?

8. Why does it mean when we say 'association is not causation'? If you needed to test whether there was a causal relationship between two variables, how would you go about it?

Chapter summary

1. Computational discovery methods take as input data from a process that needs to be understood, and they output models that may describe the process.

2. Discovery systems have three broad uses – (1) to create models that can be used within a clinical decision support system; (2) to be adjuncts in the scientific discovery process, helping scientists understand the meaning of data; and (3) in data analytics, to discover meaningful regularities in data with the goal managing a process such as running a hospital or health system.

3. Discovery systems can generate many knowledge representations including rules, networks, decision trees and deep or first-principles models.

4. Manual knowledge acquisition methods can be used when human experts are available to explain the knowledge needed for a task, and these methods are used to extract knowledge in a form useful for machine interpretation. Methods include observation, interviews, process tracing including think-aloud protocols, conceptual elicitation methods such as a repertory grid, case-driven knowledge acquisition such as Ripple-Down Rules and crowdsourcing.

5. Machine learning systems are either supervised, in which a data set comes with some class labels attached to the data, or unsupervised, in which data are unlabelled, and the learning algorithm needs to hypothesize its own classes.

6. Statistical approaches to machine learning include naïve Bayes, hidden Markov modelling and clustering.

7. Support-vector machines are an example of a non-probabilistic binary linear classifier that is capable of discovering hyperplanes that separate data with many dimensions by choosing only data points closest to the discriminating hyperplane.

8. The performance of learned models is determined by testing their ability to classify unseen examples correctly, and we measure true and false positive and negative error rates at different cut-off values of a discriminating variable. Pooling these measures creates the receiver operating characteristic (ROC) curve, and we measure the area under the curve to determine overall model performance.

9. We prefer the model that is the least complex when given two models that have the same classification performance, to minimize the risk of overfitting.

PART 8

Specialized applications for health informatics

CHAPTER 28

Patient monitoring and control

Many processes need to be observed over time, to make sure that they stay within pre-defined limits or to detect new, possibly risky states that require a response. At the level of an individual patient, we may track a patient's heart rhythm and electrocardiogram (ECG) because the patient is at risk of developing a dangerous arrhythmia. At the level of a health system, we often look for the emergence of infectious disease outbreaks or monitor the rate of adverse events across different institutions. This process of system observation and intervention is no more than the model-measure-manage cycle, which was introduced in Chapter 9.

When working at the level of patients, and especially when working with physiological signals, the tracking task is called *patient monitoring*. When we move to a population scale, it is more usual to talk about tracking as *population surveillance*. In this chapter, the focus is on monitoring patients over time, and in Chapter 29, we turn to population-level surveillance. Although the two topics have many differences, underlying both are standard statistical and biomedical engineering approaches to detecting time-varying events and triggering control responses.

Patient monitoring systems measure clinical parameters such as the ECG or oxygen saturation. They are clinically commonplace devices found in many acute care settings. Rather than simply displaying measurements for clinicians to interpret, these devices often employ computational reasoning methods to assist in the task of signal interpretation. Similar methods are used to design intelligent therapeutic devices such as patient ventilators or drug delivery systems. These devices first monitor patient status and then control the delivery of therapy to a patient automatically.

This chapter first covers the basic concepts underlying the analysis of time-varying signals. The various levels at which interpretation needs to occur are then reviewed, along with an introduction to the idea of statistical process control (SPC). The different roles intelligent monitoring and control systems have to play in healthcare are reviewed, and a discussion of the cognitive benefits and risks of relying on monitoring systems closes the chapter.

28.1 Dynamic signals can vary in both the time and frequency domains

The essence of any dynamic signal is that when we measure it at different points in time, the measured value changes. If that varying signal is plotted over time, a *waveform* is the result. Most dynamic signals of interest have the important property of *periodicity* – the waveform increases and decreases in value according to some regular cycle.

There are three basic attributes of any time-varying signal (Figure 28.1):

1. Amplitude – The greatest value the signal achieves as it varies over a cycle.
2. Frequency – The time it takes to complete one cycle.
3. *Phase* – The state a system is in at any point in time.

When comparing two otherwise identical repeating signals (e.g. sine waves) that are just offset from each other in time, we say they are 'out of phase' with each other. As shorthand, sometimes phase is recorded simply as the degree of offset between the two signals, usually measured from the origin.

Each of these properties can be analyzed, in different combinations, to provide three different views of a dynamic signal. Each view reveals different aspects of the process producing the signal, and it can be used to reason about what is happening to the process at any point in time and what may be done to keep it well controlled. The *time domain* provides the first and most natural view of a dynamic signal, by recording simply how a measured signal varies over time.

To obtain the second view of a signal we note that although most waveforms have a complex shape, for practical purposes any such complex can be deconstructed into a set of simpler component sine waves, a discovery made by the famous French mathematician Fourier (1768–30). Each such component sine wave has its own intrinsic frequency. Understanding this allows us to unpack any waveform into its component sign waves and record their unique frequencies. This frequency 'fingerprint' of a waveform provides us with our second view – the *frequency domain* – a time- and phase-free view of the signal (Figure 28.2). The mathematical process for converting a waveform into the frequency domain is known as a *Fourier transform*.

The third view typically used is of the changing phases of a signal over time – its *phase portrait*. In this time- and frequency free-free view, we graph the different values a system takes over repeated cycles. Consider, for example, a frictionless pendulum as it swings toward and then away from a central or zero point (Figure 28.3). In the time domain, it looks like a sine wave. In the frequency domain, we see a single frequency band, associated with that sine

Figure 28.1 Dynamic signals in the time domain are characterized by the duration of an individual cycle of the signal – its frequency, and the maximum value over the cycle – the amplitude. *t*, time.

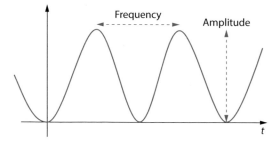

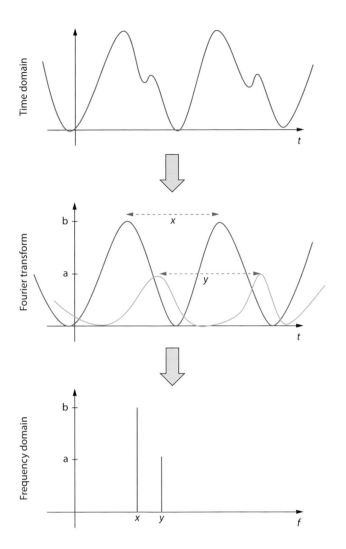

Figure 28.2
A complex waveform in the time (*t*) domain can be decomposed into its component sine waves, each with its own frequency (*f*) and amplitude. These different frequencies and their corresponding amplitude are then represented in the frequency domain.

wave. In the phase portrait, the pendulum's different states are captured by graphing its distance from the middle point and its velocity at that point. At some part of its cycle, it is moving toward the middle point, and at the opposite end of the cycle it moves away. The resulting phase portrait is circular, describing this ever-repeating motion. In a world with friction, the pendulum loses energy. Its phase portrait spirals toward the zero middle point, as the pendulum slowly loses velocity, and displacement from the middle point, as it comes to rest.

Examination of phase portraits is crucial to understanding the nature of a dynamic system. We can tell whether system states recur regularly, moving in a tightly defined band, and whether this recurrence has natural limits to the values the state can take. We can tell whether system states vary around a particular value – called an *attractor*. Independently of where a system starts in its phase space, its tendency is to be attracted toward the attractor value(s) (Figure 28.4). The portrait can also help tell whether a dynamic system is chaotic, which means both that initial conditions have a significant effect on final outcome, and also that it eventually traverses all its operating space at some point in time.

Figure 28.3
A frictionless repeating system such as a pendulum or a spring will produce a sine wave when we plot the distance it moves toward and away from a central zero point. To describe fully the state or phase of the system at any moment, we also need to describe how its velocity changes in the time (*t*) domain – another sign wave, half a cycle out of phase with the distance curve. Plotting the relationship between these two variables of distance and velocity, completely describes all the states the system can take – its *phase portrait*.

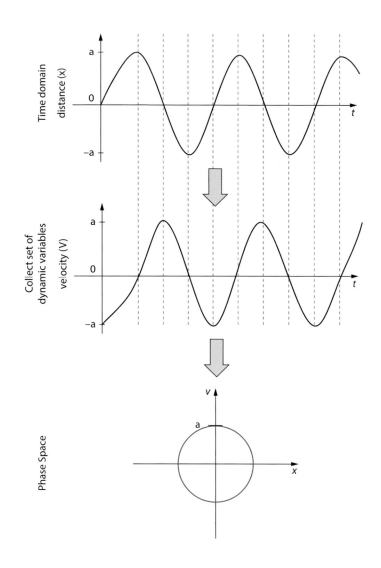

Figure 28.4
As a physical system such as a pendulum or spring slows down under friction, its phase portrait will circle the eventual position of rest, which is an *attractor* point for the system. *v*, velocity; *x*, distance.

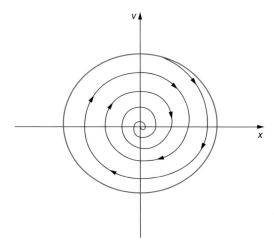

The ability to separate a complex dynamic signal into time and frequency domains, as well as into phase space, is crucial to informing our understanding of the processes that generate a signal. It is also significant because we can use time, frequency and phase information to help us monitor changes over time and interpret the changes that are observed.

28.2 Statistical control charts are a way of detecting when a dynamic system moves from one state to another

Most patients' tests, such as a blood test or blood pressure reading, are taken only sporadically. If we were to plot them in time, the graph would be very sparse. In a patient monitoring setting, the same measures are taken repeatedly, often for practical purposes continuously, thus producing a dense time line. For sporadic measures, such as blood test for cholesterol, it is typical to define a normal or abnormal value based on the population distribution of the measure in question (often normally distributed). Any reading within two standard deviations of the population mean is considered normal, and beyond that we define the test result as abnormal.

In the data-dense domain of patient monitoring, the task is a little different. Because we are gathering many data from a single individual, we are now able to compute statistics on what is 'normal' for that the individual alone. For example, we can repeatedly sample a measure over time, and as long as we are happy that the measure is stable, we can calculate what is called a *patient-specific normal range* (Harris *et al.,* 1980). This range allows us to detect when a new value falls out of the patient's own normal distribution of results. It is a good way of determining whether anything significant has changed significantly from previous measures over weeks or months. Importantly, a value in the patient-specific range does not mean that the patient is well, but only that the patient is stable.

The next feature of time-dense data is that we see much more moment-to-moment variation. The time plot of very normal patient measures thus is anything but a straight line. If we monitor such dynamic physiological signals, it is important to separate two sources of signal variation:

- The first is intrinsic or natural to any stable system that is being monitored and is often called *common cause variation*. Thus, a heart rate varies with level of exertion, body position and sleep. Blood pressures also vary over a day for similar reasons. Variation may also occur from noise on the signal, small variations in how a measurement is taken or indeed changes to the measurement system itself, such as different length leads, replaced skin transducers and so forth.
- New events can be imposed on top of a stable system, or the system can shift from normal to abnormal, with a resultant deviation in performance. Such changes are sometimes called *special cause variation*. For example, a patient may move from normal cardiac function into heart failure, with resultant significant changes in the patterns and values of cardiac function metrics. Equally, a pulmonary embolus would be a new event that would immediately cause changes to a patient's physiology.

When the monitoring task is to detect special cause variation (as opposed to fine-grained analysis of a signal), a standard approach is to build an *SPC chart* for the signal you wish to track.

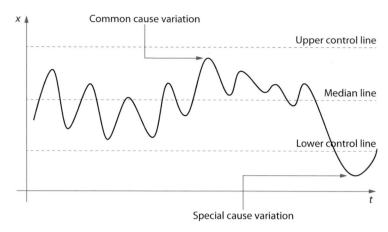

Figure 28.5   A statistical process control chart defines normal and abnormal boundaries for a time-varying signal, based upon historical data of signal variation. It ideally tolerates natural or common cause variation and should trigger an alert only when a signal exceeds its normal dynamic pattern because of a special cause such as a new significant event or change to underlying system behaviour. *t*, time; *x*, variable to be controlled.

The general approach to creating an SPC chart is similar to other learning approaches reviewed in Chapter 27. First, historical data are used as a training set. Rather than learning specific relationships in the data, however, analysis is limited to determining any natural (common cause) variability in the signal and to estimate some statistical boundaries of stable behaviour. Once such a statistical framework is built, it can be used prospectively to monitoring the signal and detect when special cause variation occurs. SPC has found widespread application in healthcare and has been used to monitor physiological parameters of individual patients, through to surveillance of system-wide signals of health service performance (e.g. Tennant *et al.*, 2007; Thor *et al.*, 2007) (Table 28.1).

A simple control chart consists of upper and lower bounds for a signal (its control limits) and a centre line typically based on the mean of past values (Figure 28.5). Control limits are often set at three standard deviations from the centre line, to allow for common cause variations. As long as future measures remain in the envelope of the control lines, the measure is said to be in control, or stable. There are many ways to calculate the centre line, including exponentially weighted moving averages (EWMA) and a cumulative sum (CUSUM) (Mohammed *et al.*, 2008). If the mean or centre line is calculated on a past data set only, then the control and centre lines will be straight. If, however, they are constantly recalculated as new data arrive, then they will drift as new measurements come in.

When a signal strays outside these control boundaries, this triggers a search for special cause variations that may need attention. The actual rule for triggering such an alert depends on the application and time available for recovery if an unexpected event occurs. Alerts may trigger after a number of measures repeatedly fall outside a control limit (to avoid triggering a false alarm from a transient variation), or they may trigger much earlier if there is clear movement of values toward the control limit (e.g. a trend line forms in the band between two and three standard deviations).

Table 28.1   Example variables that can be tracked by statistical process control

Biomedical and physiological variables

- Cardiovascular metrics e.g. heart rate, blood pressure, central venous pressure.
- Blood glucose and HbA1c.
- Peak expiratory flow rates.
- Urinary output.
- Oxygen saturation.

Biomedical instrumentation metrics

- Error in blood pressure measurements.

Other patient health variables

- Patient fall rate.
- Daily pain scales.
- Days between asthma attacks.
- Incontinence volume.
- Nausea after chemotherapy.

Clinical management variables

Time to complete a process element

- 'Door to needle' time (time from admission to thrombolytic therapy for acute myocardial infraction).
- 'Vein to brain' time (time from a blood test being taken to a clinician reading the reported test result).
- Average length of stay or mortality per patient diagnosis group in hospital, or in the intensive care unit.
- Time from discharge to general practitioner receiving a discharge summary.

Process event (and defect) rates

- Compliance with defined clinical indicators of care quality, e.g. measure the blood pressure of hypertensive patients in primary care.
- Percentage of stroke patients receiving a brain scan within 2 days.
- Days since last infection for patients with central venous lines.
- Number of operations since last complication.
- Days since last adverse event in a unit.
- Documentation of specific information items in the record, e.g. allergy, presenting condition.
- Place in record where specific information items are documented e.g. free text versus coded field.
- Deviations from protocol or guideline.
- Monthly medication errors.
- Out of hour "stat" blood test orders.
- Monthly cases of MRSA.
- Monthly admission rate for diarrhoea cases.
- Number of diabetic patients having an HbA1c test.
- Mortality after coronary artery bypass graft.

Clinical decision-making

- Number of patients with tonsillitis and without tonsillitis who were receiving antibiotics.

Patient experience

- Patient satisfaction or complaints.
- Staff ratings.
- Quality rankings for process of care.

Financial resources

- Average cost per procedure.
- Staff cost per shift.
- Number of support staff versus providers.

HbA1c, glycosylated haemoglobin; MRSA, methicillin-resistant Staphylococcus aureus.
After Thor et al., *2007.*

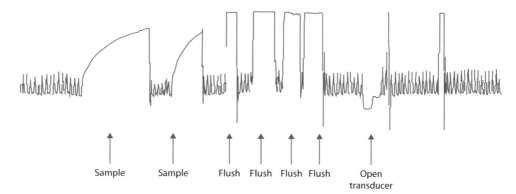

Figure 28.9
Examples of artefact
on the arterial blood
pressure channel.

blood pressure catheter line, can be detected by their unique shape (see Figure 28.9). Other artefacts can be managed by using *Kalman filtering* which computes a weighted average of the signal over a period of time and as a result smoothes out the effects of random and transient noise in the signal.

As we saw earlier, a Fourier transform can deconstruct a complex time-varying signal into a series of sine waves of different frequencies and allow us to manipulate a signal in the frequency domain. If noise is known mainly to distort a signal in certain parts of its frequency spectrum, then only that part of the spectrum can be attenuated or completely filtered out. A *low-pass filter* would eliminate components in the low-frequency range, to some cut-off point, and a *high-pass filter* achieves the reverse. A signal can then be reconstructed in the time domain and should now be much cleaner and better represent just the physiological measure we are after.

It is also possible to analyze frequency components of a signal to obtain information about the performance of the measurement system. When measuring a waveform such as arterial pressure, the signal may be *overdamped,* meaning the high-frequency signal components are attenuated compared with lower frequencies (similar to a sound wave being muffled in a padded room) (Figure 28.10). Damping may be caused by problems

Figure 28.10
The shape of arterial
pressure waves
varies with the
dynamic response of
the catheter
transducer. Analysis
of the waveform
frequency
components
following a fast flush
can assist in
detecting system
damping and assist
in optimizing
pressure
measurements.
(Adapted from
Gardner, 1981.)

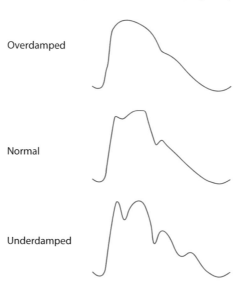

in the pressure measurement system, such as tubes that are too long, or air bubbles that are trapped in them. An overdamped blood pressure measurement underestimates systolic pressures and overestimates diastolic pressures. A pressure measurement can also be *underdamped* (similar to hearing sounds in a tiled room), in which high-frequency components are enhanced compared with lower frequencies. Overdamping overestimates systolic pressures and underestimates diastolic pressures. Analysis of a pressure signal in the frequency domain can detect these higher than normal frequency components for an underdamped system or lower than normal components in an overdamped system.

Multiple features can be extracted from a single channel to support behavioural interpretation

Having established that a signal is probably artefact free, the next stage in its interpretation is to decide whether it defines a clinically significant condition. This may be done simply by comparing the value with that of a pre-defined patient or population normal range, or using SPC lines. In most cases, simple thresholding is of limited value because clinically appropriate signal ranges can be highly context specific and require a richer model to interpret signal meaning. The notion of an acceptable range is often tied up with expectations defined by the patient's expected outcome and current therapeutic interventions. Even wildly abnormal values may have several possible interpretations.

These limitations of simple threshold based alarm techniques have spurred the development of more complex techniques capable of delivering 'smart alarms' (Gravenstein *et al.,* 1987). Much information can be extracted from a single channel if it can measure a time-varying and continuous waveform such as arterial pressure. For example, estimates of clinically useful measures such as cardiac stroke volume can be derived by analyzing the area under the curve of the wave (Figure 28.11).

Alterations in the behaviour of a repetitive signal can also carry information. Changes in the ECG are a good example. Features such as the height of the QRS peak help to label individual components within beat complexes. The presence or absence of features such as P

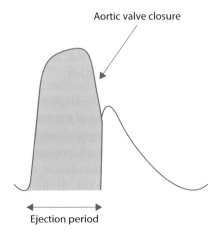

Aortic valve closure

Ejection period

Figure 28.11 Derivation of information from a waveform's shape. The systolic ejection area beneath the arterial pressure waveform gives an indirect measure of stroke volume. It is demarcated by the beginning of systole and the dicrotic notch caused by the closure of the aortic valve.

CHAPTER 29

Population surveillance and public health informatics

This chapter focusses on monitoring health events that occur across many individuals at a time. We are interested in monitoring human populations for many reasons – to make sure that they are receiving the quality of care they need, to see whether there are important changes to patterns of illness and to detect sudden and significant events that can affect health and health service delivery.

In Chapter 28, on patient monitoring, many core signal processing and interpretation concepts relevant to population surveillance were introduced. The approaches taken to capture and interpret signals at the population level are exactly the same as those for an individual patient. Signals must be acquired that are as free of noise as possible and at a sample rate that is sufficient to detect the process of interest. Statistical analyses can be used to detect important population changes, through the creation of process control charts or computational models such as neural networks and Markov models. These models need to be evaluated to ensure that they are sensitive and specific, to avoid false alarms or missed events – and the waste of public health resources associated with late detection or unnecessary investigation.

This chapter examines the way in which different informatics building blocks can come together – electronic records, decision support and communication technologies – to assist in the detection of population events such as outbreaks of infectious diseases.

29.1 Population surveillance occurs at all levels of the health system to monitor patterns of illness and the quality and safety of services and therapies

Population-level surveillance is a routine element of modern health service delivery. Monitoring may occur at any organizational level, starting internationally with authorities such as the World Health Organization (WHO), through to national and state governments, right down to the level of the practising clinician.

Public health systems have as their focus the health of the population. Surveillance is an essential precursor to any epidemiological analysis and public health response. Public health surveillance tasks include the following:

- *Biosurveillance* – The detection of new outbreaks of known diseases is a standard task for public health systems, both for those illnesses which have epidemic potential such as influenza and for sporadic outbreaks such as *Salmonella* gastroenteritis. Related tasks include the detection of emerging biothreats such as new strains of influenza, the shift of known infectious diseases to new geographical areas (perhaps because of intercontinental air travel, population shifts, climate change and immunization), the emergence of treatment-resistant strains of organisms such as methicillin-resistant *Staphylococcus aureus* (MRSA) or the intentional release of biological agents as an act of terror. Newly recognized infectious diseases are being reported at the rate of about 1 per year. More than 30 major more recent pathogens and diseases, including human immunodeficiency virus (HIV) and severe acute respiratory syndrome (SARS), have emerged since the 1970s. The number of such microbial threats continues to grow as infections cross the species barrier to people, as diseases and their vectors (e.g. ticks and mosquitos) adapt to new environments and as known organisms appear in more virulent forms.
- *Prevention and screening* – One way of reducing the burden of illness at a population level is to encourage disease prevention through vaccination (e.g. tuberculosis) and early screening for diseases (e.g. bowel and breast cancer). Tracking screening rates or lifestyle activities such as smoking rates assists in evaluating the success of public health programmes, as well as in assessing population risks.
- *Environmental health risks* – The impact of the environment on population health can be tracked by measuring water and air quality, as well as by testing for chemical traces that exceed safe standards and investigating geographical variation in measured levels. Epidemiological analyses of diagnoses at a population level, as well as local case reports, can identify geographically bounded outbreaks of illness, such as an unexpected cancer cluster in a particular locality or among employees of a particular organization. Such clusters may signal previously unidentified environmental health risks.
- Monitoring changing patterns in the *burden of disease* is another core epidemiological task. If we do not know the mix of diseases that need to be managed by a health service, then it is difficult to create the right mix of service elements to meet those needs effectively. Tracking changing patterns of illness is thus essential to developing well-targeted services that meet population disease-related priorities. For governments and for large health service delivery organizations, such data inform the allocation of existing services and resources, the development of new services and workforce recruitment and training. *Public health registries* for cancers and communicable diseases allow patients to be identified and their progress tracked over time, even if they change health providers. Chronic illnesses such as diabetes are particular foci for disease monitoring, as are predisposing conditions such as obesity, which can substantially affect health budgets, service demands and population well-being.
- *Emergency event monitoring* – Rare but predictable mass events require constant preparedness (e.g. tsunami readiness in low-lying areas that are prone to earthquakes, or

chemical spills or other large-scale hazards). This involves ongoing assessments of the readiness of emergency responders and front-line health services such as ambulance and paramedic services, emergency departments in hospitals, police or the National Guard, as well as testing civil procedures for rapidly mobilizing populations using these services.

For health service delivery organizations, monitoring *health service performance* is essential to ensure that the care that is delivered to the population is safe and effective. Surveillance takes place at all levels of service delivery, from individual clinicians who may wish to track their performance over time and benchmark themselves against others, through to small units such as primary care practices and outpatient departments, to hospitals, integrated healthcare organizations and state and national health services:

- *Quality of care* – Where standards of care exist, we can track the level of compliance with standards, using either simple indicators of the quality of care (e.g. ensuring blood pressure is measured and recorded for each primary care encounter with a patient with hypertension) or more detailed testing of conformance with clinical guidelines. Variations in compliance with such standards across different providers may be markers of differences in the burden of disease seen by them, differences in resources, education, culture and workflow or willingness to conform to the standard. At a patient level, we can monitor indicators such as adherence to treatment or health service utilization (how often patients visit a health service) and can ascertain with which section of the system they engage (e.g. primary care practice or the emergency department).
- *Safety of care* – Adverse events, in which a patient has been unintentionally harmed or was nearly harmed because of care delivered, may be reported to a central registry by either clinical staff or patients. These events are markers of the safety of care. Event rates and types can indicate the type of risks associated with different health services, and clusters of similar events are likely to indicate systematic problems requiring attention. Event reports, however, are not designed to collect statistically meaningful or representative samples of safety risks. Hospital records containing diagnostic codes that are assigned after discharge (e.g. International Classification of Diseases [ICD] codes) can provide more robust and statistically valid population-level estimates of harm suitable for epidemiological analyses. More general statistics such as hospital-acquired infection rates, surgical complication rates, length of stay and death rates can also indicate when a particular health service or provider is performing less safely than their peers. Such calculations are often confounded by local variations such as population age, ethnicity or socioeconomic status, and epidemiological analysis requires significant adjustments to try to account for such sources of variation.
- *Monitoring service effectiveness* is another core function for service delivery organizations. Data gathered from electronic records systems and computerized physician order entry systems allow the calculation of important metrics such as the turnaround time from an order being placed to a laboratory returning a result and to the result's being reviewed by the ordering clinician. Clinical processes are also trackable, and measurements of waiting time for a booking or to be seen in an emergency department, as well as metrics such as the time to create and receive a discharge summary, are key performance indicators of a clinical service (see Table 28.1). Measuring performance such as computer network downtimes or computer response

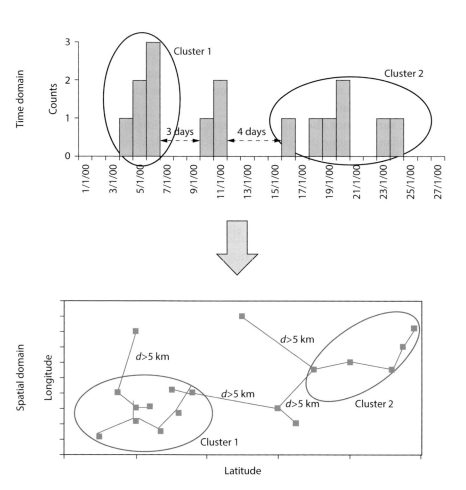

Figure 29.2 Counts of infected cases over time may be unable to resolve whether there is a new outbreak of an infection or not. Transforming data from the time domain into a spatial or map view may show cases clustering in space around particular locations, which is much more suggestive of an outbreak. *d*, distance. (Adapted from Gallego *et al.*, 2009.)

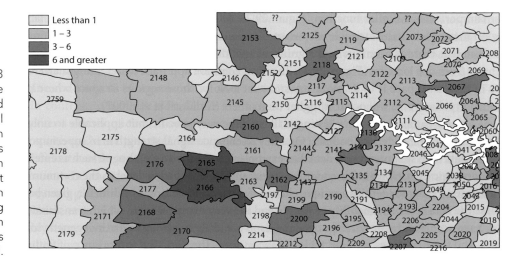

Figure 29.3 Mapping case counts onto defined geographical regions assists in identifying areas with higher infection rates and can direct public health resources to tracking down sources of an infection, as well as mapping the spread.

Multiple data sources are used for biosurveillance to ensure that early signals of outbreaks are available

The rapid identification of outbreaks and the implementation of control measures are crucial in limiting the impact of epidemics, both in preventing more casualties and in shortening the period during which stringent control measures are needed. One of the specific challenges faced by public authorities is the short window of opportunity between cases first being identified and a second wave of the population becoming ill through person-to-person transmission. During that window, public authorities need to identify the organism or agent and may need to commence prevention strategies such as mass vaccination, isolation procedures or administration of prophylaxis.

Yet many recent infectious disease outbreaks have been characterized by delayed recognition or public health response. Such delays diminish the window of opportunity to mount effective response measures and are likely to be costly to society. It was estimated that, in Canada, a 1-week delay in the implementation of control measures for SARS resulted in a 2.6-fold increase in the mean epidemic size and a 4-week extension of the mean epidemic duration (Wallinga and Teunis, 2004). Deaths from anthrax would be expected to double if the recognition delay for an attack with this agent increased from 2 to 4.8 days (Wein *et al.*, 2003).

Traditional infectious disease surveillance systems are vulnerable to incomplete and delayed reporting of public health threats (Box 29.1). Given the potential for widespread and large-scale civilian casualties in the event of an emerging disease or other large-scale event, much effort is thus focussed on developing surveillance systems that use multiple data sources to detect and report suspected outbreaks rapidly.

In one study, callers to the UK National Health Service (NHS) help line provided the earliest reports of the influenza season and augmented community-based surveillance programmes (Cooper *et al.*, 2008). Laboratory reporting of notifiable diseases can be speeded up by the introduction of automated data extraction and electronic communication to public health departments. Electronic laboratory reporting (ELR) can double the number of reports received. One study detected 91 per cent of 357 illness reports, compared with 44 per cent through the manual system (Effler *et al.*, 1999). Further, electronic reports arrived an average of 3.8 days earlier than manual laboratory reports. Electronic reporting thus significantly increases the total number of notifications and improves their timeliness and completeness (Panackal *et al.*, 2002).

Pooling records from emergency departments at different hospitals allows automated surveillance of chief complaints and provisional diagnoses. Other clinical reporting sources that can be used include primary care and outpatient presentations, intensive care or general hospital admission and discharge data. Laboratory process data are also valuable. For example, the number of laboratory requests for cerebral fluid microbiology can be used as an early surrogate indicator of a potential outbreak of encephalitis and meningitis.

Non-clinical data sources can also provide early indication of an outbreak, such as absenteeism in schools and childcare centres or patterns of over-the-counter sales of cough or anti-diarrhoeal medications from pharmacies and supermarkets. Social media, microblogging reports and Internet search logs for a specific symptom or syndrome from a given location are also very useful adjuncts to traditional laboratory or clinical case reporting (Figure 29.4).

from a hospital laboratory reporting system can be monitored to see whether they trigger criteria for infections that need to be reported to a public health authority. Such alerts can inform local infection control staff to attend to potentially significant infection and can also be sent to public health authorities. A similar approach can apply to hospital policy rules for laboratory data, to identify potentially significant hospital-acquired infections (Kahn *et al.*, 1993).

Detection and response to an infectious outbreak depend on multiple communication pathways and channels

No two outbreaks are likely to unfold in the same way because of variations in the organism, the health of the population and the state of civil, emergency and health services in geography. There are, however, clear communication pathways that would typically be used. Clinicians who have identified a potential case must communicate this to public health organization capable of initiating a population response. Government public health regulations usually specify which conditions should be notified to authorities immediately by telephone and which diseases require only standard laboratory reporting. Once alerted, public health authorities must rapidly communicate with all clinicians working in the community, the public health system and the public, to raise the level of awareness so that clinicians and the public are able to commence responding in an appropriate manner. The execution of such a communication strategy requires both a robust communication infrastructure and a well-organized plan for sending the right messages to the right individuals.

We can deconstruct this process into a series of interconnecting communication flows that evolve as an outbreak or an epidemic unfolds and a biosurveillance system comes into action (Figure 29.5):

1. A sentinel presentation of patient(s) to a clinician occurs in the absence of prior evidence of an outbreak.
2. The clinician consults colleagues or evidence resources such as an online system of journals, texts and paper guidelines.
3. The clinician sends appropriate patient specimens to the laboratory for testing.
4. The clinician sends a report to the public health authority before the laboratory result is received.
5. The SSS identifies signal of a potential (pre-diagnostic) outbreak from clinical records or from less specific population data sets such as social media.

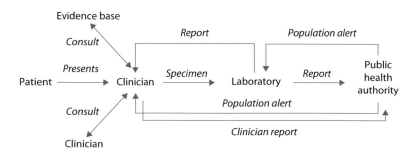

Figure 29.5
Biosurveillance and infection outbreak response rely on multiple communication flows.

6. The laboratory identifies an infectious disease agent of public health concern in a patient's specimen.
7. The laboratory notifies the referring clinician.
8. The laboratory notifies the public health authority.
9. The public health authority rapidly develops a message, which contains instructions that are as clear as possible and sends out a communication to laboratories and clinicians in the geographical region considered under threat, to warn of a potential outbreak or epidemic and to indicate clinical and laboratory signs to scan for, as well as to commence the disaster response and management plan. There is always a challenge of balancing the content of this communication to alert the professionals against creating alarm in the community. When required, the jurisdictional public health agency notifies the WHO about public health emergencies, according to the International Health Regulations.
10. New patients present to the clinician after the public health authority warning.

If we consider clinicians to be an event detection system, then in normal circumstances their likelihood of suspicion of an emerging infectious disease is typically low. Consequently, it is the role of public health authorities to 'calibrate' physicians to a higher degree of suspicion during periods of suspected or confirmed outbreaks. In such cases, the need is to maximize the reach of communication, by aiming to maximize the audience reached without raising undue public concern.

The United Kingdom has an emergency 'cascade' system called Public Health Link, which operates in this way. Public Health Link is an electronic urgent communication system to health professionals that is initiated in the office of the Chief Medical Officer (CMO) (similar to the Surgeon General in the United States). Messages cascade from the broadcasting health authority to a set of regions, each with the responsibility of contacting the clinicians in their area, by using the channels designated by clinicians ahead of time. Thus, urgent messages are sent to health authorities for onward cascade to nominated professionals, who may include general practitioners, practice nurses, community services pharmacists, medical directors in NHS Trusts and so forth.

The system contains a pager alert mechanism so that health authorities are aware when a message has been sent. Messages are classified for cascade within either 6 (immediate) or 24 hours (urgent). The system aims to reach every clinician in the NHS in 24 hours. Urgent and immediate communications from the CMO on public health are transmitted on average 15 times a year and are most likely to be connected with issues about drugs, infections, vaccines or other public health matters. As well as being cascaded, the health link messages are archived at a Web site, where they can be viewed.

Social media are powerful communication channels for public health messaging and co-ordination of responses to events of pubic importance such as outbreaks or emergencies. Social media can be used for one-way public broadcasting of health messages and as emergency broadcast channels (Thackeray *et al.,* 2012). They can also be used as a mechanism to track first-hand accounts of citizens, enriched with video, audio and GPS location data (Merchant *et al.,* 2011). Social media sites can help establish emergency communication cascades and buddy networks or communicate emergency department locations and current waiting times. The Red Cross has developed smart phone apps that help people create an emergency plan and share it with others. During the 2010 Haiti earthquake, social media

Box 30.2
(Contd.)

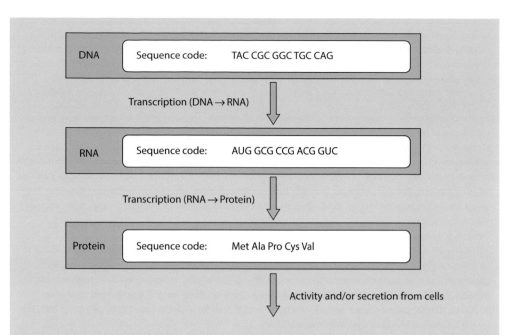

Figure 30.1
The flow of genetic information from DNA to RNA to protein. This simplified diagram shows how the production of specific proteins is determined by a DNA sequence and mediated by the production of RNA.

(T). In addition, RNA forms a single strand, not a helix. Thus, the basic RNA alphabet is *ACUG* instead of the DNA alphabet *ACTG*. The specific form of RNA that codes for proteins is called *messenger RNA* (mRNA). A diagram of the genetic information flow, from DNA to RNA to protein, is illustrated in Figure 30.1.

Structure and processing of RNA transcripts

Genes are not necessarily continuous on a DNA strand. Instead, most genes are made of both *exons* (the portions of the gene that will be translated into mRNA) and *introns* (portions that will not appear in the mRNA, but are 'spliced out' during transcription). Introns are not inert, however. They can have functions including control of the transcription process through promoter regions that can turn transcription on or off. Thus, the existence of a gene in an organism's DNA does not mean that the gene will actually be expressed as a protein because the process of transcription is regulated. This explains why different tissues in the same body can behave differently, as well as why possession of a gene does not mean that an organism will exhibit the gene in action. Further, introns are not always spliced consistently. If an intron is left in the mRNA, an *alternative splicing product* is created. Various tissue types can flexibly alter their gene products through alternative splicing. In fact, some cells can use the ratio of one alternative splicing to another to govern cellular behaviour.

The mRNA molecule that has been generated is then exported through nuclear pore complexes into the cell's cytoplasm, where cellular machinery generates the protein described in the mRNA code. Specifically, a ribosomal complex, built from hundreds of proteins and special transfer RNA (t-RNA), undertakes the protein manufacture. Each sequence of three DNA or RNA base pairs (known as triplets or *codons*) codes an amino acid. A protein is thus built up from individual amino acids, which are added one at a time in a chain, as the ribosome reads along the mRNA sequence. Shorter sequences of up to about 70 amino acids are known as polypeptides.

Triplet codons exist for each of 20 amino acids (Table 30.2), and there is redundancy in this code because amino acids can be coded by different but unique codons. For example, there are 4 codes for alanine, and the initial GCU and the final GCG always code for alanine.

A ribosome need not start reading mRNA at the beginning of a sequence or only in one direction. This means that the actual protein built depends on where one starts to read the code and on the direction in which it is read. Depending on whether one starts at the first, second or third base pair of a triplet, there are three different *reading frames* possible in one direction (Figure 30.2). The translation of a DNA code

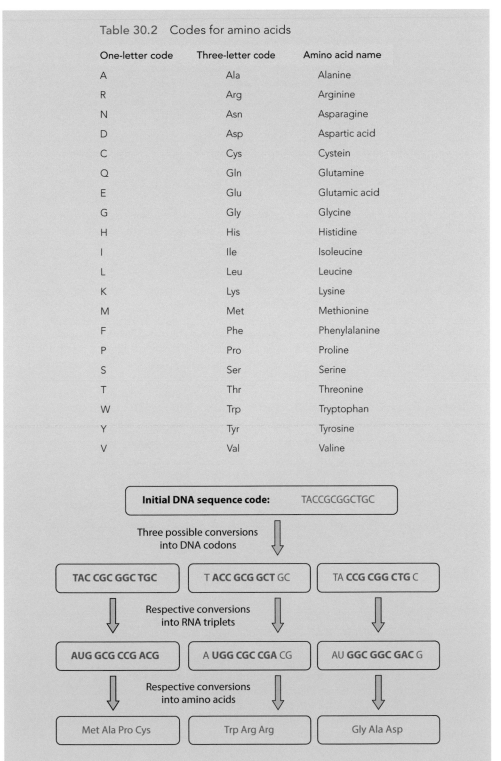

Table 30.2 Codes for amino acids

One-letter code	Three-letter code	Amino acid name
A	Ala	Alanine
R	Arg	Arginine
N	Asn	Asparagine
D	Asp	Aspartic acid
C	Cys	Cystein
Q	Gln	Glutamine
E	Glu	Glutamic acid
G	Gly	Glycine
H	His	Histidine
I	Ile	Isoleucine
L	Leu	Leucine
K	Lys	Lysine
M	Met	Methionine
F	Phe	Phenylalanine
P	Pro	Proline
S	Ser	Serine
T	Thr	Threonine
W	Trp	Tryptophan
Y	Tyr	Tyrosine
V	Val	Valine

Initial DNA sequence code: TACCGCGGCTGC

Three possible conversions
into DNA codons

TAC CGC GGC TGC   T ACC GCG GCT GC   TA CCG CGG CTG C

Respective conversions
into RNA triplets

AUG GCG CCG ACG   A UGG CGC CGA CG   AU GGC GGC GAC G

Respective conversions
into amino acids

Met Ala Pro Cys   Trp Arg Arg   Gly Ala Asp

Figure 30.2
Open reading
frames. There are
three possible ways
to read a sequence
of DNA into different
codons, and each
leads to translation
into one of three
different proteins.

(Contd.)

Box 30.2
(*Contd.*)

into amino acids, and hence the resulting protein, can be completely different in each of the three cases. A gene often specifies its reading frame by starting with a start codon for amino acid methionine, or AUG, to initiate transcription. In much the same way, codons TGA, TAA and TAG often act as stop codons. Thus, if you know where a protein-coding region starts (i.e. start codon) in a DNA sequence, we can build bioinformatics-enabled techniques to translate this DNA sequence into a corresponding amino acid sequence.

Processing of amino acid chains

Once a protein is formed, it has to find the right place to perform its function. It may be a structural protein that forms part of a cell's own cytoskeleton, as a cell membrane receptor or as a hormone that is secreted by the cell. A complex cellular apparatus determines this translocation process. One determinant of location and handling of a polypeptide comes from the structure of its final or *signal peptide*. The cellular translocation machinery recognizes this header sequence of amino acids. The ribosomal-mRNA complex can be directed to stop temporarily, move to a specific location and then resume protein assembly. Alternatively, some proteins are delivered after they are fully assembled, and chaperone molecules can prevent proper folding until the protein reaches its correct destination.

Epigenetic factors alter gene expression in normal development and disease

Whether a gene is expressed in an organism (i.e. is transcribed and leads to the creation of a protein) is partly regulated by the genetic structure itself, with structures such as promoter sites shaping whether a particular gene is active. There are also *epigenetic* processes (external to DNA) that can affect gene expression and are potentially inheritable. For example, *DNA methylation* (the addition of a methyl group to cytosine or adenine) affects whether a gene can be transcribed. Changing patterns of methylation are a normal part of the process of organism development, and they help explain how the same genome can differentiate into functionally different tissues. Methylation can also be altered by environmental factors, and aberrant methylation patterns may underpin the abnormal behavior of some cancer cell lines, independent of any mutation in the underlying genetic sequence (Craig and Wong, 2011). Aberrant

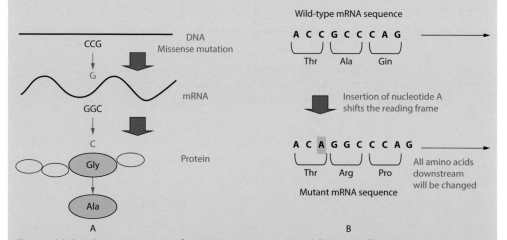

Figure 30.3 Consequences of missense mutations and frame-shift mutations. (a) A mutation change of C to G in a DNA strand will result in a G-to-C change in the mRNA. The mutant codon GCC will be translated as alanine instead of glycine. (b) The wild-type mRNA is translated to threonine (Thr), alanine (Ala), glutamine (Gln), etc. Insertion of the nucleotide A into the third position of the sequence would shift the entire reading frame by one base, so that the codons would now be translated as threonine (Thr) – arginine (Arg) – proline (Pro), with the ongoing amino acid changes continuing downstream.

methylation of RNA may also be associated with conditions such as obesity (Jia *et al.*, 2011). Histones, which are the proteins responsible packaging DNA into chromosomal structures, can also influence gene transcription and are altered according to their own 'histone code' by several biochemical processes including methylation.

Mutation is the cause of both normal variations and genetic disease

Mutations in DNA sequences occur all the time (Figure 30.3). The most common type of mutation is a simple replacement of one base pair in DNA with another (a *missense mutation*). Not all mutations affect protein assembly. If the original and new amino acids have similar properties, the change in amino acid sequence may have little effect on the activity of a protein. Mutations that delete nucleotides or insert new nucleotides into a sequence can have much more far-reaching consequences. For example, ribosomes may read all succeeding codons in the wrong reading frame (a frame-shift mutation), and all the amino acids attached to the growing protein will be changed.

Further reading

Craig, J. and N. C. Wong (2011). *Epigenetics: A Reference Manual*. Norwich, United Kingdom, Horizon Scientific Press.

Jia, G., Y. Fu, X. Zhao, Q. Dai, G. Zheng, Y. Yang, C. Yi, T. Lindahl, T. Pan and Y.-G. Yang (2011). N6-methyladenosine in nuclear RNA is a major substrate of the obesity-associated FTO. *Nature Chemical Biology* **7**(12): 885–887.

- Given the effect of a drug on various cancer cell lines, which gene or gene set is most predictive of the responsiveness of the cell line to the chemotherapeutic agent?
- Given a known clinical distinction, such as that between acute lymphocytic leukaemia and acute myelogenous leukaemia, what is the minimal set of genes that can most reliably distinguish these two diseases?

Bioinformatics has even enabled the re-synthesis of genomes and live organisms. In a seminal study, a 582 970–base-pair (bp) genome of *Mycoplasma genitalium,* the smallest prokaryotic pathogen, was synthesized. This synthetic genome contained all the genes of wild-type organisms, but researchers removed one gene that was responsible for virulence to block pathogenicity. They also inserted 'watermarks' between genes to identify the genome as synthetic (Gibson *et al.,* 2008).

30.2 High-throughput sequencing has allowed the large-scale discovery of genes and genomes

DNA sequencing was invented by Fred Sanger in 1975, and the number of human gene sequences that have been identified since has grown exponentially. The development of *high-throughput sequencing* in 2000 dramatically reduced the cost of sequencing, by moving the technology from a few major international research centres to being a routine pathology service (Mardis, 2008; Metzker, 2010; Shendure and Ji, 2008). We have full sequence data for many thousands of species and many human genomes (Kahn, 2011), and this production of gene data outstrips our ability to carry out functional assessments of the meaning of genes and genomes.

Figure 30.4
The cumulative
growth of
biomedical and
genetics literature
(dark purple) is
compared with DNA
sequences (light
purple) and the
relative cost of
sequencing 1 million
base pairs (black).

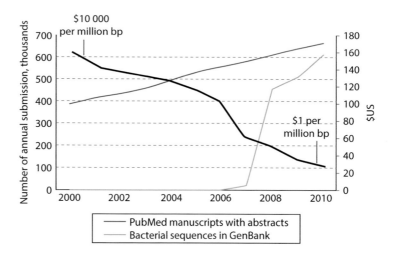

Figure 30.4 illustrates how the number of entries in one major international public gene sequence repository called GenBank is rapidly outstripping the growth of publications in PubMed/Medline, driven by a reduction in the cost of sequencing. It is a pointed demonstration of the great gap between our knowledge of the functioning of the genome and raw genomic data.

This volume of data must somehow be sifted and linked to human biology before it can have any meaning. Doing so exhaustively, reliably and reproducibly is plausible only with the use of sophisticated algorithms and computer technology. Even the storage, aggregation and access to such large volumes of sequencing data have become significant informatics challenges (Schatz *et al.*, 2010). As a benchmark, the *1000 Genomes Project* pilot data exceeded 7 Terabytes of sequences (Kahn, 2011).

30.3 Gene sequence alignment methods are needed to assemble DNA fragments into plausible sequences as well as to compare sequences

Neither conventional Sanger sequencing nor high-throughput sequencing can decode a whole genomic sequence at once. Both produce pieces or 'reads' of DNA that have to be joined together. Because the various sequencing techniques rely on different biochemical methods, they produce different types of raw data. Sanger sequencing produces high-quality reads about 1000 bp in length. Newer, more rapid methods produce much shorter and slightly lower-quality reads of 100 to 500 bp. Many billions of such short sequences can be produced during the sequencing of a single genome. Such massively parallel sequencing is a very cost-effective way to decode large numbers of genomes. Given these variations in measurement, different computational tools are needed for each. In particular, the assembly of huge numbers of short reads into longer and high-quality genomes is not a trivial task.

Sequence assembly has a number of basic steps (Scheibye-Alsing *et al.*, 2009). First, the degree of alignment or overlap between every fragment needs to be calculated. Next, we

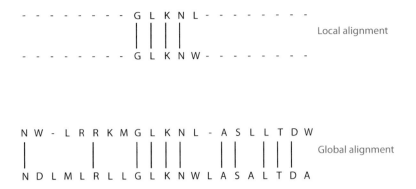

Figure 30.5
Global and local
alignments of two
hypothetical protein
sequences. Vertical
bars between
sequences indicate
the presence of
identical amino acids.
Dashes indicate
sequences not
included in the
alignment.

recognize that the process of creating the gene fragments involves breaking up and then read-ing multiple copies of the same genome. This means that the same information is repeated across different fragments, but each fragment may start and end in a different place. Thus, we choose two candidate fragments with the largest degree of overlap and assume that they both come from the same sequence, and we merge them, assuming the overlapping portion is a single and common sequence. The process is repeated until we have assembled what is known as the shortest common super-sequence.

Sequence alignment is the basic process that underpins assembly, and it can involve compar-ing two (pair-wise alignment) or more (multiple sequence alignment) DNA or protein sequences and searching for regions of similarity. Sequence alignment is useful not just for assembly, but also for discovering functional and structural information from sequences. Sequences that are similar probably have the same function or have a common ancestor. There are two forms of pair-wise alignment – global and local (Figure 30.5). With global alignment, an attempt is made to align the entire sequence. This may include gaps either in the middle of the alignment or at either end of one or both sequences. Sequences that are similar and of simi-lar in length are most suitable for this type of comparison. In contrast, local alignment looks for shorter stretches of two sequences with the highest density of matches.

Global and local alignments are accomplished by different algorithms. In local alignment, the alignment process stops at the end of regions of strong similarity, and higher priority is given to finding these local regions. *Sequence similarity* scores are calculated from the sum of the number of identical matches or conservative (high-scoring) substitutions, divided by the total number of aligned sequence characters. Gaps are usually ignored, but some algorithms employ penalties for gaps. *Percent identity* is the proportion of aligned positions in which sequence characters are identical.

Typical examples of global and local alignment algorithms are the Needleman-Wunsch and Smith-Waterman algorithms, respectively. The computational cost of such algorithms is in order of O *(nm)*, meaning that the amount of time required to complete the alignment grows linearly with the product of two sequence lengths *n* and *m*. It makes the task of search-ing for exact matches in a database containing hundreds of billions of bases of DNA sequence such as GenBank rather unwieldy. Not surprisingly, heuristic methods of approximate align-ment that may not guarantee an optimal solution but deliver faster results are often favoured. The classic approximate alignment method is BLAST or Basic Logical Alignment and Search Tool. BLAST looks for common patterns shared by two sequences and tries to extend these

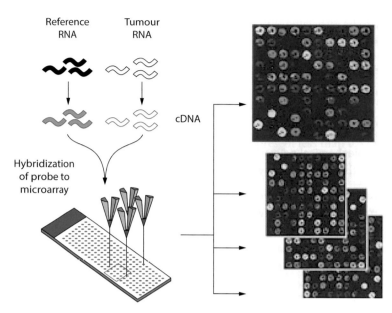

Reference RNA Tumour RNA

cDNA

Hybridization of probe to microarray

Figure 30.6   An overview of procedures for preparing and analysing cDNA microarrays and tumour tissue, using robotically spotted microarray hybridized to two samples, each stained with two coloured dyes. Reference RNA and tumour RNA are labelled with different fluorescent dyes (dark purple for the reference and light purple for tumour) and hybridized to a microarray. The slides are scanned with a confocal laser-scanning microscope, and colour images are generated. Genes that have been upregulated in the tumour appear light purple, whereas those with decreased expression appear dark purple. Genes with similar levels of expression in the two samples appear grey.

microarray is lit under a laser light and scanned. To determine the actual level of expression or concentration of DNA at a given probe, a digital image scanner records the brightness level at each grid location on the microarray. Studies have demonstrated that the brightness level is correlated with the absolute amount of RNA in the original sample and, by extension, the expression level of the gene associated with this RNA (Figure 30.6).

A characteristic of microarray technologies is that they enable the comprehensive measurement of the expression level of many genes simultaneously. For example, the level of RNA expression of a biological system can be measured under different control and test experimental conditions. Similarly, one can compare the expression profile of two such biological systems (two different tissues from one individual, or perhaps two different strains of an infectious organism) under one or several conditions.

Hybridization is the interaction of complementary nucleic acid strands. Because DNA is a double-stranded structure held together by complementary interactions (in which C always binds to G and A to T), complementary strands favourably bind or 'hybridize' to each other when separated.

30.6 Machine learning methods can assist in the discovery of associations between genetic and phenotypic data

Microarray data generate potentially many thousands of gene expression measurements from a few tissue samples, in contrast to typical clinical studies, which measure few variables over many cases (Figure 30.7). This high *dimensionality* of gene expression data poses

A typical clinical study
Variables (10s–100s)

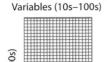

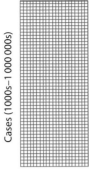

A typical genomic study
Variables (10 000s–100 000s)

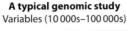

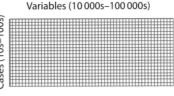

Figure 30.7
Although clinical studies typically measure few variables over many patients, gene studies typically measure many variables over few cases.

problems for standard analysis because not enough data may be available to solve all the 'variables' in the data set, thus leaving it relatively undetermined. For example, to solve a linear equation of one variable $4x = 5$, we need only one equation to find the value of the variable. To solve a linear equation of two variables, e.g. $y = 4x+b$, two equations are required. If we have tens of thousands of variables, but only hundreds of equations, then there will be thousands of potentially valid solutions. This is the essence of what constitutes an underdetermined system. In this context, we must use techniques that inform us most about the relationships among the variables of interest (and find out which ones are of interest). High-dimensionality data sets are well known in machine learning, so it is not surprising that these techniques have found their way into functional genomics.

Machine learning techniques can be either *supervised learning* or *unsupervised learning* techniques (see Chapter 27). In supervised learning, the goal is to find a set of variables (e.g. expressed genes measured with a microarray) that can best be used to a categorize data as belonging to a class of interest (e.g. a given disease). In unsupervised learning, the typical application is to 'data mine' either to find a completely novel cluster of genes with a hypothesized common function or, more commonly, to obtain a cluster of genes that appear to have patterns of expression that are similar to an already known gene (Figure 30.8). These techniques are thus distinguished by the presence or absence of external labels on the data being examined:

- *Supervised learning* – Before applying a supervised learning technique, each datum needs to be assigned a label. For example, we would label a tissue as coming from a case of acute myeloid leukaemia or acute lymphoblastic leukaemia before trying to learn which combinations of variables predict these diagnoses. Neural networks and decision tree learning systems fall into this category.
- *Unsupervised learning* – Here, data patterns must be analyzed without labels. For example, we may wish to find those genes that are co-regulated across all tissue samples. The variables (or *features*) can include measures of clinical outcome, gene expression, gene sequence, drug exposure and proteomic measurements. Unsupervised techniques include relevance networks, dendrograms and self-organizing maps that analyze every possible pair of genes to determine whether a functional relationship exists between them. The end result of such analysis may be a ranked list of hypotheses about which pairs of genes work together.

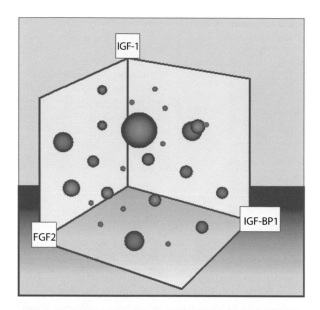

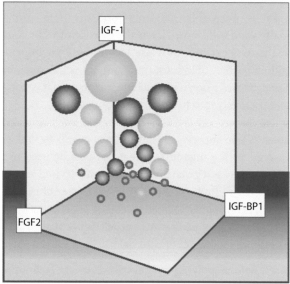

Figure 30.8   Clustering studies seek to determine whether genes are loosely or tightly coupled. If genes are tightly coupled, they will tend to form a tight cluster over any set of experiments (bottom figure). If genes are loosely coupled or even causally unrelated (top figure), then their expression levels will have little relation to one another and therefore tend to be scattered over a greater volume of the expression space. BP, binding protein; FGF, fibroblast growth factor; IGF, insulin-like growth factor.

However, the strengths of relationships found by clustering algorithms are not all necessarily novel or illuminating. A case could include several thousand gene expression measurements and several hundred phenotypic measurements, such as blood pressure or the response to a chemotherapeutic agent (Figure 30.9). A clustering algorithm may reveal significant relationships between non-genomic rather than genomic variables. For example, if one looks at

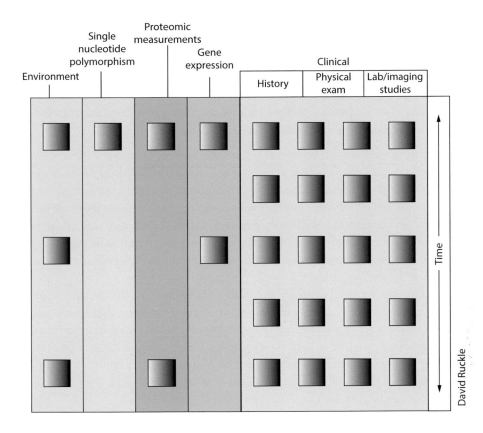

Figure 30.9
Clustering studies can involve phenotypic and genetic data sets. A full-fledged functional genomic study with clinical relevance involves multiple and quite heterogeneous data types, with missing data at different time points.

David Ruckle

the effect of different drugs on a cancer cell line, then these drug effects may be tightly clustered around drugs that are derived from one another. Similarly, phenotypic features that are highly interdependent, such as height and weight, also cluster together. These obvious clusters can dominate those that contain gene expression measurements.

30.7 Gene networks are responsible for many biological processes

Sometimes we can identify that alteration in a single gene is responsible for a particular disease. More frequently, however, genes do not work in isolation, but rather interact with each other to shape biological processes. Indeed, scientists now talk about the *interactome*, which represents all the different genetic and molecular network interactions that shape a biological process (Ito *et al.*, 2001).

It is not unusual in a genetic study to find that large numbers of genes are associated with a specific disease. The challenge is to understand in what way each gene may contribute to the end state.

There are several different reasons that two genes may be highly correlated with a disease:

● *Structural colocation exists* – 'Driver' mutations, which directly alter biochemistry and cause disease, may be collocated with more common 'passenger' mutations, which are often found with driver mutations but appear to have no biochemical role in disease. They are fellow travellers but not functionally related.

- *Both are members of a gene regulatory network* – One gene may create a protein that binds to the promoter site of another gene and turns it on.
- *Both create gene products that are part of a shared biochemical pathway* – Many biochemical reactions involve multiple molecules, and as a result several genes will need to be active for a biochemical pathway to be active.

Bioinformatics methods can be used to try to infer likely gene networks from expression data (Hecker *et al.*, 2009). Biological experiments provide both initial data about gene co-expression and additional data that come from experiments that try to understand the nature of gene relationships. Perturbations of the gene set can test to see which genes are related to a process and which are not. For example, gene deletion of 'knock-out' studies can be conducted to see how removal of a gene affects the expression and function of others. Typically, such experiments can be carried out only on model organisms such as yeast or mice, and they are not suitable for studying human biology.

An alternate experimental approach is to carry out expression studies over a period of time because a time series of gene studies can show evolving changes in gene expression as a biological pathway is activated. Different genes and their products become active at different times, and temporal ordering of such events gives us strong clues about the causal relationships among the biological entities being measured. When genes are annotated according to biological function, for example, using the Gene Ontology (GO), then the nature of functional relationships in a network can become clearer (Figure 30.10).

Machine learning methods can be used to infer the networks generated by such experimental data. Boolean networks (in which entities are either 'on' or 'off'), Bayesian networks and Markov models are all used for gene network representations. Given the large number of possible genes and proteins that may be candidates for a network, the task of feature selection (deciding which biological entities to include in the model) has a major impact on the accuracy of any model learned (Hecker *et al.*, 2009).

30.8 Bioinformatics analyses are limited by our understanding of biological contexts as well as computational complexity

There is little doubt that one of the tremendous accomplishments of the Human Genome Project is that it has enabled a rigorous computational approach to identifying many questions of interest to the biological and clinical community at large, and it has led to new ways to create therapies. However, the danger of this success is a kind of computational triumphalism, which believes that all the problems of disease will now rapidly be solved. Such a view is founded on several risky assumptions, mostly based upon a misunderstanding of the nature of models and, in particular, the complexity of biological models.

The first misunderstanding is that of genetic or sequence level reductionism. Most bioinformaticians understand that physiology is the product of the genome and its interaction with the environment. In practice, however, a computationally oriented investigator often assumes that all regulation can be inferred from a DNA sequence. It is assumed that one can

NP computability – Some problems are more difficult for computers to solve than others. The time it takes for a computer to solve a problem can be characterized by the shape of the 'time it takes to solve it' function. Some problems can be solved in linear time, thus making them easy to solve. More difficult problems are said to take polynomial time because the time to solve them is a function of polynomial form. A further class of potentially intractable problems has super-polynomial or exponential time solutions. These are known as non-deterministic polynomial time (NP) problems because it cannot be said ahead of time how long it may take to solve them once you start or even whether an answer will be found (although by luck you may just solve it).

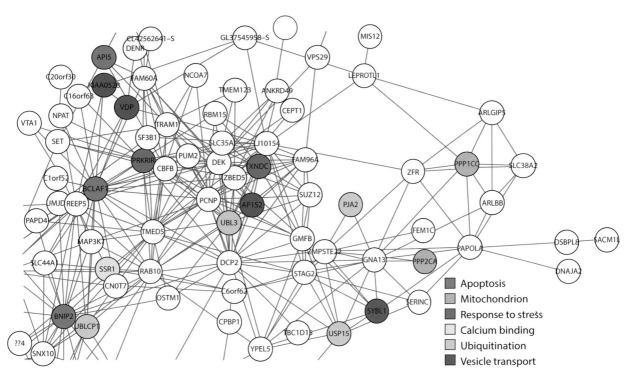

Figure 30.10   A portion of a gene-network from patients with amyotrophic lateral sclerosis. Genes are connected by an edge if the correlation of their expression profiles is significant, and genes are colour coded according to their biological function by using the Gene Ontology. (Adapted from Saris *et al.*, 2009.)

predict whether a change in nucleotide sequence will result in different physiology. However, cellular metabolic pathways are substantially more complicated than this and involve many levels of interaction among molecules.

The second dubious assumption is the computability of complex biochemical phenomena. One of the oldest branches of bioinformatics seeks to model molecular interactions such as the thermodynamics of protein folding. Studies by computer scientists suggest that the protein-folding problem is 'NP hard'. That is, the computational task belongs to a class of problems that are believed to be computationally unsolvable. Therefore, it seems overly ambitious to imagine that we will be able to generate robust models that can accurately predict the interactions of thousands of molecules from the transcription of RNA through to protein manufacture and function. We could call this ambition 'interactional reductionism'.

The final questionable assumption is the *closed-world assumption*. Both sequence-level reductionism and interactional reductionism are based upon the availability of a reliable and complete mechanistic model. That is, if a fertilized ovum can follow the genetic programme to create a full human being after 9 months, then surely a computer program should be able to follow the same genetic code to infer all the physiological events determined by the genetic code. Indeed, there have been several efforts, such as the E-cell effort (Takahashi *et al.*, 2003), which aim to provide robust models of cellular function based on the known regulatory behaviour of cellular systems. Although such models are important, our knowledge of all the relevant parameters for these models is still grossly incomplete. We now know, for example, that environmental factors can alter epigenetic controls (see Box 30.2), and they have a significant influence on the risk of disease. In recognition of this knowledge, the interaction of biological and environmental factors to cause disease is sometimes called the *diseasome* (Barabási, 2007).

Conclusions

Bioinformatics is a rapidly moving field, and although it is technically a subspecialty of health informatics, it has developed relatively independently of health informatics. However, as we have seen, the only way the functional genomic research programme can proceed is through the use of computational tools such as machine learning and through the use of phenotypic data, which are stored in the electronic health record. As such, it is inconceivable that clinically oriented bioinformatics will drift farther away from health informatics. Rather, the two are deeply entwined. Bioinformatics researchers depend on health terminologies, ontologies and electronic health records. Similarly, health informatics must contend with genetic and other '-omic' data in the clinical record and support genetically informed decision-making as routine. Thus, clinical decision support systems, protocol systems, clinical vocabularies and the patient record all must incorporate the fruits of the bioinformatics revolution and genomic medicine – a theme that is explored in Chapter 31, which looks at personalized medicine.

Discussion points

1. Could the Human Genome Project have succeeded without computer technology?

2. What is 'shotgun' sequencing?

3. What is a gene chip?

4. How reliable is BLAST as an alignment method?

5. What are the potential impacts of sequencing errors on genome analyses?

6. Describe how you think bioinformatics will alter the path of health informatics.

7. Describe how you think health informatics will alter the path of bioinformatics.

8. Explain how the temporal sequence in which different genes are expressed in a tissue can be used to infer a gene network.

9. What role did the Internet play in the development of bioinformatics?

10. Are your genes your destiny?

Further reading

Cristianini, N. and M. Hahn (2007). *Introduction to Computational Genomics: A Case Studies Approach.* Cambridge, Cambridge University Press.

Pevzner, P. and R. Shamir (2011). *Bioinformatics for Biologists.* New York, Cambridge University Press.

Chapter summary

1. Bioinformatics is the name given to the collection, organization and computational analysis of large biological data sets from genomics, proteomics and biochemistry.

2. Since DNA sequencing techniques were invented, the number of human gene sequences that have been identified through experiments has grown exponentially. In contrast, our knowledge of what these genes actually do has grown at a much slower rate, demonstrating the large gap that has now opened up between our knowledge of the functioning of the genome and raw genomic data.

3. Bioinformatics tools are needed to assemble fragments of gene sequences into plausible DNA strands and to align different fragments to determine their degree of similarity or overlap.

4. Heavily annotated reference DNA sequences are stored in archival databases and serve as gold standard comparators for future genetic studies. Draft sequence data are of lower quality, are typically unannotated and constitute the bulk of stored sequence information.

5. Functional genomics is concerned with identifying the biological function of genes, or groups of genes, to answer broad questions about the role of specific genes in health and disease.

6. Functional genomics is made possible by several measurement and analysis technologies:

   a. Methods to measure gene sequences and their expression rapidly in bulk. In particular, microarrays have enabled large-scale measurement of gene activity.

   b. Methods to collect clinically relevant (phenotypic) data that measure human disease states.

   c. Methods that correlate the gene and phenotype data and identify relevant associations.

   d. Methods that store and disseminate these biological data, such as gene sequence data sets.

7. Machine learning methods can assist in the discovery of associations between genetic and phenotypic data, and both supervised or unsupervised learning techniques play a major role.

8. Gene networks describe the way in which different genes interact or collaborate to produce a particular biochemical pathway. Machine learning methods can use temporal expression data to infer such networks by using binary, Bayesian and Markov models.

9. Although the Human Genome Project has been tremendously successful, there is danger of computational triumphalism, which believes that all the problems of disease will now be rapidly solved. However, such a view is based on several dubious assumptions, most founded upon a misunderstanding of the nature of models and, in particular, the complexity of biological models.

CHAPTER 31

Clinical bioinformatics and personalized medicine

I am not my genome.

Coiera, 2012

Every one of us is unique. That uniqueness has many sources – our personal context, hopes and desires. We are also biologically unique – although we share a common core genome, different racial groups have their own genetically distinguishing signatures, and each individual will likely have both small (single nucleotide polymorphisms or SNPs) and large genetic variations or mutations. Some mutations occur as a result of environmental damage – for example, chemical exposure or radiation – and can lead to cellular variants that cause cancer.

When we look at diseases such as cancer, genetics has made clear that what once were considered to be single diseases are in fact much more diverse, with many different genetic sub-types all leading to the same 'cancer' behaviour. We also know that as individuals, we respond to treatments in different ways. Some patients experience adverse drug reactions, some obtain little benefit and others benefit greatly – all the result of differences in our biochemistry that affect how a drug is transported, metabolized or excreted through the body.

The promise of *personalized medicine* (sometimes called *precision medicine*) is that a molecular understanding of these different sources of individual variation can lead to the development of targeted molecular therapies, as well as tests to determine which type of therapy is most appropriate for an individual (Burke and Psaty, 2007; Ruano, 2004).

Clinical bioinformatics (also known as *translational bioinformatics*) seeks to bridge the world of clinical practice and the world of molecular biomedicine and bioinformatics. Through the development of tools and technologies such as decision support systems, this sub-discipline is focussed on helping clinicians use our knowledge of genetics and biological processes to select the most appropriate therapies for disease groups, and ultimately, through personalized medicine, tailor treatment to the individual patient. In this chapter, we build on the concepts developed in Chapter 30, on bioinformatics, and show that these concepts can be harnessed in clinical practice.

31.1 Genomic data can improve diagnosis, prognosis and therapeutic choice

Decoding of the human genome is driven by the hope that it will result in new ways of treating patients. Specifically, using the methods described in Chapter 30, we can identify genes that indicate a patient's susceptibility to disease, as well as infer the cellular pathways involved in producing an illness. As a consequence, we have many different opportunities to develop highly targeted or personalized therapies.

For example, a seminal analysis of large B-cell lymphoma saw researchers, using DNA microarray technology, measure the expression level of thousands of genes in the lymphatic tissues of patients with this deadly malignant disease of the lymphatic system (Alizadeh *et al.*, 2000). When a clustering analysis was performed to see which patients resembled one another the most based on their gene expression pattern, two distinct clusters of patients were found. When the investigators examined the patients' histories, it became apparent that the clusters corresponded to two distinct populations of patients with dramatically different mortality rates, as evidenced by a statistically significant difference in survival curves (Figure 31.1). The implications of these two distinct mortality rates are profound. First, these investigators have discovered a new sub-category of large B-cell lymphoma, a new diagnosis with clinical significance. Second, they have generated a tool that identifies a new *prognosis,* and as a result patients can be given much more precise estimates of their longevity. Third, it provides a new *therapeutic opportunity,* because the patients with an expression pattern predicting a poor response to standard therapy may be treated with different chemotherapy. Fourth, it presents a new *biomedical research* opportunity to uncover what it is about these two sub-populations that makes them so different in outcome and how that can be related to the differences in gene expression.

There is a wide range of clinical applications for which bioinformatics methods are used:

- *Disease diagnosis and monitoring* – The genomes of most tumours carry unique re-arrangements detectable by sequencing methods, and these sequences could be used

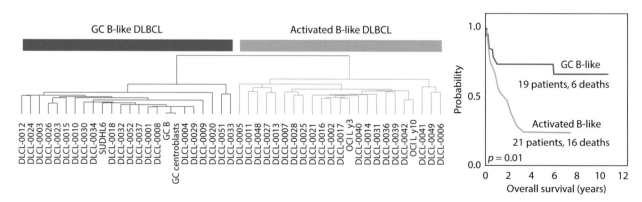

Figure 31.1   Sub-categories of diffuse large B-cell lymphoma (DLBCL) determined by microarrays correspond clinically to the duration of survival. On the left is a dendrogram or tree constructed from samples of B-cell lymphoma that uses an unsupervised learning technique. The top branch defines an even split between the two that was never before made clinically. On the right are survival curves of the patients. Patients whose cancer matched the Activated B-like DLBCL gene expression profile had a significantly worse prognosis. (From Alizadeh *et al.*, 2000.)

as biomarkers. Many types of solid organ tumours release DNA fragments into the blood. These fragments can be detected by laboratory tests, for example, using a purpose-built microarray. The level of expression of such genes can be used to quantify the level of post-treatment residual disease and help detect early disease recurrence, thus shaping decisions about surgery, radiotherapy and chemotherapy.

- *Near patient testing for infectious diseases* – The identification of infectious diseases has historically relied on culturing organisms or on morphological identification in specialized laboratories. However, the ability to identify micro-organisms genetically enables the detection, identification and characterization of infective pathogens to be performed near the patient, whether at the hospital bedside, in general practice or at home (Borriello, 1999). Testing kits provide rapid analysis of a drop of blood, saliva or urine to detect whether an infective pathogen is present and to provide an indication of its antimicrobial resistance potential. The technologies that make such test kits possible include microarrays. Identifying genetic resistance markers allows a clinician to predict an organism's susceptibility to antimicrobial drugs and the selection of appropriate chemotherapy. The ability to identify how virulent an infection is likely to be, based upon genetic markers, should allow clinicians to predict clinical outcomes (Jenks, 1998). The detection of the human influenza virus or respiratory syncytial virus should reduce inappropriate antibiotic prescriptions. Near patient testing should also assist in controlling infectious diseases in the community through rapid detection.

- *Pharmacogenomics* – Bioinformatics analysis of genomic, pathological and clinical data from clinical trials can identify which sub-populations react well or poorly to a given drug. Simple genetic tests can then be used on patients to determine whether they belong to a sub-population that is genetically predisposed to respond well or poorly with that drug. Pharmacogenomics is thus likely to bring about a new age of personalized 'molecular' medicine in which a patient's unique genetic profile will be determined for certain drugs, with the aim of providing therapy that is targeted to the patient's specific biological needs and is free of side effects. Unfortunately, the uptake, impact and excretion mechanisms for many drugs depend on multiple genes, and finding simple biomarkers for drug efficacy can be maddeningly difficult. Warfarin, for example, is an anticoagulant drug characterized by a narrow range of blood concentration within which it is effective, and overdosage brings significant risks of bleeding. The genes *CYP2C9* (associated with cytochrome P450) and *VKORC1* (linked to the vitamin K epoxide reductase complex) are known to affect warfarin dose requirements. Patients with particular variants should be given reduced doses of warfarin because their metabolism of the drug is slightly different, and the genes also shape the time required to attain therapeutic anticoagulation levels and the risk of excessive anticoagulation or hemorrhage. Although these genotype and associated clinical factors can explain about 50 to 60 per cent of the variance in warfarin dose requirements in Caucasians and Asians, they explain only 25 to 40 per cent in African Americans (Cavallari and Limdi, 2009).

- *Drug discovery* – Genetic knowledge is enhancing our ability to design new drug therapies. Bioinformatics data help us understand the relationships between a cancer patient's genes and the molecular pathways that have been altered to produce their tumour. They offer clues for new ways of disrupting aberrant biomedical pathways with new molecules. For example, once the entire genome of an infective micro-organism is available, it can be examined for potential molecular target sites for attack by specially designed drugs (Fischbach and Walsh, 2009). Novel designer drugs such as *imatinib mesylate*, which interferes with the abnormal protein made in chronic myeloid leukaemia, have been developed using bioinformatics methods to identify and target specific human genetic markers (Wood *et al.*, 2002). New classes of chemotherapy for malignant melanoma have revolutionized the treatment of what once was too often a lethal disease (Eggermont and Robert, 2011). Similar methods can be used to create new vaccines based on a molecular understanding of the antigen proteins associated with an infective organism (Box 31.1).

Box 31.1
Reverse vaccinology–using informatics to discover new vaccines

One of the success stories in translational bioinformatics has been the application of whole genome analysis to reverse engineer proteins that could be successful vaccines to protect against infectious diseases (Figure 31.2).

With the availability of multiple completely sequenced genomes of pathogens, it is now possible to run comparative genomics analyses to find vaccine targets shared by many pathogens. The existence of high-quality and high-volume databases with structural and functional information on microbial proteins enables 'reverse vaccinology', which combines available genomic data, computational data analysis and biotechnology to construct synthetic proteins (Sette and Rappuoli, 2010).

During computational analysis, researchers first identify dozens of candidate proteins (antigens located on the outer layers of bacteria that are exposed to the host immune system) from hundreds of proteins predicted in the microbial genome. The initial protein list is trimmed by further genome-wide screens of multiple genomes to confirm these proteins that are broadly conserved and are not unique to a single genome. The successful development of the vaccine against *Neisseria meningitidis* serogroup B has provided the proof for this novel approach.

Figure 31.2
Conventional (left) and computational (right) approaches to the design of vaccines against infectious diseases. Computational selection of candidate vaccine molecules with high-throughput screening algorithms has offered an alternative to a slow and laborious trial and error of the consecutive laboratory testing of microbial proteins.

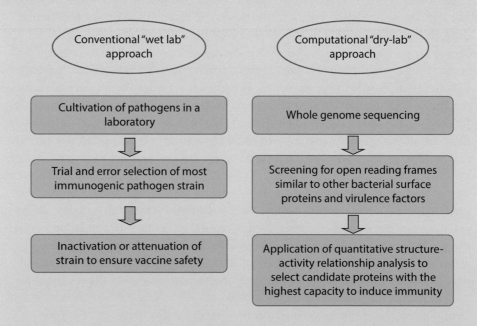

Further reading
Sette, A. and R. Rappuoli (2010). Reverse vaccinology: developing vaccines in the era of genomics. *Immunity* **33**(4): 530–541.

- *Gene therapies* – For patients with genetically based chronic illnesses such as cystic fibrosis, gene therapies are being pursued that should eventually offer the possibility of directly interacting with the defective genes to moderate, repress or disable the biochemical processes that result in the disease state (Griesenbach *et al.*, 2006).

31.2 Genomic data undergo a series of interpretive stages before the data are ready for clinical use

Large-scale genetic sequencing projects have created reference catalogues of many of the common genetic variants found in the human populations, as well as the genomic changes associated with different diseases. As we saw in Chapter 30, two broad types of genetic study are possible to determine gene–disease associations:

- Whole genome studies, *or genome-wide association studies* (GWAS), analyze genetic data from individuals with and without a condition and identify the genetic differences between the two populations. GWAS can suggest genes of interest, whether their function was previously known or not, by comparing newly identified genes with structurally similar genes that have known function.
- Targeted or *candidate gene* studies look for the presence and activity levels of a predefined gene set, for example, using a microarray. These studies, by definition, are not capable of discovering new genes or gene combinations.

If a genetic study has a particular question it is seeking to answer, then the degree to which we need to analyze the data further will depend on the type of study done and on whether an answer is immediately obvious from what is well known. This stage can present significant challenges if the role of mutations in biological processes is unclear.

The informatics pipeline for genome sequencing and analysis can be broadly divided into two analytical stages. The first step, consisting of sequence assembly and alignment, is the domain of bioinformatics. In this step, a sequence of nucleotides is mapped to an annotated reference genome, and the extent of variation from the reference is determined. Next, the sequence data are structurally and functionally *annotated* with biological information, and the location of genome variants is identified and, if need be, visualized using genome browsers (Figure 31.3). Such browsers can be linked to external reference databases. One successful approach to this cognitively demanding task is the *ideogram,* which is a standardized way to represent the presence of genes and variants on top of a standard chromosome map (Figures 31.4 and 31.5).

31.3 Gene set enrichment with additional information from the literature can significantly enhance the accuracy of gene–disease associational data

Genomes, as we saw, are annotated to show the presence of known genes of specific function, as well as structural variations. For many diseases, more than one gene is identified in GWAS as being associated with a disease. We can rank the likelihood that a gene is truly

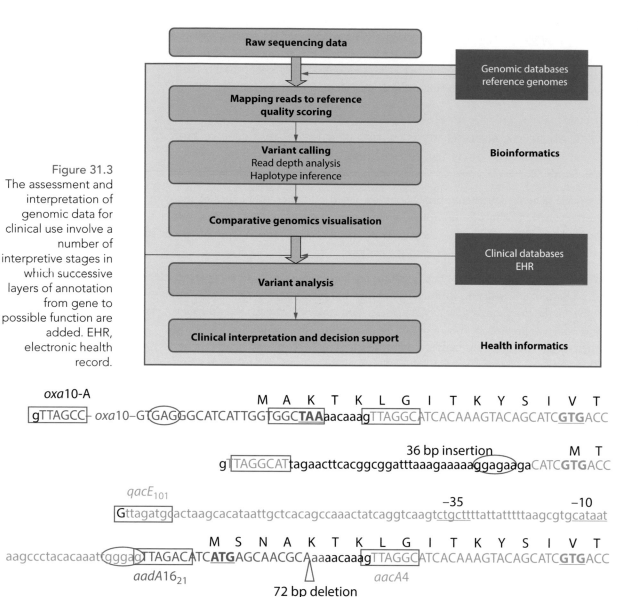

Figure 31.3 The assessment and interpretation of genomic data for clinical use involve a number of interpretive stages in which successive layers of annotation from gene to possible function are added. EHR, electronic health record.

Figure 31.4   Raw gene sequences are annotated with the names of known genes from reference databases. Alignment algorithms can identify variations such as insertions and deletions in the DNA base-pair sequence. This figure demonstrates different versions of the beginning of the *aacA4* gene cassette, which is a genetic structure responsible for transferring antibiotic resistance from one bacterium to another. (Adapted from Partridge *et al.*, 2009.)

associated with a disease state by turning to microarray gene expression studies that compare the level of activation or signal strength of these genes in disease. A higher gene rank can be given to genes that are most strongly expressed. This process may not always be reliable, however. Different studies of the same disease may find very little correlation among their results (Fortunel *et al.*, 2003). The reasons could be individual variations in disease or in the timing of gene activation in a disease process or the protocol used in tissue preparation or the type of microarray used (Dupuy and Simon, 2007).

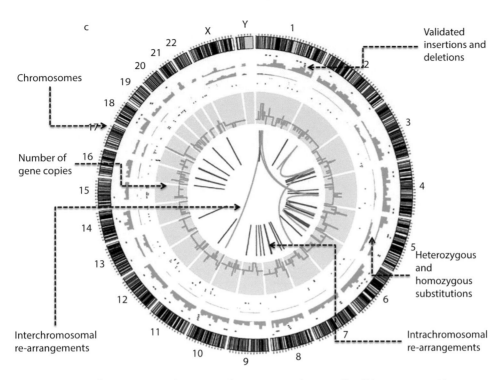

Figure 31.5 A chromosome ideogram of a patient with a small cell lung cancer. The ideogram represents identified mutations in a patient's genome and correlates them with known disease risks. Chromosomes are placed on the circumference. The next tracks moving from outside to in show validated genome insertions, deletions, and heterozygous and homozygous substitutions, all recorded as density per 10 megabases. The number of copies of a gene is shown toward the middle, followed by intrachromosomal re-arrangements and inter chromosomal rearrangements at the centre. (Adapted from Pleasance *et al.*, 2010.)

Gene expression analyses may also fail to detect biological processes that are distributed across a network of genes. To circumvent this, one approach to increasing the disease signal in microarray data is to annotate such data sets with additional information about biological function (Ashburner *et al.*, 2000). Functional annotation can provide insights into which biochemical pathways may be activated or de-activated by genes in an array. Later in this chapter, we discuss the Gene Ontology (GO), which can be used at this stage in annotation to provide information on the location in the cell where a protein coded by a gene carries out its function and the pathways in which the protein has a role. Genes that are either strongly expressed or downregulated and inactive may share a common pathway and provide clues to the biological process changes associated with a disease.

Gene Set Enrichment Analysis (GSEA) uses a catalogue of genes developed from the biological knowledge accumulated in public databases, also grouped by functional labels (Subramanian *et al.*, 2005). The catalogue enriches the microarray data to help identify gene sets rather than individual genes. The performance of GSEA largely depends on the enrichment catalogue used. Many such catalogues are available, e.g. from the Molecular Signatures Database (MSigDB) (Liberzon *et al.*, 2011). These catalogues are derived using a combination

Figure 31.6   The likelihood that a gene is associated with a disease can be initially obtained with a rank based on strength of expression in microarray experiments. These ranks can be improved by adding in additional information on gene–disease associations extracted by text mining the research literature, searching for gene names and biological functions and utilizing terminologies and ontologies to group together those cases in which a gene–disease association is expressed in a slightly different way in natural language. MeSH, Medical Subject Heading; UMLS, Unified Medical Language System. (Adapted from Tsafnat *et al.*, 2014.)

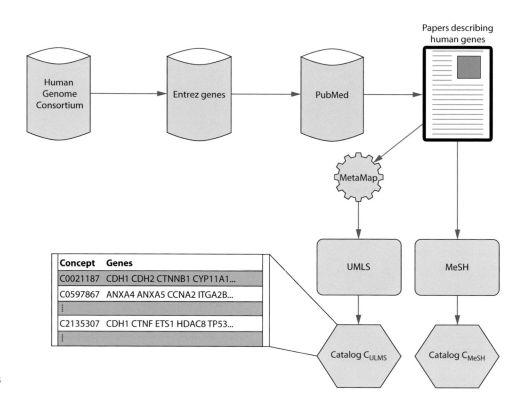

of expert knowledge and automatic mining of manually collected databases such as the GO. GSEA has been shown to produce higher inter-study agreement than single gene comparisons (Subramanian *et al.*, 2005). Text mining the scientific literature has also been proposed as a source of additional information to enrich microarray data annotation (Rubinstein and Simon, 2005). Gene–disease associational data can be calculated from the published research literature by counting the number of times a gene is mentioned in texts in association with a disease (Figure 31.6) (Sintchenko *et al.*, 2010). Literature-derived data can be combined with gene expression data to arrive at modified gene rank scores, which appear to improve the quality of gene–disease association ranks significantly (Tsafnat *et al.*, 2014).

31.4 Genome data can contribute to personalized risk assessment for diseases but need to be interpreted in association with multiple other factors

We all have different approaches to risk and to whether we even wish to be told of our risks of disease. James Watson, the first human to have his whole genome sequenced, was initially given his entire genome on a hard disk. He declined the offer of genetic counselling to assist in its interpretation and specifically chose to suppress (not have analyzed or disclosed to him) any information about apolipoprotein E, which is linked to Alzheimer's disease. Apart from this one omission, he then made his genome publicly available.

For a given individual, genome sequencing captures the full genetic signature. This individual-level data can be annotated with known gene functions and with those genes associated with increased risk of different diseases. The end result is a genetically defined disease risk profile. Alternatively, using a measurement technology such as a microarray, one could create a personalized report on the expression of a defined subset of human genes, for example the genes known to shape an individual's suitability for a particular form of treatment.

Today it is possible for anyone to take a simple sample such as a buccal swab, send it off for testing and then receive an extensive personal genetic analysis, potentially linked to research evidence about the associated disease risks of each identified gene. Although some individuals would rather not know their risks, others wish to be told of risks for important conditions such as coronary artery disease, sudden cardiac death and genetic conditions, so that they can undertake appropriate preventive actions or receive genetic counselling.

Although such analyses can tell us much about the probability of a disease given the gene across a population, it does not follow that the population risk is the same as our individual risks. Disease risk is multifactorial, influenced both by genetic and environmental factors. For example, genes shape how we metabolize cholesterol, and diet shapes how much of it we ingest. Developing models that integrate genotypic and phenotypic risks is not trivial because risk estimates change over time and among different populations. It is also clear that genes interact with each other, just as do the environment and genes through epigenetic modification. These networks of gene–gene and gene–environment interactions create a further level of complexity in determining whether the presence or absence of a gene is a true risk for a patient.

Bayes' theorem helps calculate the true risk of having a disease based upon its known prevalence in the population

Genetic risk modelling thus requires several stages of analysis. Firstly, risk markers are determined from GWAS, which can survey thousands or millions of biological data points across control and diseased patients. GWAS can identify the gene variants or *alleles* that are strongly associated with a disease state. The alleles that occur most frequently in diseased patients (i.e. with an odds ratio greater than 1) when compared with well patients are identified as *risk alleles*. For example, among patients with Alzheimer's disease, 38 per cent of *ApoE* gene's alleles are the *ApoE4* variant, but this variant occurs in only 14 per cent of normal controls (Ng *et al.,* 2009), thus making it a marker of increased risk. However, many markers discovered by GWAS are not strong enough on their own to account fully for the risks of disease. For example, approximately 65 per cent of the heritability of coeliac disease remains unexplained. Therefore, using risk alleles alone to screen for this disease will miss many cases (Ng *et al.,* 2009).

The next step in assigning risk is to adjust the odds ratios for a disease obtained from GWAS with environmental risk factors. One method to make such adjustments is to use Bayes' theorem (see Chapter 8). For a given patient, we first calculate their pre-test probability of disease based, for example, on the disease's prevalence in the population. Next, we adjust that risk with the new genetic information to arrive at a post-test probability for the disease (Figure 31.7). This approach allows a patient's *additional risk* of disease, given the presence of a risk allele, to be calculated. It is an important adjustment, because it can substantially change how a risk is managed.

Figure 31.7 Bayes' theorem is used to combine the baseline population of risks with the implied disease risks associated with the possession of a genetic variant, to calculate an individual's risk of disease. (Adapted from Ng *et al.*, 2009.)

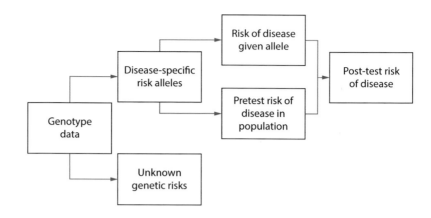

For example, assume we have a genetic test for an SNP that is 99.9 per cent sensitive (true-positive rate) and 99.9 per cent specific (true-negative rate). If we give this test to a population that we know has a family history of this disease, say with 1 in 1000 chance of having the disease, then the pre-test probability of disease is 0.001, and the post-test probability of having the disease rises to 0.5 if you test positive (Figure 31.8). In other words if we tested 1000 people, there would be 1 false-positive and 1 true-positive result, and these 2 individuals together have a 50 per cent chance of the disease. More testing would make sense to rule out the disease. Assume we now apply the same test to the general population, with no family history, whose risk of disease is 1 in 100 000. The pre-test probability of disease is now 0.00001, and the post-test probability of disease if you test positive rises to only 0.0099. If we gave this test to 10 million people in the general population, we would have 10 000 positive results, but only 100 individuals will actually have the disease. These 10 100 would then require further testing to identify the 100 individuals with risk and set the minds at ease for the remaining 10 000 – thus making this a potentially very expensive screening exercise in this population.

Multiple genetic tests increase the risk of a false-positive finding

Genetic assays may screen individuals for many hundreds of thousands of known SNPs. Although such tests are incredibly powerful, they suffer from a statistical problem associated with multiple testing. In other words, if you repeatedly test for a number of independent measures, then the chance of incidentally making a false-positive finding increases as the number of tests increases. These spurious false-positive genetic test results have been called the *incidentalome* (Kohane *et al.*, 2006).

Consider, for example, what will happen if we have 10 000 genetic tests available in a panel. The tests are superbly accurate, with a 100 per cent sensitivity and a 0.01 per cent false-positive rate. This means that in a population of 100 000, there will be 10 people who register as false positive for any individual test in the panel. The risk of a false-positive test result rises to more than 60 per cent by the time all 10 000 tests have been applied to every member of the population (Kohane *et al.*, 2006) (Figure 31.9).

To reduce the likelihood of such high false-positive rates (Pe'er *et al.*, 2008; Westbrook *et al.*, 2012), several different strategies are employed, for example, limiting testing to only

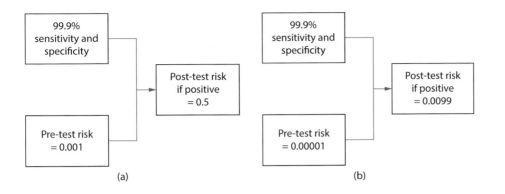

Figure 31.8 The post-test risk of disease following a genetic test depends on the prevalence of disease in the population. Using Bayes' theorem, (a) the application of a very precise test to a population with high risk can be worthwhile, but (b) its use in the general population where disease prevalence is lower may not be cost-effective.

clinically relevant tests, as well as improving the statistical sophistication of risk assignment (Berg *et al.*, 2012; Rice *et al.*, 2008).

Combining multiple sources of risk information can improve the quality of personal risk assessment

There are wide variations in estimates of disease risk for some genetic markers, and caution is needed when interpreting such risks. The accuracy of genetic risk assessments heavily depends on a number of factors:

- *The precision with which we can assign an initial risk of disease to an individual, ahead of any genetic testing* – The quality of population disease records and the quality of disease coding are known to be variable, and they were designed to be good enough for tracking the population burden of disease. Many population data sets were never intended for use in individual risk prediction and so were never calibrated to the correct level of precision for this task.
- *The precision of our estimates of the risk that possession of a given genetic marker or marker set brings* – This risk depends on the quality of the population data used (how well the data identify patients with and without a disease), as well as the accuracy of the genetic assays on this population and any bioinformatics methods used to infer the presence or absence of a genetic marker.

Figure 31.9 The chance of a false-positive test result increases with the number of independent tests. With 10 000 independent tests with 100 per cent sensitivity but a 0.01 per cent false-positive rate, there is greater than 60 per cent chance of a false-positive reading after testing 10 000 individuals. (After Kohane *et al.*, 2006.)

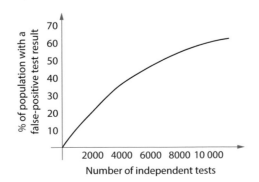

One way of dramatically improving disease risk assessment is to use an individual's phenotype data alongside their genotype data. We saw in Chapter 25 that electronic health record (EHR) data can be used to generate individual risk assessments and guide therapeutic decisions. Clinical trial data have traditionally been used to determine the likely benefits of a treatment, for example, but they exclude patients with multiple diseases. This means that it is difficult to determine whether an individual patient with multi-morbidity will truly benefit from a drug, based solely on clinical trial data. EHR data allow us to identify a patient cohort that is similar to a given patient, and the comparative effectiveness of different treatments within this matched cohort is likely to be a better predictor of therapeutic response than are general population data or even clinical trial data (Gallego *et al.*, 2013). Historical data from matched cohorts also allow us to estimate the risk of disease progression or appearance of new diseases for an individual (Figure 31.10). For example, there are increased risks of diseases such as stroke associated with heart disease and hypertension. Record data can also contain family history of disease, important environmental information, such as geography, and history of exposure to substances or radiation.

31.5 Analyzing genome and clinical data enables new decision support systems

Given that most clinicians will not be expert in the deep genetic biology of disease or have the capacity to track the progress in our understanding of biology, clinical decision support systems (CDSSs) have a major role to play in clinical bioinformatics. CDSSs can assist clinicians by prompting them when a genetic test can help in the selection of one pharmacological agent over another or determining when a patient is likely to benefit from genetic screening, or they can advise on a patient's risks of disease so that preventive actions can be taken.

Bioinformatics-guided decision support for therapy for human immunodeficiency virus (HIV) provides an excellent example of what is possible through such an approach. Since its recognition in 1981, HIV has been responsible for the deaths of millions of people worldwide, and significant research and public health efforts have been devoted to control the destructive pandemic of HIV infection. A great many antiviral drugs with different mechanisms of action have been approved for use in HIV infection and are usually prescribed in combination to minimize the risk of drug resistance, as well as contributing to delay disease progression, prolonging survival and maintaining quality of life. Sequencing and genotyping resistance testing are routine practice in HIV medicine and have led to the discovery of many drug-resistance genes in the HIV genome. Interpreting the role of different mutational patterns on HIV drug resistance is a complicated task that requires predictive models that relate genotype to phenotype.

These models are built using machine learning on data sets that match viral genotype with resistance (Lengauer and Sing, 2006) (Figure 31.11). HIV continues to mutate and evolve while it is within a single host, and resistance mutations accumulate as a patient is being treated – those members of the infecting virus population that are susceptible to a drug die, but those that are resistant remain in tissues and eventually return in numbers to cause disease. Understanding the genetic mutational pathways that lead to the creation of resistant

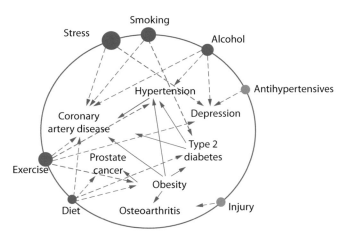

Figure 31.10 A conditional dependency diagram for one patient relates how the patient's risk of disease is shaped by environmental factors, as well as genetic risks and phenotypic risks extracted from the patient's health record. Diseases with post-test risk probabilities greater than 10 per cent are shown, with text size proportional to the post-test risk. Arrows indicate that one disease predisposes to another. Modifiable environmental factors are shown at the circumference with circles. Dashed lines link environmental factors associated with the cause of a disease. Text and circle sizes for environmental factors are proportional to the number of diseases with which each factor is associated. Color intensity represents the maximum post-test risk probability for diseases directly associated with a factor. (Adapted from Ashley *et al.*, 2010.)

Figure 31.11 Machine learning can classify human immunodeficiency virus (HIV) genomes into those that are susceptible or resistant to an antiviral drug or drug combination. Training data in the form of matched genotype–phenotype pairs are used to develop models that treat prediction of drug resistance from viral sequences as either a regression or a classification problem. Once validated, the rules that are derived can be used classify a new patient's viral sequences into drug-susceptible or drug-resistant categories with associated probability estimates. Machine learning approaches can further rank drug combinations by their likely antiviral activity, human toxicity and cost.

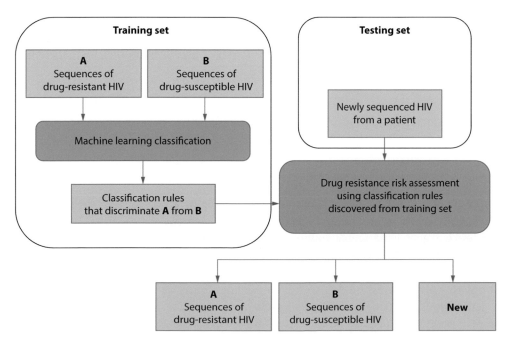

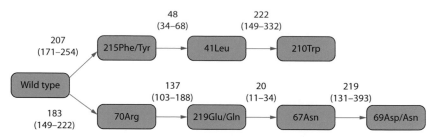

Figure 31.12   An evolutionary model of human immunodeficiency virus (HIV) mutagenesis. This tree depicts the development of HIV resistance against zidovudine along two different mutation pathways for the viral protein reverse transcriptase. The lower pathway starts with the mutation 70Arg and continues with the mutations 219 Glu or Gln. A drug resistance mutation can emerge only if all parent mutations on the way to the root are present. The numbers on the links between mutations represent the expected time in weeks for acquiring the respective mutation, and numbers in brackets reflect 95 per cent confidence intervals. (Adapted from Lengauer and Sing, 2006.)

viruses is important because it not only helps to determine which drugs are best for a patient now, but also can highlight the risk that giving a drug will push a viral population along the way to evolving a resistance pattern (Figure 31.12). Evolutionary models that incorporate such pathways are thus used to rank different combination therapies and appear to give the most reliable predictions of drug responses (Lengauer and Sing, 2006).

Similar applications for CDSSs exist in a wide variety of diseases, such as the management of cancer, in which drug resistance is also a constant problem because cancer cells that are resistant to a drug are differentially selected by treatment. The most appropriate management plan for a patient with cancer can thus be informed by assessing a patient's normal genome and the mutated genome of the tumour. For example, inhibitor drugs for protein kinases can be prescribed if mutations in the genes encoding these enzymes are detected. The dosage of toxic and expensive anticancer chemotherapy can also be adjusted by measuring the expression of genes associated with drug-metabolizing enzymes, thus ensuring that a patient is exposed to as low a dose as is necessary.

31.6 Phenotype data are stored in the patient record and require standard terminologies and ontologies for the data to be meaningful

Genomic data can have clinical relevance only if the data are assessed with respect to phenotypic information. The only way we found genes that distinguish between acute myeloid leukaemia and acute lymphoid leukaemia (Golub *et al.*, 1999), refined our understanding of prognosis with large B-cell lymphoma (Alizadeh *et al.*, 2000) or made pharmacogenomic predictions of gene targets for chemotherapy (Butte *et al.*, 2000) was by correlating gene expression data with biological or clinical data. If we want to know how a gene expression pattern predicts mortality, the risk of a particular disease or drug responsiveness, we need to be as meticulous in characterizing patients, their histories, their tissues and their environmental context as we are in obtaining their gene expression profile. It follows that the functional genomic enterprise strongly depends on the quality of non-genetic data.

Standardized vocabularies are needed for clinical phenotypes

GenBank and many related genomic and protein databases are major assets to functional genomics, by providing reference genomes and gene–disease association data. The Human Genome Project benefits from the elegant simplicity of the genetic code, and there are relatively few data types that are needed for a GenBank entry to be valid. Electronic patient records are an invaluable source of phenotypic data and as we have seen are also crucial to understanding genetic risk. The types of data recorded in the EHR are, however, far more complicated. As we saw in Chapter 23, the number of concepts that can be covered in a clinical terminological system is vast, and concepts can appear in multiple different hierarchies.

Standardized clinical vocabularies such as the International Classification of Diseases (ICD), Unified Medical Language System (UMLS) or Systematized Nomenclature of Medicine Clinical Terms (SNOMED-CT) are thus essential to developing standardized phenotypic data models. That these terminological systems overlap and compete with each other makes it more difficult to integrate clinical records across a population or from different disease registries, each of which may adopt one or another standard and indeed one or another version of a standard. For example, if a set of expressed genes is thought to be associated with a particular set of cardiac arrhythmias, this association will be found only if the nomenclature used to describe the arrhythmias in the clinical databases is drawn from a standardized vocabulary.

Similar problems exist in bioinformatics. Many microarray and sequencing technologies use their own system of gene accession numbers, which must then be translated into a more widely used nomenclature such as LocusLink (Pruitt and Maglott, 2001).

Bio-ontologies are essential to identify which gene associations are likely to have clinical relevance and which are spurious

Simply tagging clinical records with recognized terms or concepts allows for associational studies to be conducted. However, just because two entities are associated statistically, we know that they may not have a causal relationship. Experts in a specific area are often able to recognize potentially meaningful correlations among genes, proteins or phenotypic features. However, population-wide studies can generate vast numbers of candidate associations, and sorting these out manually is not really feasible, especially when the goal is a data mining exercise to discover novel associations.

We have already encountered *ontologies* several times in this book. Ontologies provide a conceptual map of a domain that explains the different classes of concept that are to be found and how concepts can relate to each other. Ontology can be modelled implicitly (e.g. in the axes of a multiaxial terminology) or may be explicitly described as a stand-alone structure. An ontology allows a computer to recognize that, although osteomyelitis and penicillin are

provider resulted in a significant reduction of unexplained medication discrepancies from 51 to 42 per cent (Schnipper *et al.,* 2012).
● A diabetes mellitus tailored PHR that provided patient decision support and enabled the patient to author and submit a diabetes care plan before upcoming appointments resulted in an increased number of treatment regimen adjustments (Grant *et al.,* 2008).

Personal health record usage appears to be associated with dose-response effects

Given that the benefit of a PHR is going to increase with the level of usage of the system (as the number of interactions increase, there is a resulting increased likelihood that some interactions will provide important information with an impact on decisions, processes or outcomes), obtaining robust levels of PHR usage seems critical to obtaining any benefit. When levels of usage are low, it has indeed proved difficult to demonstrate any real benefits (Wagner *et al.,* 2012).

There does appear to be a clear dose-response effect between PHR use and detectable behaviour or process outcome changes. In other words, increased use of a PHR is associated with increased benefits. In the PCHMS trial of influenza vaccination, greater use of the PCHMS was associated with higher rates of vaccination and health service provider visits (Lau *et al.,* 2012). In another study, when compared with low users or non-users, high PHR users reported significantly more changes in medication use and improved medication reconciliation behaviours, and they recognized significantly more side effects (Chrischilles *et al.,* 2013).

PHRs that come with additional tools form a care bundle, and as we saw in Chapter 11, it is important to try to understand which particular bundle elements have the most influence on a particular outcome because this can shape future system design, as well as explain usage patterns. Through analysis of the patterns of frequency and duration of bundle element uses within a PHR, it is possible to identify which elements are most likely to be used together and which may as a group be most likely to cause observed changes (Lau *et al.,* 2013).

32.3 Consumer decisions can be supported by tools from question asking through to decision-making

It should not be surprising that the basic information tasks for a consumer the same ones we find for professionals – asking the right and well-structured question, searching for answers to the question and then assembling information such as likelihoods and personal preferences to make a decision (see Chapters 6 to 8). Although there are often differences between health professionals and consumers in their understanding of biomedical terminology and the nature of disease processes, many consumers are highly informed and want access to high-quality information when they are faced with questions about illness.

Informatics provides tools to consumers to help them make informed choices. These consumer decision support systems (DSS) come in many forms, ranging from patient education pamphlets to summarized guides (similar to clinical pathways), decision aids, health risk calculators and interactive tools to aid in screening, diagnosis and therapy selection.

There are however significant differences in the context in which such information and support is sought. Consumers are not disinterested parties. The decision context is thus likely to be one in which there is uncertainty, anxiety and stress, which can all inhibit information seeking, understanding and processing. There is thus a clear need for professionals to ensure that what has been read is appropriately interpreted and its meaning accurately personalized and that judgements are as informed as possible.

Interview tools can encourage consumers to ask questions

Consumers may need to be reminded or even given permission to ask questions, especially if there are cultural barriers that give health professionals asymmetrical power and status. Asking basic questions such as 'What are my options?', 'What are the benefits and harms?' and 'How likely are these?' appears to lead clinicians to provide more information and engage in more behaviour that supports patient involvement (Shepherd et al., 2011).

Simple methods that can help patients identify and ask questions before or during consultations include coaching sessions, written materials such as question checklists and prompt sheets and videos. A systematic review of these methods found positive but small effects on the number of questions asked and patient satisfaction, but no impact on patients' anxiety, knowledge or consultation length (Kinnersley et al., 2008). One likely explanation for these modest results is that these interventions target only the patient. It may be that support for question asking needs to occur within the dialogue that occurs between patients and their carers, rather being isolated from it.

Computerized interview tools provide a more interactive form of support to consumers, by programmatically guiding them through a specific set of questions and then allowing clinicians to discuss their answers with them. These disease- or context-specific questions can be designed to make sure that all clinically relevant information has been provided, and the use of such tools does seem to have a positive impact on patient assessment. The idea of computers as a tool to guide patients through a structured interview is actually one of the oldest concepts in health informatics (Peckham et al., 1967), and the capability of computers to 'take' patients' histories before consultation, even in the home, has been studied extensively (Slack et al., 2012). The apparent results of the use of such tools are that more patient symptoms are addressed, and symptom distress levels and the need for longer-term symptom management are reduced (Ruland et al., 2010).

Information retrieval tools can assist consumers to structure questions when searching on the Internet and improve decision quality as a result

One of the most likely places that consumers will first turn to for information is the Internet, and health-related searches are among the most common of all search topics. The most common searches for health information relate to treatment or therapy (62 per cent), disease information (58 per cent), drug information (51 per cent) and side effects (51 per cent) (Pletneva and Vargas, 2011).

ARPAnet: Advanced Research Projects network. A computer network developed by the United States Department of Defense in the late 1960s and the forerunner of today's Internet.

Artificial intelligence (AI): Any artefact, whether embodied solely in computer software or a physical structure such as a robot, that exhibits behaviours associated with human intelligence. Also the study of the science and methods for constructing such artefacts. *See also* Turing test.

Artificial intelligence in medicine: The application of artificial intelligence methods to solve problems in medicine, e.g. developing expert systems to assist with diagnosis or therapy planning. *See also* Artificial Intelligence, Expert system.

Assembly: Construction of longer sequences, such as contigs or genomes, from shorter sequences, such as sequence reads with or without prior knowledge on the order of the reads or reference to a closely related sequence.

Asynchronous communication: A mode of communication between two parties when the exchange does not require both to be active participants in the conversation at the same time, e.g. sending a letter. *See also* Synchronous communication, Isochronous communication, E-mail.

ATM: Asynchronous transfer mode. A packet-based communication protocol that provides the high bandwidth transmission rates required for multimedia communication. *See also* Packet-switched network, Circuit-switched network.

Augmented reality: The overlay of additional information onto human sense data, e.g. overlaying labels onto images seen by a human.

Bandwidth: Amount of data that can be transmitted across a communication channel over a given period of time. *See also* Bits per second, Channel capacity.

Base pair: The chemical structure that forms the units of DNA and RNA and that encode genetic information. The bases that make up the base pairs are adenine (A), guanine (G), thymine (T), cytosine (C) and uracil (U). *See* DNA.

Base-pair (bp): Pair of complementary nucleotides. Specific pairing of these bases (adenine with thymine and guanine with cytosine) facilitates accurate DNA replication; when quantified (e.g. 120 bp), bp refers to the physical length of a sequence of nucleotides.

Bayes' theorem: Theorem used to calculate the relative probability of an event given the probabilities of associated events. It is used to calculate the probability of a disease given the frequencies of symptoms and signs within the disease and within the normal population. *See also* Conditional probability, Prior Probability, Posterior Probability.

Bioinformatics: A sub-discipline of health informatics concerned with the application of molecular biology to biomedical science and translational medicine, especially the use of computational tools and algorithms in genomics and proteomics research. Historically, bioinformatics concerned itself with the analysis of the sequences of genes and their products (proteins), but the field has since expanded to the management, processing, analysis and visualization of large quantities of data from genomics, proteomics, drug screening and pharmacology.

Biomarker: A biological characteristic that is objectively measured and evaluated as an indicator of normal or pathological processes or host responses to a therapeutic intervention.

B-ISDN: Broadband ISDN. A set of communication system standards for ATM systems. *See also* ATM, ISDN.

Bit: One binary digit, in base 2. The basic unit for electronically stored or transmitted data. *See also* Byte.

Bits per second: A measure of data transmission rate. *See also* Bit.

BLAST (Basic Logical Alignment Search Tool): A computer program for finding sequences in databases that have identity to a query sequence.

Bluetooth: Wireless communication system designed to allow many personal devices such as computers, mobile phones and digital cameras to communicate with each other over a short range.

Boolean logic: A system of logic devised by Georges Boole that defined the meaning of linguistic notions such as *and, or* and *not* to produce 'laws of thought' that had a clear syntax and semantics.

Broadband network: General term for a computer network rated capable of high-bandwidth transmission. *See also* ATM.

Browser: A program used to view data, e.g. examining the contents of a database or knowledge base or viewing documents on the World Wide Web. *See also* Mosaic, World Wide Web, Internet.

Byte: Eight bits. Bytes are usually counted in kilobytes (1024 bytes), megabytes and gigabytes. *See also* Bit.

Candidate gene study: A study of specific genetic loci in which a phenotype–genotype association may exist (hypothesis-led genotype experiment).

Care pathway: Describes the expected course of the patient's management and what actions need to be taken at every stage. *See also* Algorithm, Protocol, Guideline.

Case-based reasoning: An approach to computer reasoning that uses knowledge from a library of similar cases, rather than by accessing a knowledge base containing more generalized knowledge, such as a set of rules. *See also* Artificial intelligence, Expert system.

Causal reasoning: A form of reasoning based on following from cause to effect, in contrast to other methods in which the connection is weaker, such as probabilistic association.

CDSS: Clinical decision support system.

Centrality: Family of social network metrics based on number or type of connections between an individual and others, to estimate degree of influence or location in the network.

CERN: Conseil Européan pour la Recherche Nucléaire. The European Particle Physics Laboratory. It was here that the initial set of standards was developed to create the World Wide Web. *See also* HTML, HTTP, World Wide Web.

Channel: The connection between two parties that transports their messages, such as a telephone or e-mail.

Channel capacity: Amount of data that can be transmitted per unit time along a communication channel. Synonym: Bandwidth.

Checklist: An ordered list of items that must be 'ticked off' as they are completed. *See also* Protocol.

Chromosome: One of the physically separate segments that together forms the genome, or total genetic material, of a cell. Chromosomes are long strands of genetic material, or DNA, that have been packaged and compressed by wrapping around proteins. The number and size of chromosomes vary from species to species. In humans, there are 23 pairs of chromosomes (a pair has one chromosome from each parent). One pair forms the sex chromosomes because they contain genes that determine sex. The chromosome carrying the male determining genes is designated Y and the corresponding female one is the X chromosome. The remaining pairs are called autosomes. Chromosome 1 is the largest and chromosome 22 the smallest. Each chromosome has two 'arms' designated p and q.

Circuit-switched network: A communication network that connects parties by establishing a dedicated circuit between them. *See also* Packet-switched network.

Client: A computer connected to a network that does not store all the data or software it uses, but retrieves it across the network from another computer that acts as a server. *See also* Client-server architecture, Server.

Client-server architecture: A computer network architecture that places commonly used resources on centrally accessible server computers, which can be retrieved as they are needed across the network by client computers on the network. *See also* Client, Server.

Closed-loop control: Completely automated system control method in which no part of the control system need be given over to humans. *See also* Open-loop control.

Clustering: Algorithm that puts similar things together and different things apart.

Code: In medical terminological systems, the unique numeric identifier associated with a medical concept, which may be associated with a variety of terms, all with the same meaning. *See also* Term.

Cognitive science: A multidisciplinary field studying human cognitive processes, including their relationship to technologically embodied models of cognition. *See also* Artificial Intelligence.

Communication protocol: The rules governing how a conversation may proceed between well-behaved agents. *See also* OSI seven-layer model.

Complementary DNA (cDNA): DNA that is synthesized from a messenger RNA template; the single-stranded form is often used as a probe in physical mapping or for detecting RNA. Because cDNA is constructed from messenger RNA (after introns have been spliced out), it does not contain introns.

Complex adaptive system: A system characterized by high complexity and the ability to alter structure based upon a source of variation and a fitness function.

Complexity: The degree of connection among different component elements in a system.

Computer network: For computers, any collection of computers connected together so that they are able to communicate, permitting the sharing of data or programs.

Computerized protocol: Clinical guideline or protocol stored on a computer system, so that it may be easily accessed or manipulated to support the delivery of care.

Conditional probability: The probability that one event is true, given that another event is true. *See also* Bayes' theorem.

Connectionism: The study of the theory and application of neural networks. *See also* Neural network.

Consent: Explicit agreement to allow another party to carry out an action on our behalf. *See also* E-Consent.

Control system: A system that uses measurement of its output and feedback to influence future behaviour based upon a measurement of past performance. *See also* System, Feedback, Cybernetics.

CPOE: Computerized physician order entry. Clinical information system designed to support tasks such as ordering tests or medications.

CPR: Computer-based patient record. *See also* Electronic health record.

CSCW: Computer-supported co-operative work. The study of computer systems developed to support groups of individuals work together. *See also* Groupware.

Cybernetics: A name coined by Norbert Weiner in the 1950s to describe the study of feedback control systems and their application. Such systems were seen to exhibit properties associated with human intelligence and robotics and were early contributors to the theory of artificial intelligence.

Cyberspace: Popular term now associated with the Internet, which describes the notional information 'space' that is created across computer networks. *See also* Virtual reality.

Data: Any and all complex data entities from observations, experiments, simulations, models and higher-order assemblies, along with the associated documentation needed to describe and interpret them.

Data integration: The process of combining disparate data and providing a unified view of these data.

Data mining: Automatically searching large volumes of data for patterns or associations.

Data warehouse: An information infrastructure that enables researchers and clinicians to access and analyze detailed data and trends. It is created by collecting databases and linking them using common data elements.

Database: A structured repository for data, consisting of a collection of data and their associated data model and usually stored on a computer system. The existence of a regular and formal indexing structure permits rapid retrieval of individual elements of the database. *See also* Model, Knowledge base.

Decision support system: General term for any computer application that enhances a human's ability to make decisions.

Decision tree: A method of representing knowledge that structures the elements of a decision into a tree-like fashion. Chance nodes in a decision tree represent alternative possibilities, and decision nodes represent alternative choices. The leaf nodes of the tree represent outcomes, which may be assigned a numeric utility. *See also* Utility.

DECT: Digital European Cordless Telephony standard, which defines the architecture for wireless voice and data communication systems restricted to campus-size areas, rather than wide-area systems that would be publicly available.

Deduction: A method of logical inference. Given a cause, deduction infers all logical effects that may arise as a consequence. *See also* Inference, Abduction, Induction.

Deoxyribonucleic acid (DNA): The chemical that forms the basis of the genetic material in virtually all living organisms. Structurally, DNA is composed of two strands that intertwine to form a spring-like structure called the double helix. Attached to each backbone are chemical structures called bases (or nucleotides), which protrude away from the backbone toward the centre of the helix and which come in four types: adenine, cytosine, guanine and thymine (designated A, C, G and T). In DNA, cytosine only forms optimal hydrogen bonding with guanine, and adenine only with thymine. These interactions across the many nucleotides in each strand hold the two strands together.

Distributed computing: Term for computer systems in which data and programs are distributed across different computers on a network and are shared.

DNA sequencing: Biochemical methods for determining the order of the nucleotide bases, adenine, guanine, cytosine and thymine, in a DNA oligonucleotide.

DTMF: Dial tone multifrequency. The tones generated by punching in numbers on a telephone key pad.

E-Consent: Explicit agreement from a patient to allow another party to view the patient's data captured in an electronic health record. *See also* Consent.

EDI: Electronic data interchange. General term describing the need for healthcare applications to be able to exchange data and requiring the adoption of agreed-on common standards for the form and content of the messages passing between applications. *See also* HL7.

Electronic health record (EHR): A general term describing computer-based patient record systems. It is sometimes extended to include functions such as order entry for medications and tests, among others. *See also* Electronic medical record, Electronic nursing record, Summary care record.

Electronic mail: *See* E-mail.

Electronic medical record (EMR): A general term describing computer-based patient record systems designed mainly for the use of doctors.

Electronic nursing record (ENR): A general term describing computer-based patient record systems designed mainly for the use of nurses.

Electrophoresis: The use of electrical fields to separate charged biomolecules such as DNA, RNA and proteins. DNA and RNA carry a net negative charge because of the numerous phosphate groups in their structure. In the process of gel electrophoresis, these biomolecules are put into wells of a solid matrix typically made of an inert substance such as agarose. When this gel is placed into a bath and an electrical charge applied across the gel, the biomolecules migrate and separate according to size in proportion to the amount of charge they carry. The biomolecules can be stained for viewing and isolated and purified from the gels for further analysis. Electrophoresis can be used to isolate pure biomolecules from a mixture or to analyze biomolecules (e.g. for DNA sequencing).

E-mail: Electronic mail. Messaging system available on computer networks and providing users with personal mail boxes from which electronic messages can be sent and received.

EMR: *See* Electronic medical record.

Enzyme: A protein that catalyzes chemical reactions in a living cell. Enzymes are protein molecules whose function it is to speed the making and breaking of chemical bonds required for essential physiochemical reactions.

Epigenetics: Heritable influence on gene activity that does not involve changes to the DNA sequence itself.

Epistemology: The philosophical study of knowledge.

Epitope: The regions of an antigen that bind to antigen-specific membrane receptors on lymphocytes.

EPR: Electronic patient record. *See* Electronic medical record.

Evidence-based medicine: A movement advocating the practice of medicine according to clinical guidelines, developed to reflect best practice as captured from a meta-analysis of the clinical literature. *See also* Guideline, Meta-analysis, Protocol.

Exon: The protein-coding DNA sequences of a gene. *See* Intron.

Expected utility: In decision theory, the expected utility of a decision is the sum of the utilities of the same decision repeated over multiple trials. At the limit, with an infinite number of decisions, it is the sum of the utilities of each different possible outcome of that option, each weighted by its own probability. *See also* Decision tree, utility.

Expected value: In probability theory, the expected value of variable is the sum of all its values over multiple trials. The expected value of the mean value of a normally distributed binary variable that can either be 0 or 1 is 0.5.

Expert system: A computer program that contains expert knowledge about a particular problem, often in the form of a set of if–then rules that is able to solve problems at a level equivalent or greater than human experts. *See also* Artificial intelligence.

FAQ: Frequently asked questions. Common term for information lists available on the Internet that have been compiled for newcomers to a particular subject and answering common questions that would otherwise often be asked by submitting e-mail requests to a newsgroup.

Feedback: Taking some or all of the output of a system and adding it to a system's own input. *See also* System.

Finite state machine: A knowledge representation that makes different states in a process explicit and connects them with links that specify some transition condition that specifies how one traverses from one state to another.

Firewall: A security barrier erected between a public computer network such as the Internet and a local private computer network.

First principles, reasoning from: Use of a model of the mechanisms that control a system to predict or simulate the likely outcome if some of the inputs or internal structure of the system is altered. *See also* System.

Fitness landscape: A mathematical surface representing the relationship between phenotype and fitness for an organism, technology, organization or other construct existing within a complex adaptive system.

Formative assessment: Evaluation of the performance of an information system against user needs. *See also* Summative assessment.

FTP: File transfer protocol. A computer protocol that allows electronic files to be sent and received in a uniform fashion across a computer network.

Functional genomics: Exploration of the function of genes and other parts of the genome.

Fuzzy logic: An artificial intelligence method for representing and reasoning with imprecisely specified knowledge, e.g. defining loose boundaries to distinguish 'low' from 'high' values. *See also* Qualitative reasoning, Artificial intelligence.

Gene: An ordered sequence of nucleotides located in a particular position on a particular chromosome that encodes a specific functional product such as a protein.

Gene ontology: A set of controlled vocabularies in molecular function, biological process and cellular component for the standardized annotation of genes and gene products across all species.

other documents through hyperlinks, permitting 'non-linear' reading following concepts of interest to the reader. *See also* Hyperlink, HTML, World Wide Web.

ICD-9: *The International Classification of Diseases,* ninth revision, published by the World Health Organization.

ICD-10: *The International Classification of Diseases,* tenth revision, published by the World Health Organization.

Implementation: The act of fitting a technological construct such as an information system into a working setting such as an organization. Also the act of taking a design and translating it into a working system.

Implementation science: The study of the process of implementation.

Indicator: A measurable event or quantity that can be used to monitor a system, such as progress of a disease or quality, efficiency or safety of a health service process.

Indifference probability: The probability at which a decision maker is indifferent to the present outcome (status quo) or taking a gamble that could improve or worsen the situation. It is used to determine utilities in the standard gamble method. *See also* Standard gamble, Utility.

Induction: A method of logical inference used to suggest relationships from observations. This is the process of generalization we use to create models of the world. *See also* Deduction, Abduction, Inference.

Infectome: System of networks of interacting host and pathogen's genes, proteins and metabolites involved in a process of infection and disease.

Inference: A logical conclusion drawn using one of several methods of reasoning, knowledge and data. *See also* Abduction, Deduction, Induction.

Information superhighway: A popular term associated with the Internet that is used to describe its role in the global mass transportation of information.

Information theory: Initially developed by Claude Shannon, describes the amount of data that can be transmitted across a channel given specific encoding techniques and noise in the signal. *See also* Channel.

Internet: Technically, a network of computer networks. Today, it is associated with a specific global computer network that is publicly accessible and upon which the World Wide Web is based. *See also* ARPAnet, World Wide Web.

Intranet: A computer network, based upon World Wide Web and Internet technologies, but whose scope is limited to an organization. An intranet may be connected to an Internet, so that there can be communication and flow of information between it and other intranets. *See also* Internet, World Wide Web.

Intron: Non-coding portion of the gene that is spliced out from the nascent RNA transcript in the process of making an mRNA transcript. It frequently includes regulator elements (i.e. binding sites) in addition to those of the promoter.

IP (internetworking protocol): Communication protocol to allow different individual networks to communicate with each other. IP is the basis of the Internet's communication infrastructure.

IP address: The address of a computer on the Internet that permits it to send and receive messages from other computers on the Internet.

ISDN: Integrated Services Digital Network. A digital telephone network that is designed to provide channels for voice and data services.

Isochronous communication: A communication process that operates at a regular interval to provide a certain minimum data rate, e.g. sending a communication with a guaranteed regularity in ATM. *See also* Synchronous communication, Asynchronous communication, ATM.

Knowledge acquisition: Sub-speciality of artificial intelligence, usually associated with developing methods for capturing human knowledge and of converting it into a form that can be used by computer. *See also* Machine learning, Expert system, Heuristic.

Knowledge base: A structured repository for knowledge, consisting of a collection of knowledge elements such as rules and their associated data model, or *ontology*. A knowledge base is a core component of an *expert system*. *See also* Database, Model, Ontology, Expert system.

Knowledge-based system: *See* Expert system.

LAN: Local area network. A computer network limited to servicing computers in a small locality. *See also* Intranet.

Language: A formal language specifies a way of constructing messages. A language is built from an alphabet of allowed symbols, which can be arranged according to rules, which define the syntax of the language. *See also* Grammar.

Machine learning: Sub-speciality of artificial intelligence concerned with developing methods for software to learn from experience or to extract knowledge from examples in a database. *See also* Artificial intelligence, Knowledge acquisition.

Mailing list: A list of e-mail addresses for individuals. It is used to distribute information to small groups of individuals, who may, for example, have shared interests. *See also* E-mail.

Medline: Bibliographic database maintained by the National Library of Medicine in the United States that indexes articles published by most of the major biomedical journals.

Megabyte: 1 048 576 or 2^{20} bytes. *See also* Byte.

Messenger RNA (mRNA): The RNA that codes for proteins and is active in the cellular cytoplasm.

Meta-analysis: A statistical method that pools the results from multiple similar experiments, in the hope that the improved power obtained from the combined data sets will identify statistically significant patterns that cannot be identified within the smaller sample sizes of individual studies.

Metagenomics: The high-throughput study of sequences from multiple genomes recovered from samples that contain mixed microbial populations.

Microarray: A technology used to study many genes at once. Hundreds of samples containing DNA or RNA are deposited as dots on the slide. The binding of complementary base pairs from the sample and the gene sequences on the slide can be measured with the use of fluorescence.

Microbiome: Collective system of genomes of all microbial flora of the human.

Model: Any representation of a real object or phenomenon or template for the creation of an object or phenomenon.

Model-based reasoning: Approach to the development of expert systems that uses formally defined models of systems, in contrast to more superficial rules of thumbs. *See also* Heuristic, Artificial intelligence.

Modem: Modulator–demodulator. Device used for converting a digital signal into tones that can be transmitted down a telephone wire.

Mosaic: The first commonly available World Wide Web browser for viewing hypertext documents, developed at CERN.

Multidimensional data: Data spanning multiple levels or context of granularity or scope while maintaining one or more common linkages that span such levels.

Multimedia: Computer systems or applications that are able to manipulate data in multiple forms, including still and video images, sound and text.

Mutation: Any alteration to DNA that can potentially result in a change in the function of one or more genes. Mutations can be a change in a single base of DNA (point mutation) or a loss of base pairs (deletion) affecting a single gene or a movement of chromosomal regions (translocation) affecting many genes. Some changes in DNA occur naturally and lead to no harmful effects; these changes in a population are called polymorphisms.

Network: Series of points or nodes interconnected by edges. Edges can have direction or different weights.

Neural computing: *See* Connectionism.

Neural network: Computer program or system designed to mimic some aspects of neurone connections, including summation of action potentials, refractory periods and firing thresholds.

Newsgroup: A bulletin board service provided on a computer network such as the Internet, where messages can be sent by e-mail and be viewed by those who have an interest in the contents of a particular newsgroup. *See also* E-mail, Internet.

Next-generation sequencing: Novel approaches to DNA sequencing that dispense with the need to create libraries of clone sequences in bacteria and provide faster and less expensive sequencing.

Noise: Unwanted signal that is added to a transmitted message while being carried along a channel and that distorts the message for the receiver. *See also* Channel.

Northern blot: RNA from a sample is spatially separated and distributed by mass on a gel. Radioactively labelled DNA or RNA strands with sequence complementary to the RNA segments from the sample are used to locate the position of those RNA segments.

Object-oriented programming: Computer languages and programming philosophy that emphasizes modularity among the elements of a program and their sharing of properties and intercommunication.

Oligonucleotide: A short molecule consisting of several linked nucleotides (typically between 10 and 60) chained together and attached by covalent bonds.

Ontology: A formal and rigorous description of the set of concepts entities within a body of knowledge and the relationships between them. An ontology can help reason about the entities by identifying legal and nonsense relationships and inferences. It is usually represented as a hierarchy and often as a richly interconnected set of objects, concepts and other entities that embody knowledge about a given field. *See also* Knowledge base, Language.

Open-loop control: Partially automated control method in which a part of the control system is given over to humans.

Open reading frame: Regions in a nucleotide sequence that are bounded by start and stop codons and are therefore possible gene coding regions.

Open system: Computer industry term for computer hardware and software that are built to common public standards, thus allowing purchasers to select components from a variety of vendors and use them together.

Orthologous: Homologous genes in two or more organisms that are related only by lineage splitting and not by gene duplication.

OSI seven-layer model: International Organization for Standardization (ISO) model that defines the protocol layers for communicating between heterogeneous computers. *See also* Communication protocol.

PABX: Public area branch exchange. Telecommunication network switching station that connects telephones in an area with the wider telephone network.

Packet-switched network: Computer network that exchanges messages among different computers not by seizing a dedicated circuit, but by sending a message in a number of uniformly sized packets along common channels, shared with other computers. *See also* Circuit-switched network.

Personal health record (PHR): View of the electronic health record designed for patients that also may include patient-created records. *See also* Electronic health record.

Personally controlled health management systems (PCHMS): A set of consumer tools designed to support management of health conditions. Typically includes a PHR. Tools may support organizational aspects of care (e.g. appointment booking, vaccine reminders), social media links to peer support groups, communication with clinicians, decision aids and access to shared care plans with clinicians.

Personally controlled health record: A PHR in which consumers are able to place access controls on who can see aspects of their record.

Pharmacogenomics: The study of the pharmacological response to a drug by a population based on the genetic variation of that population. It has long been known that different individuals in a population respond to the same drug differently and that these variations result from variations in the molecular receptors affected by the drug or from differences in metabolic enzymes that clear the drug. Pharmacogenomics is the science of studying these variations at the molecular level. Applications of pharmacogenomics include reducing side effects, customizing drugs, improvement of clinical trials and the rescue of some drugs that have been banned because of severe side effects in a small percentage of the eligible population.

Phenotype: The observable traits of an individual person. Some traits are determined largely by genotype (e.g. blood type), whereas others (e.g. height) are determined by environmental factors.

Physician's workstation: A computer system designed to support the clinical tasks of doctors. *See also* Electronic medical record.

Polymerase chain reaction (PCR): A technique used to amplify or generate large amounts of replica DNA or a segment of any DNA whose 'flanking' sequences are known. Oligonucleotide primers that bind these flanking sequences are used by an enzyme to copy the sequence in between the primers. Cycles of heat to break apart the DNA strands, thus cooling to allow the primers to bind, and heating again to allow the enzyme to copy the intervening sequence lead to doubling of the DNA present at each cycle.

Polymorphism: Common variation in a region of DNA sequence.

Posterior probability: The probability that an event occurs with evidence both about the prior probability and also about the current case in question. *See also* Bayes' theorem, Prior probability.

Postscript: Commercial language that describes a common format for electronic documents that can be understood by printing devices and converted to paper documents or images on a screen.

Post-test probability: Posterior probability of an event after a test to see whether the event is true. *See also* Posterior probability, Pre-test probability.

Practice parameter: *See* Care pathway.

Precision: The percentage of elements correctly matching a given attribute, out of all the elements identified as matching by a procedure.

Pre-test probability: Prior probability of an event ahead of a test. *See also* Prior probability, Post-test probability.

Prior probability: The probability that an event occurs in a population, with no evidence about the current case in question. *See also* Bayes' theorem.

Probe: Any biochemical agent that is labelled or tagged in some way so that it can be used to identify or isolate a gene, RNA or protein. Typically refers to the immobilized specified nucleic acid in a detection system.

Proteomics: The study of the entire protein complement or 'protein universe' of the cell. Mirroring genomics, proteomics aims to determine the entire suite of expressed proteins in a cell. This includes determining the number, level and turnover of all expressed proteins, their sequence and any post-translational modifications to the sequence and protein–protein and protein–other molecule interactions within the cell, across the cell membrane and among (secreted) proteins.

Protocol: A set of instructions that describe the procedure to be followed when investigating a particular set of findings in a patient or the method to be followed in the management of a given disease *See also* Algorithm, Care pathway, Checklist, Guideline.

PSTN: Public switched telephone network, providing ordinary voice-based telephone services.

Qualitative reasoning: A sub-speciality of artificial intelligence concerned with inference and knowledge representation when knowledge is not precisely defined, e.g. 'back of the envelope' calculations.

Randomized controlled trial (RCT): A form of scientific study that randomly allocates patients either to a group receiving a new treatment or to a control group. If patients or scientists do not know which group patients are allocated to, the trial is a randomized blinded controlled trial. *See also* Systematic review.

Read codes: Medical terminology system, developed initially for primary care medicine in the United Kingdom. It was subsequently enlarged and developed to capture medical concepts in a wide variety of situations. *See also* Terminology.

Reading frame: The succession of codons determined by reading nucleotides in groups of three from a specific starting position.

Reasoning: A method of thinking. *See also* Inference.

Representation: The method chosen to model a process or object, e.g. a building may be represented as a physical scale model, drawing or photograph. *See also* Reasoning, Syntax.

Ribonucleic acid (RNA): RNA is generated from the DNA template in the nucleus of the cell through a process called transcription and is then exported into the cell cytoplasm from the nucleus where it begins the process of protein synthesis.

Rule-based expert system: *See* Expert system.

Search engine: Computer program capable of seeking information on the World Wide Web (or indeed any large database) based upon search criteria specified by a user. *See also* World Wide Web.

Semantics: The meaning associated with a set of symbols in a given language that is determined by the syntactic structure of the symbols, as well as knowledge captured in an interpretative model. *See also* Syntax.

Sequence alignment: The comparison of two or more sequences by searching for a series of individual characters or patterns that are in the same order in the sequence.

Server: A computer on a network that stores commonly used resources such as data or programs and makes these available on demand to clients on the network. *See also* Client, Client-server architecture.

SGML: Standard General Mark-up Language. Document definition language used in printing and used as the basis for the creation of HTML. *See also* HTML.

Shared decision-making (SDM): A collaborative process between patient and health professional that explores both what is known from best scientific evidence but also explores a patient's values and preferences.

Signal to noise ratio: Measure of the amount of noise that has been added to a message during transmission. *See also* Channel, Information theory.

Single nucleotide polymorphism (SNP): Sites in the genome where individual organisms differ in their DNA sequence, often by a single base, usually with very low population frequencies.

SNOMED: Systematized Nomenclature of (Human and Veterinary) Medicine. A commercially available general medical terminology, initially developed for the classification of pathological specimens. *See also* Terminology.

Social contagion: The transmission of behaviours or beliefs across a social network.

Social network: The collection of strong and weak ties that link individuals into a social group.

Social media: A software application designed to support interactions among a group of individuals, as well as manage the creation of new ties among individuals.

Sociotechnical system: The system is created when people and technology together interact in an organization, emphasizing that both the human social and technological features contribute to the overall behaviour of the system.

Software: Synonym for computer program. *See also* Application.

Southern blot: DNA from a sample is cut with restriction enzymes and the position of the fragments (e.g. on a gel) is determined by the fragment's molecular weight. Complementary strands of radioactively labelled DNA are used to identify the position of the DNA fragments on the gel.

Standard gamble: A method to persuade an individual to express a preference for an outcome where the value is unknown as a preference for a gamble where the value for the outcomes are known. *See also* Indifference probability, Utility.

Summary care record (SCR): A general term describing a high-level view of the computer-based patient record, typically restricted to a small number of information items considered most useful in quickly gaining an overview of a patient's health circumstance. *See also* Electronic health record.

Summative assessment: Evaluation of an information system against formal functional metrics or organizational outcome measures. *See also* Formative assessment.

Symbol: A representation that is used to signify a more complex concept. *See also* Model.

Synchronous communication: A mode of communication in which two parties exchange messages across a communication channel at the same time, e.g. telephones. *See also* Asynchronous communication, Isochronous communication.

Syntax: The rules of grammar that define the formal structure of a language. *See also* Semantics.

System: A collection of component ideas, processes or objects that has an input and an output. *See also* Feedback.

Systematic review: A formal process for searching for and then summarizing the evidence contained in scientific papers, to obtain an aggregate view. The review process uses statistical techniques appropriately to combine the individual statistical results of each paper, which ideally is a randomized trial. *See also* Randomized controlled trial.

Systematized Nomenclature of Medicine (SNOMED): A standard vocabulary system for medical databases. It contains more than 144 000 terms and is available in at least two languages. It was developed by the College of American Pathologists.

Telco: Abbreviation for telecommunication company.

Teleconsultation: Clinical consultation carried out using a telemedical service. *See also* Telemedicine.

Telemedicine: The delivery of healthcare services between geographically separated individuals by using telecommunication systems, e.g. video-conferencing.

Term: In medical terminologies, an agreed-on name for a medical condition or treatment. *See also* Code, Terminology.

Terminal: A screen and keyboard system that provides access to a shared computer system, e.g. a mainframe or mini-computer. In contrast to computers on a modern network, terminals are not computers in their own right.

Terminology: A standard set of symbols or words used to describe the concepts, processes and objects of a given field of study. *See also* Term.

Transcription: The synthesis of RNA from DNA.

Transcription factor: A molecule, typically a protein, that binds to DNA binding sites with some regulatory role in transcription. The binding (or unbinding) of a transcription factor from a promoter eventually leads to a change of transcription activity in the gene controlled by that promoter.

Translation: The process of reading of sequence bases in messenger RNA to create a sequence of amino acids, i.e. protein.

True-negative rate (specificity): The percentage of elements correctly detected as not matching a given attribute by a procedure, out of all the possible non-matching elements.

True-positive rate (sensitivity): The percentage of elements correctly detected as matching a given attribute by a procedure, out of all the possible correct elements.

Turing test: Proposed by Alan Turing, the test suggests that an artefact can be considered intelligent if its behaviour cannot be distinguished by humans from other humans in controlled circumstances. *See also* Artificial intelligence.

Unified Medical Language System (UMLS): A comprehensive metavocabulary maintained by the US National Library of Medicine that combines more than 100 individual standardized vocabularies. The UMLS is composed of the Metathesaurus, the Specialist Lexicon and the Semantic Network. The largest component of the UMLS is the Metathesaurus, which contains the term string, concept grouping of terms and concept interrelationships.

Universal genetic code: A misnomer based on an earlier, incorrect belief that all genomes share the same code for specifying amino acids from triplets of nucleotides.

URL: Universal Resource Locator. The address for a document placed on the World Wide Web. *See also* World Wide Web.

User interface: The view a user has of a computer program, usually understood to mean the visual look and feel of a program, but also extending to other modes of interaction, e.g. voice and touch.

Utility: A quantitative measure assigned to an outcome, expressing the preference for that outcome compared with others. *See also* Decision tree.

Value of information (VOI): The economic value that can be placed on receiving particular data before making a decision. VOI is sometimes measured as the *difference* between two outcomes measured as expected utilities. *See also* Expected utility.

Virtual reality: Computer-simulated environment within which humans are able to interact in some manner that approximates interactions in the physical world.

Virulence factor: A protein or a gene that is required for a pathogen to cause disease.

Vocabulary: *See* Terminology.

Voicemail: Computer-based telephone messaging system, capable of recording and storing messages, for later review or other processing, e.g. forwarding to other users. *See also* E-mail.

W3: *See* World Wide Web.

WAN: Wide area network. Computer network extending beyond a local area such as a campus or office. *See also* LAN.

Whole-genome shotgun sequencing: An approach to determine the sequence of a genome in which the genome is broken into numerous small fragments. These fragments are then assembled *en masse*. The individual sequences are assembled into larger sequences (known as contigs) that correspond to substantial portions of the genome.

Workaround: A routine, behaviour or process created to bypass or augment a design element of a pre-existing system.

World Wide Web: An easy-to-use hypertext document system developed for the Internet that allows users to access multimedia documents. *See also* Internet, CERN, HTTP, HTML, URL.

WWW: *See* World Wide Web.

References

Chapter 1

Einstein, A. (1935). *The World as I See it*. London, John Lane, The Bodley Head Limited.

Kafka, F. (1931). *Investigations of a Dog*. London, Martin Secker.

Kent, W. (1978). *Data and Reality*. Amsterdam, North Holland.

Korzybski, A. (1948). *Science and Sanity: An Introduction to Non-Aristotelian Systems and General Semantics*. San Francisco. Institute of General Semantics.

Leveson, N. G. and C. S. Turner (1993). An investigation of the Therac-25 accidents. *Computer* **26**(7): 18–41.

Popper, K. (1976). *Unended Quest*. London, Fontana Collins.

Schafer, E. A. and G. D. Thane (1891). *Quain's Elements of Anatomy*, Vol 1, Part III. London, Longmans, Green and Co.

Skolimowski, H. (1977). The twilight of physical descriptions and the ascent of normative models. In: Laszlo E. (ed.). *The World System: Models, Norms, Variations*. New York, George Braziller.

Sterman, J. D. (2002). All models are wrong: reflections on becoming a systems scientist. *System Dynamics Review* **18**: 501–531.

Chapter 2

Dawkins, R. (1982). *The Extended Phenotype: The Long Reach of the Gene*. Oxford, Oxford University Press.

Lewontin, R. C. (1993). *The Doctrine of DNA: Biology as Ideology*. London, Penguin Books.

Steels, L. and R. A. Brooks. (1995). *The Artificial Life Route to Artificial Intelligence*. Mahwah, NJ, Lawrence Erlbaum Associates.

Chapter 3

Babbage, C. (1833). *On the Economy of Machinery and Manufactures*. London, Charles Knight.

Bean, N. (1996). Secrets of network success. *Physics World* **February**: 30–34.

Chapter 11

Bagozzi, R. P. (2007). The legacy of the technology acceptance model and a proposal for a paradigm shift. *Journal of the Association for Information Systems* **8**(4): 3.

Berg, M. (1997). *Rationalizing Medical Work: Decision Support Techniques and Medical Practices.* Cambridge, MA, MIT Press.

Beuscart-Zéphir, M.-C., F. Anceaux, V. Crinquette and J.-M. Renard (2001). Integrating users' activity modeling in the design and assessment of hospital electronic patient records: the example of anesthesia. *International Journal of Medical Informatics* **64**(2): 157–171.

Boehm, B. W. (1988). A spiral model of software development and enhancement. *Computer* **21**(5): 61–72.

Braithwaite, R. S. and M. Scotch (2013). Using value of information to guide evaluation of decision supports for differential diagnosis: is it time for a new look? *BMC Medical Informatics and Decision Making* **13**(1): 105.

Chuttur, M. (2009). Overview of the technology acceptance model: origins, developments and future directions. *Sprouts Working Papers on Information Systems* **9:** 37.

Cohen, B., W. T. Harwood and M. I. Jackson (1986). *The Specification of Complex Systems.* Boston, Addison-Wesley Longman Publishing.

Coiera, E. (1995). Medical informatics. *BMJ* **310**(6991): 1381.

Coiera, E. (2001). Mediated agent interaction. In: Quaglini S., P. Barahona and S. Andreassen, editors. *8th Conference on Artificial Intelligence in Medicine.* Springer Lecture Notes in Artificial Intelligence No. 2101. Berlin, Springer, pp 1–15.

Coiera, E. (2003). Interaction design theory. *International Journal of Medical Informatics* **69:** 205–222.

Davis, F. D., R. P. Bagozzi and P. R. Warshaw (1989). User acceptance of computer technology: a comparison of two theoretical models. *Management Science* **35**(8): 982–1003.

Downs, S. M., C. P. Friedman, F. Marasigan and G. Gartner (1997). A decision analytic method for scoring performance on computer-based patient simulations. In: *Proceedings of the AMIA Annual Fall Symposium.* Nashville, TN, American Medical Informatics Association.

Fafchamps, D., C. Young and P. Tang (1991). Modelling work practices: input to the design of a physician's workstation. In: *Proceedings of the Annual Symposium on Computer Application in Medical Care.* Washington, D.C., American Medical Informatics Association.

Fenwick, E., K. Claxton and M. Sculpher (2008). The value of implementation and the value of information: combined and uneven development. *Medical Decision Making* **28**(1): 21–32.

Friedman, C. and J. Wyatt (2005). *Evaluation Methods in Biomedical Informatics.* New York, Springer.

Gosling, A., J. Westbrook and J. Braithwaite (2003). Clinical team functioning and IT innovation: a study of the diffusion of a point-of-care online evidence system. *Journal of the American Medical Informatics Association* **10**(3): 246–253

Hogarth, R. M. (1986). Generalization in decision research: the role of formal models. *IEEE Transactions on Systems, Man and Cybernetics* **16**(3): 439–449.

Holden, R. J. and B.-T. Karsh (2010). The technology acceptance model: its past and its future in health care. *Journal of Biomedical Informatics* **43**(1): 159–172.

Howard, R. A. (1966). Information value theory. *IEEE Transactions on Systems, Science and Cybernetics* **2**(1): 22–26.

Larman, C. and V. R. Basili (2003). Iterative and incremental development: a brief history. *Computer* **36**(6): 47–56.

Lau, A., J. Proudfoot, A. Andrews, S. Liaw, J. Crimmins, A. Arguel and E. Coiera (2013). Which bundles of features in a web-based personally controlled health management are associated with consumer help-seeking behaviors for physical and emotional wellbeing? *Journal of Medical Internet Research* **15**(5): e79.

Lilford, R. J., J. Foster and M. Pringle (2009). Evaluating eHealth: how to make evaluation more methodologically robust. *PLoS Medicine* **6**(11): e1000186.

Littlewood, B. and L. Strigini (2000). Software reliability and dependability: a roadmap. In: *Proceedings of the Conference on the Future of Software Engineering*. New York, Association for Computing Machinery.

Lorenzi, N. M., R. T. Riley, A. J. Blyth, G. Southon and B. J. Dixon (1997). Antecedents of the people and organizational aspects of medical informatics review of the literature. *Journal of the American Medical Informatics Association* **4**(2): 79–93.

Markus, M. L. (1994). Electronic mail as the medium of managerial choice. *Organization Science* **5**(4): 502–527.

Nisbett, R. E. and T. D. Wilson (1977). Telling more than we can know: verbal reports on mental processes. *Psychological Review* **84**(3): 231.

Parnas, D. L. and P. C. Clements (1986). A rational design process: how and why to fake it. *IEEE Transactions on Software Engineering* **SE-12**(2): 251–257.

Patel, V. L., D. R. Kaufman and T. Cohen (2013). *Cognitive Informatics in Health and Biomedicine*. London, Springer.

Pearce, C., M. Arnold, C. Phillips, S. Trumble and K. Dwan (2011). The patient and the computer in the primary care consultation. *Journal of the American Medical Informatics Association* **18**(2): 138–142.

Pluye, P., R. M. Grad, J. Johnson-Lafleur, V. Granikov, M. Shulha, B. Marlow and I. L. M. Ricarte (2013). Number needed to benefit from information (NNBI): proposal from a mixed methods research study with practicing family physicians. *Annals of Family Medicine* **11**(6): 559–567.

Pope, C. and N. Mays (2008). *Qualitative Research in Health Care*. New York, John Wiley & Sons.

Reeves, B. and C. Nass (1996). *The Media Equation*. New York: Cambridge University Press.

Royce, W. W. (1970). Managing the development of large software systems. In: *Proceedings of IEEE WESCON*. Los Angeles, Institute of Electrical and Electronic Engineeers.

Schulz, K. F., D. G. Altman and D. Moher (2010). CONSORT 2010 statement: updated guidelines for reporting parallel group randomised trials. *BMC Medicine* **8**(1): 18.

Scott, D. and I. N. Purves (1996). Triadic relationship between doctor, computer and patient. *Interacting with Computers* **8**(4): 347–363.

Talmon, J., E. Ammenwerth, J. Brender, N. de Keizer, P. Nykänen and M. Rigby (2009). STARE-HI: Statement on reporting of evaluation studies in health informatics. *International Journal of Medical Informatics* **78**(1): 1–9.

Taylor, P. (1998). A survey of research in telemedicine. 2. Telemedicine services. *Journal of Telemedicine and Telecare* **4**(2): 63–71.

Toth, B., J. Gray and A. Brice (2005). The number needed to read: a new measure of journal value. *Health Information and Libraries Journal* **22**(2): 81–82.

Venkatesh, V., M. G. Morris, G. B. Davis and F. D. Davis (2003). User acceptance of information technology: toward a unified view. *MIS Quarterly* **27**(3): 425–478.

Westbrook, J. I. and A. Ampt (2009). Design, application and testing of the Work Observation Method by Activity Timing (WOMBAT) to measure clinicians' patterns of work and communication. *International Journal of Medical Informatics* **78**: S25–S33.

Westbrook, J. I., A. Ampt, L. Kearney and M. I. Rob (2008). All in a day's work: an observational work measurement study to quantify how and with whom doctors on hospital wards spend their time. *Medical Journal of Australia* **188**(9): 506–509.

Westbrook, J., C. Duffield, L. Li and N. Creswick (2011). How much time do nurses have for patients? A longitudinal study of hospital nurses' patterns of task time distribution and interactions with other health professionals. *BMC Health Services Research* **11**: 319.

Westbrook, J. I., M. Reckmann, L. Li, W. B. Runciman, R. Burke, C. Lo, M. T. Baysari, J. Braithwaite and R. O. Day (2012). Effects of two commercial electronic prescribing systems on prescribing error rates in hospital in-patients: a before and after study. *PLoS Medicine* **9**(1): e1001164.

Wickens, C., J. Hollands, R. Parasuraman and S. Banbury (2012). *Engineering Psychology and Human Performance.* Upper Saddle River, NJ, Pearson.

Wicker, A. W. (1969). Attitudes versus actions: the relationship of verbal and overt behavioral responses to attitude objects. *Journal of Social Issues* **25**(4): 41–78.

Winograd, T. (1997). *The Design of Interaction: Beyond Calculation.* New York, Springer, pp 149–161.

Winograd, T. and F. Flores (1986). *Understanding Computers and Cognition: A New Foundation for Design.* Bristol, United Kingdom, Intellect Books.

Chapter 12

Albert, R., H. Jeong and A. Barabasi (2000). Error and attack tolerance of complex networks. *Nature* **406**(6794): 378–382.

Albertos, R., B. Caralt and J. Rello (2011). Ventilator-associated pneumonia management in critical illness. *Current Opinion in Gastroenterology* **27**(2): 160–166.

Barochia, A. V., X. Cui, D. Vitberg, A. F. Suffredini, N. P. O'Grady, S. M. Banks, P. Minneci, S. J. Kern, R. L. Danner, C. Natanson and P. Q. Eichacker (2010). Bundled care for septic shock: an analysis of clinical trials. *Critical Care Medicine* **38**(2): 668–678.

Bogers, M., A. Afuah and B. Bastian (2010). Users as innovators: a review, critique, and future research directions. *Journal of Management* **36**(4): 857–875.

Braithwaite, J. and E. Coiera (2010). Beyond patient safety Flatland. *Journal of the Royal Society of Medicine* **103**(6): 219–225.

Braithwaite, J., W. B. Runciman and A. F. Merry (2009). Towards safer, better healthcare: harnessing the natural properties of complex sociotechnical systems. *Quality and Safety in Health Care* **18**(1): 37–41.

Braithwaite, J., J. Westbrook and R. Iedema (2005). Restructuring as gratification. *Journal of the Royal Society of Medicine* **98**(12): 542–544.

Classen, D. C., A. J. Avery and D. W. Bates (2007). Evaluation and certification of computerized provider order entry systems. *Journal of the American Medical Informatics Association* **14**(1): 48–55.

Coiera, E. (2000). When conversation is better than computation. *Journal of the American Medical Informatics Association* **7**(3): 277–286.

Coiera, E. (2009). Building a national health IT system from the middle out. *Journal of the American Medical Informatics Association* **16**(3): 271–273.

Coiera, E. (2011). Why system inertia makes health reform so hard. *BMJ* **343**(7813): 27–29.

Coiera, E. (2014). Communication spaces. *Journal of the American Medical Informatics Association* **21**(3): 414–422.

Connolly, C. (2005). Cedars-Sinai doctors cling to pen and paper. *Washington Post* March 21.

Cresswell, K. M., A. Worth and A. Sheikh (2012). Integration of a nationally procured electronic health record system into user work practices. *BMC Medical Informatics and Decision Making* **12**(1): 15.

Dishaw, M. T. and D. M. Strong (1999). Extending the technology acceptance model with task–technology fit constructs. *Information and Management* **36**(1): 9–21.

Dunn, A. G., M.-S. Ong, J. I. Westbrook, F. Magrabi, E. Coiera and W. Wobcke (2011). A simulation framework for mapping risks in clinical processes: the case of in-patient transfers. *Journal of the American Medical Informatics Association* **18**(3): 259–266.

Eccles, M. and B. Mittman (2006). Welcome to implementation science. *Implementation Science* **1**(1): 1.

Ferneley, E. H. and P. Sobreperez (2006). Resist, comply or workaround? An examination of different facets of user engagement with information systems. *European Journal of Information Systems* **15**(4): 345–356.

Fullbrook, P. and S. Mooney (2003). Care bundles in critical care: a practical approach to evidence-based practice. *Nursing in Critical Care* **8**(6): 249–255.

Gaver, W. W. (1996). Situating action. II. Affordances for interaction: the social is material for design. *Ecological Psychology* **8**(2): 111–129.

Genschel, P. (1997). The dynamics of inertia: institutional persistence and change in telecommunications and health care. *Governance* **10**(1): 43–66.

Goodhue, D. L. and R. L. Thompson (1995). Task-technology fit and individual performance. *MIS Quarterly* **19**(2): 213–236.

Grant, R. W., K. E. Lutfey, E. Gerstenberger, C. L. Link, L. D. Marceau and J. B. McKinlay (2009). The decision to intensify therapy in patients with type 2 diabetes: results from an experiment using a clinical case vignette. *Journal of the American Board of Family Medicine* **22**(5): 513–520.

Grimshaw, J. M. and M. P. Eccles (2004). Is evidence-based implementation of evidence-based care possible? *Medical Journal of Australia* **180**(6 Suppl): S50–S51.

Hannan, M. and J. Freeman (1984). Structural inertia and organisational change. *American Sociological Review* **49**(April): 149–164.

Helfrich, C. D., L. J. Damschroder, H. J. Hagedorn, G. S. Daggett, A. Sahay, M. Ritchie, T. Damush, M. Guihan, P. M. Ullrich and C. B. Stetler (2010). A critical synthesis of literature on the promoting action on research implementation in health services (PARIHS) framework. *Implementation Science* **5:** 82.

Hofer, T., J. Zemencuk and R. Hayward (2004). When there is too much to do. *Journal of General Internal Medicine* **19**(6): 646–653.

Jaén, C., H. McIlvain, L. Pol, R. Phillips, S. Flocke and B. Crabtree (2001). Tailoring tobacco counseling to the competing demands in the clinical encounter. *Journal of Family Practice* **50**(10): 859.

Jaén, C., K. Stange and P. Nutting (1994). Competing demands of primary care: a model for the delivery of clinical preventive services. *Journal of Family Practice* **38**(2): 166–171.

Kahneman, D. and A. Tversky (1979). Prospect theory: an analysis of decision under risk. Econometrica **47**: 263–291.

Kauffman, S. (1993). *The Origins of Order: Self-Organization and Selection in Evolution.* New York, Oxford University Press.

Kauffman, S. (1995). *At Home in the Universe: The Search for the Laws of Self-Organization and Complexity.* Oxford, Oxford University Press.

Kauffman, S. and S. Levin (1987). Towards a general theory of adaptive walks on rugged landscapes. *Journal of Theoretical Biology* **128**(1): 11–45.

Kauffman, S. and W. Macready (1995). Technological evolution and adaptive organizations. Complexity **1**(2): 26–43.

Kauffman, S. A. and E. D. Weinberger (1989). The NK model of rugged fitness landscapes and its application to maturation of the immune response. *Journal of Theoretical Biology* **141**(2): 211–245.

Kerr, J. F. R., A. H. Wyllie and A. R. Currie (1972). Apoptosis: a basic biological phenomenon with wide-ranging implications in tissue kinetics. *British Journal of Cancer* **26**(4): 239–257.

Klinkman, M. S. (1997). Competing demands in psychosocial care: a model for the identification and treatment of depressive disorders in primary care. *General Hospital Psychiatry* **19**(2): 98–111.

Krasner, S. D. (1984). Approaches to the state: alternative conceptions and historical dynamics. *Comparative Politics* **16**(2): 223–246.

Lee, S. D. and J. A. Alexander (1999). Managing hospitals in turbulent times: do organizational changes improve hospital survival? *Health Services Research* **34**(4): 923–946.

Lenz, M., A. Steckelberg, B. Richter and I. Mühlhauser (2007). Meta-analysis does not allow appraisal of complex interventions in diabetes and hypertension self-management: a methodological review. *Diabetologia* **50**(7): 1375–1383.

Leonard, D. A. (1988). Implementation as mutual adaptation of technology and organization. *Research Policy* **17**(5): 251–267.

McShea, D. W. and R. N. Brandon (2010). *Biology's First Law.* Chicago, University of Chicago Press.

Metzger, J., E. Welebob, D. W. Bates, S. Lipsitz and D. C. Classen (2010). Mixed results in the safety performance of computerized physician order entry. *Health Affairs* **29**(4): 655–663.

Niazkhani, Z., H. Pirnejad, A. De Bont and J. Aarts (2010). CPOE in non-surgical versus surgical specialties: a qualitative comparison of clinical contexts in the medication process. *Open Medical Informatics Journal* **4:** 206–213.

Nutting, P. A., M. Baier, J. J. Werner, G. Cutter, C. Conry and L. Stewart (2001). Competing demands in the office visit: what influences mammography recommendations? *Journal of the American Board of Family Practice* **14**(5): 352–361.

O'Connor, P. (2005). Commentary: improving diabetes care by combating clinical inertia. *Health Services Research* **40**(6): 1854–1861.

Parchman, M. L., J. A. Pugh, R. L. Romero and K. W. Bowers (2007). Competing demands or clinical inertia: the case of elevated glycosylated hemoglobin. *Annals of Family Medicine* **5**(3): 196–201.

Phillips, L. S., W. T. Branch, C. B. Cook, J. P. Doyle, I. M. El-Kebbi, D. L. Gallina, C. D. Miller, D. C. Ziemer and C. S. Barnes (2001). Clinical inertia. *Annals of Internal Medicine* **135**(9): 825–834.

Purola, T. (1972). A systems approach to health and health policy. *Medical Care* **10**(5): 373–379.

Rammel, C., S. Stagl and H. Wilfing (2007). Managing complex adaptive systems: a co-evolutionary perspective on natural resource management. *Ecological Economics* **63**(1): 9–21.

Rice, R. E. and E. M. Rogers (1980). Reinvention in the innovation process. *Science Communication* **1**(4): 499–514.

Rivkin, J. W. and N. Siggelkow (2002). Organizational sticking points on NK landscapes. *Complexity* **7**(5): 31–43.

Rogers, E. M. (1995). *Diffusion of Innovations.* New York, Free Press.

Ruef, M. (1997). Assessing organizational fitness on a dynamic landscape: an empirical test of the relative inertia thesis. *Strategic Management Journal* **18**(11): 837–853.

Schneider, C. M., A. Moreira, J. Andrade, S. Havlin and H. J. Herrmann (2011). Mitigation of malicious attacks on networks. *Proceedings of the National Academy of Sciences of the United States of America* **108**: 10.

Shiell, A., P. Hawe and L. Gold (2008). Complex interventions or complex systems? Implications for health economic evaluation. *BMJ* **336**(7656): 1281–1283.

Simon, H. A. (1956). Rational choice and the structure of the environment. *Psychological Review* **63**(2): 1129–1138.

Stange, K. C. (2007). Is 'Clinical inertia' blaming without understanding? Are competing demands excuses? *Annals of Family Medicine* **5**(4): 371–374.

Stetler, C. B., L. J. Damschroder, C. D. Helfrich and H. J. Hagedorn (2011). A guide for applying a revised version of the PARIHS framework for implementation. *Implementation Science* **6**: 99.

Tilebein, M. (2006). A complex adaptive systems approach to efficiency and innovation. *Kybernetes* **35**(7/8): 1087–1099.

van Bruggen, R., K. Gorter, R. Stolk, O. Klungel and G. Rutten (2009). Clinical inertia in general practice: widespread and related to the outcome of diabetes care. *Family Practice* **26**(6): 428–436.

Vicente, K. J. and J. Rasmussen (1992). Ecological interface design: theoretical foundations. *IEEE Transactions on Systems, Man and Cybernetics* **22**(4): 589–606.

Westbrook, J. I., M. T. Baysari, L. Li, R. Burke, K. L. Richardson and R. O. Day (2013). The safety of electronic prescribing: manifestations, mechanisms, and rates of system-related errors associated with two commercial systems in hospitals. *Journal of the American Medical Informatics Association* **20**(6): 1159–1167.

Westbrook, J. I., M. Reckmann, L. Li, W. B. Runciman, R. Burke, C. Lo, M. T. Baysari, J. Braithwaite and R. O. Day (2012). Effects of two commercial electronic prescribing systems on prescribing error rates in hospital in-patients: a before and after study. *PLoS Medicine* **9**(1): e1001164.

Chapter 13

Adelman, J. S., G. E. Kalkut, C. B. Schechter, J. M. Weiss, M. A. Berger, S. H. Reissman, H. W. Cohen, S. J. Lorenzen, D. A. Burack and W. N. Southern (2013). Understanding and preventing wrong-patient electronic orders: a randomized controlled trial. *Journal of the American Medical Informatics Association* **20**(2): 305–310.

Ash, J. S., M. Berg and E. Coiera (2004). Some unintended consequences of information technology in health care: the nature of patient care information system-related errors. *Journal of the American Medical Informatics Association* **11**: 104–112.

Coiera, E., J. Aarts and C. Kulikowski (2012). The dangerous decade. *Journal of the American Medical Informatics Association* **19**(1): 2–5.

Coiera, E. W. and J. I. Westbrook (2006). Should clinical software be regulated? *Medical Journal of Australia* **184**(12): 600–601.

Del Beccaro, M. A., H. E. Jeffries, M. A. Eisenberg and E. D. Harry (2006). Computerized provider order entry implementation: no association with increased mortality rates in an intensive care unit. *Pediatrics* **118**(1): 290–295.

DeRosier, J., E. Stalhandske, J. P. Bagian and T. Nudell (2002). Using health care failure mode and effect analysis: the VA National Center for Patient Safety's prospective risk analysis system. *Joint Commission Journal on Quality and Patient Safety* **28**(5): 248–267.

Fernando, B., B. S. Savelyich, A. J. Avery, A. Sheikh, M. Bainbridge, P. Horsfield and S. Teasdale (2004). Prescribing safety features of general practice computer systems: evaluation using simulated test cases. *BMJ* **328**(7449): 1171–1172.

Ferreira, A., R. Cruz-Correia, L. Antunes, P. Farinha, E. Oliveira-Palhares, D. W. Chadwick and A. Costa-Pereira (2006). How to break access control in a controlled manner. In: *CBMS 2006: 19th IEEE International Symposium on Computer Based Medical Systems*. Salt Lake City, Utah, Institute of Electrical and Electronics Engineers.

Han, Y. Y., J. A. Carcillo, S. T. Venkataraman, R. S. Clark, R. S. Watson, T. C. Nguyen, H. Bayir and R. A. Orr (2005). Unexpected increased mortality after implementation of a commercially sold computerized physician order entry system. *Pediatrics* **116**(6): 1506–1512.

Hewett, R., A. Kulkarni, R. Seker and C. Stringfellow (2006). On effective use of reliability models and defect data in software development. *Region 5 Conference, 2006 IEEE*. San Antonio, TX, USA 67-71.

Hollnagel, E. (2004). *Barriers and Accident Prevention*. Aldershot, UK, Ashgate Publishing.

Horsky, J., G. J. Kuperman and V. L. Patel (2005). Comprehensive analysis of a medication dosing error related to CPOE. *Journal of the American Medical Informatics Association* **12**(4): 377–382.

Koppel, R., T. Wetterneck, J. L. Telles and B.-T. Karsh (2008). Workarounds to barcode medication administration systems: their occurrences, causes, and threats to patient safety. *Journal of the American Medical Informatics Association* **15**(4): 408–423.

Kushniruk, A. W., D. W. Bates, M. Bainbridge, M. S. Househ and E. M. Borycki (2013). National efforts to improve health information system safety in Canada, the United States of America and England. *International Journal of Medical Informatics* **82**(5): e149–e160.

Lau, A. Y. and E. W. Coiera (2007). Do people experience cognitive biases while searching for information? *Journal of the American Medical Informatics Association* **14**(5): 599–608.

Lau, A. Y. S. and E. W. Coiera (2009). Can cognitive biases during consumer health information searches be reduced to improve decision making? *Journal of the American Medical Informatics Association* **16**(1): 54–65.

Leveson, N. G. (2011). *Engineering a Safer World: Systems Thinking Applied to Safety.* Cambridge, MA, MIT Press.

Magrabi, F., J. Aarts, C. Nohr, M. Baker, S. Harrison, S. Pelayo, J. Talmon, D. F. Sittig and E. Coiera (2013). A comparative review of patient safety initiatives for national health information technology. *International Journal of Medical Informatics* **82**(5): e139–e148.

Magrabi, F., M.-S. Ong, W. Runciman and E. Coiera (2010). An analysis of computer-related patient safety incidents to inform the development of a classification. *Journal of the American Medical Informatics Association* **17**(6): 663–670.

Magrabi, F., M. Baker, I. Sinha, M.-S. Ong, S. Harrison, M. R. Kidd, W. B. Runciman and E. Coiera (2015). Clinical safety of England's national programme for IT: A retrospective analysis of all reported safety events 2005 to 2011. *International Journal of Medical Informatics* **84**(3): 198–206.

McLaughlin, M., Y. Nam, J. Gould, C. Pade, K. A. Meeske, K. S. Ruccione and J. Fulk (2012). A videosharing social networking intervention for young adult cancer survivors. *Computers in Human Behavior* **28**(2): 631–641.

Nielsen, J. (1993). *Usability Engineering.* San Francisco, Morgan Kaufmann.

Ong, M. S., F. Magrabi and E. Coiera (2010). Automated categorisation of clinical incident reports using statistical text classification. *Quality and Safety in Health Care* **19**(6): e55.

Ong, M. S., F. Magrabi and E. Coiera (2012a). Automated identification of extreme-risk events in clinical incident reports. *Journal of the American Medical Informatics Association* **19**(1e): e110–e118.

Ong, M. S., F. Magrabi and E. Coiera (2012b). Syndromic surveillance for health information system failures: a feasibility study. *Journal of the American Medical Informatics Association* **20**(3): 506–512.

Runciman, W. B., M. T. Kluger, R. W. Morris, A. D. Paix, L. M. Watterson and R. K. Webb (2005). Crisis management during anaesthesia: the development of an anaesthetic crisis management manual. *Quality and Safety in Health Care* **14**(3): e1.

Runciman, W. B., J. A. H. Williamson, A. Deakin, K. Benveniste, K. Bannon and P. D. Hibbert (2006). An integrated framework for safety, quality and risk management: an information and incident management system based on a universal patient safety classification. *Quality and Safety in Health Care* **15**(Suppl 1): i82–i90.

Sheehy, A., D. Weissburg and S. Dean (2014). The role of copy-and-paste in the hospital electronic health record. *JAMA Internal Medicine* **174**(8): 1217–1218.

Singh, H., J. S. Ash and D. F. Sittig (2013). Safety assurance factors for electronic health record resilience (SAFER): study protocol. *BMC Medical Informatics and Decision Making* **13**(1): 46.

Singh, H., D. C. Classen and D. F. Sittig (2011). Creating an oversight infrastructure for electronic health record-related patient safety hazards. *Journal of Patient Safety* **7**(4): 169–174.

Sittig, D. F. and D. C. Classen (2010). Safe electronic health record use requires a comprehensive monitoring and evaluation framework. *JAMA* **303**(5): 450–451.

Sittig, D. F. and H. Singh (2010). A new sociotechnical model for studying health information technology in complex adaptive healthcare systems. *Quality and Safety in Health Care* **19**(Suppl 3): i68–i74.

Sparnon, E. (2013). Spotlight on electronic health record errors: paper or electronic hybrid workflows. *Pennsylvania Patient Safety Advisory* **10**(2): 55–58.

Sparnon, E. and W. Marela (2012). The role of the electronic health record in patient safety events. *Pennsylvania Patient Safety Advisory* **9**(4): 113–121.

Steinberg, R. A. (2011). *ITIL Service Operation.* London, United Kingdom, The Stationery Office.

Stringfellow, C., A. Andrews, C. Wohlin and H. Petersson (2002). Estimating the number of components with defects post-release that showed no defects in testing. *Software Testing, Verification and Reliability* **12**(2): 93–122.

Sweidan, M., J. F. Reeve, J. E. Brien, P. Jayasuriya, J. H. Martin and G. M. Vernon (2009). Quality of drug interaction alerts in prescribing and dispensing software. *Medical Journal of Australia* **190**(5): 251–254.

Thomas, E., D. Studdert, W. Runciman, R. Webb, E. Sexton, R. Wilson, R. Gibberd, B. Harrison and T. Brennan (2000). A comparison of iatrogenic injury studies in Australia and the USA. I. Context, methods, casemix, population, patient and hospital characteristics. *International Journal for Quality in Health Care* **12**(5): 371–378.

Walker, J. M., P. Carayon, N. Leveson, R. A. Paulus, J. Tooker, H. Chin, A. Bothe, Jr. and W. F. Stewart (2008). EHR safety: the way forward to safe and effective systems. *Journal of the American Medical Informatics Association* **15**(3): 272–277.

Chapter 14

Antelman, K. (2004). Do open-access articles have a greater research impact? *College and Research libraries* **65**(5): 372–382.

Balakrishnan, H., M. F. Kaashoek, D. Karger, R. Morris and I. Stoica (2003). Looking up data in P2P systems. *Communications of the ACM* **46**(2): 43–48.

Brousseau, E. and N. Curien (2007). *Internet and Digital Economics: Principles, Methods and Applications.* Cambridge, Cambridge University Press.

Cimino, J. J. (2006). Use, usability, usefulness, and impact of an infobutton manager. In: *AMIA Annual Symposium Proceedings.* Washington, DC, American Medical Informatics Association.

Coiera, E. (2000). Information economics and the Internet. *Journal of the American Medical Informatics Association* **7**: 215–221.

Davis, J. and M. Stack (1997). The digital advantage. In: Davis, H. T. and M. Stack, editors. *Cutting Edge: Technology, Information, Capitalism and Social Revolution.* London, Verso, pp 121–144.

Dunn, A. G., R. O. Day, K. D. Mandl and E. Coiera (2012). Learning from hackers: open-source clinical trials. *Science Translational Medicine* **4**(132): 132–135.

Fishburn, P. C., A. M. Odlyzko and R. C. Siders (2000). Fixed fee versus unit pricing for information goods: competition, equilibria, and price wars. In: Kahin, B. and H. R. Varian, editors. *Internet Publishing and Beyond: The Economics of Digital Information and Intellectual Property.* Information Infrastructure Project at Harvard University. Cambridge, MA, MIT Press, pp 167–189.

Frank, R. H. (1997). *Microeconomics and Behavior.* New York, McGraw-Hill.

Gaynor, M., L. Lenert, K. D. Wilson and S. Bradner (2014). Why common carrier and network neutrality principles apply to the Nationwide Health Information Network (NWHIN). *Journal of the American Medical Informatics Association* **21**(1): 2–7.

Kelley, K. (1999). *New Rules for the New Economy: 10 Radical Strategies for a Connected World.* London, Penguin Books.

Kephart, J. O. and A. R. Greenwald (2002). *Shopbot Economics: Game Theory and Decision Theory in Agent-Based Systems.* London, Springer, pp 119–158.

Krämer, J., L. Wiewiorra and C. Weinhardt (2013). Net neutrality: a progress report. *Telecommunications Policy* **37**(9): 794–813.

Ku, R. S. R. (2002). The creative destruction of copyright: Napster and the new economics of digital technology. *University of Chicago Law Review* **69**: 263–324.

Mandl, K. D. and I. S. Kohane (2008). Tectonic shifts in the health information economy. *New England Journal of Medicine* **358**(16): 1732–1737.

Saroiu, S., K. P. Gummadi and S. D. Gribble (2003). Measuring and analyzing the characteristics of Napster and Gnutella hosts. *Multimedia Systems* **9**(2): 170–184.

Shapiro, C., H. R. Varian and W. Becker (1999). Information rules: a strategic guide to the network economy. *Journal of Economic Education* **30**: 189–190.

Simon, H. A. (1971). Designing organizations for an information-rich world. *Computers, Communications, and the Public Interest* **72**: 37.

Stigler, G. J. (1961). The economics of information. *Journal of Political Economy* **69**(3): 213–225.

Varian, H. R. (1996). Pricing electronic journals. *D-Lib Magazine* **2**(6).

Varian, H. R. (1999). Market structure in the network age. In: *Understanding the Digital Economy: Data, Tools, and Research.* Cambridge, MA, MIT Press, pp 137–150.

Varian, H. R. and N. Ginkō (1999). *Markets for Information Goods.* Tokyo: Institute for Monetary and Economic Studies, Bank of Japan.

Chapter 15

Allen, D., E. Gillen and L. Rixson (2009). Systematic review of the effectiveness of integrated care pathways: what works, for whom, in which circumstances? *International Journal of Evidence-Based Healthcare* **7**(2): 61–74.

Antman, E. M., J. Lau, B. Kupelnick, F. Mosteller and T. C. Chalmers (1992). A comparison of results of meta-analyses of randomized control trials and recommendations of clinical experts: treatments for myocardial infarction. *JAMA* **268**(2): 240–248.

Arndt, K. A. (1992). Information excess in medicine: overview, relevance to dermatology, and strategies for coping. *Archives of Dermatology* **128**(9): 1249–1256.

Beller, E. M., J. K.-H. Chen, U. L.-H. Wang and P. P. Glasziou (2013). Are systematic reviews up-to-date at the time of publication? *Systematic Reviews* **2**: 36.

Bergs, J., J. Hellings, I. Cleemput, Ö. Zurel, V. De Troyer, M. Van Hiel, J. L. Demeere, D. Claeys and D. Vandijck (2014). Systematic review and meta-analysis of the effect of the World Health Organization surgical safety checklist on postoperative complications. *British Journal of Surgery* **101**(3): 150–158.

Cutler, P. (1979). *Problem Solving in Clinical Medicine: From Data to Diagnosis.* Baltimore, Williams & Wilkins.

Darling, G. (2002). The impact of clinical practice guidelines and clinical trials on treatment decisions. *Surgical Oncology* **11**(4): 255–262.

Deneckere, S., M. Euwema, P. Van Herck, C. Lodewijckx, M. Panella, W. Sermeus and K. Vanhaecht (2012). Care pathways lead to better teamwork: results of a systematic review. *Social Science and Medicine* **75**(2): 264–268.

Elstein, A. S., L. S. Shulman and S. A. Sprafka (1978). *Medical Problem Solving: An Analysis of Clinical Reasoning.* Cambridge, MA, Harvard University Press.

Feinstein, A. R. (1967). *Clinical Judgment.* Baltimore, Williams & Wilkins.

Gallego, B., A. G. Dunn and E. Coiera (2013). Role of electronic health records in comparative effectiveness research. *Journal of Comparative Effectiveness Research* **2**(6): 529–532.

Grimshaw, J. M. and I. T. Russell (1993). Effect of clinical guidelines on medical practice: a systematic review of rigorous evaluations. *Lancet* **342**(8883): 1317–1322.

Guyatt, G., J. Cairns, D. Churchill, Evidence Based Medicine Working Group, *et al.* (1992). Evidence-based medicine: a new approach to teaching the practice of medicine. *JAMA* **268**(17): 2420–2425.

Hales, B. M. and P. J. Pronovost (2006). The checklist: a tool for error management and performance improvement. *Journal of Critical Care* **21**(3): 231–235.

Haynes, A. B., T. G. Weiser, W. R. Berry, S. R. Lipsitz, A.-H. S. Breizat, E. P. Dellinger, T. Herbosa, S. Joseph, P. L. Kibatala and M. C. M. Lapitan (2009). A surgical safety checklist to reduce morbidity and mortality in a global population. *New England Journal of Medicine* **360**(5): 491–499.

Heathfield, H. A. and J. Wyatt (1993). Medical informatics: hiding our light under a bushel, or the emperor's new clothes? *Methods of Information in Medicine* **32**(2): 181–182.

Kinsman, L., T. Rotter, E. James, P. Snow and J. Willis (2010). What is a clinical pathway? Development of a definition to inform the debate. *BMC Medicine* **8**(1): 31.

Klein, G. A. and R. Calderwood (1991). Decision models: some lessons from the field. *IEEE Transactions on Systems, Man, and Cybernetics* **21**(5): 1018–1026.

Krall, L. P. and R. S. Beaser (1989). *Joslin Diabetes Manual.* Philadelphia, Lea & Febiger.

Kwan, J. and P. Sandercock (2003). In-hospital care pathways for stroke: a Cochrane systematic review. *Stroke* **34**(2): 587–588.

Kwan, J. and P. Sandercock (2005). In-hospital care pathways for stroke: an updated systematic review. *Stroke* **36**(6): 1348–1349.

McCue, J. D., A. Beck and K. Smothers (2009). Quality toolbox: clinical pathways can improve core measure scores. *Journal for Healthcare Quality* **31**(1): 43–50.

McGlynn, E. A., S. M. Asch, J. Adams, J. Keesey, J. Hicks and A. DeCristofaro (2003). The quality of health care delivered to adults in the United States. *New England Journal of Medicine* **348**(26): 2635–2645.

Mulrow, C. D. (1994). Systematic reviews: rationale for systematic reviews. *BMJ* **309**(6954): 597–599.

Patel, V. L., D. R. Kaufman and J. F. Arocha (2002). Emerging paradigms of cognition in medical decision-making. *Journal of Biomedical Informatics* **35**(1): 52–75.

Roper, W. L., W. Winkenwerder, G. M. Hackbarth and H. Krakauer (1988). Effectiveness in health care: an initiative to evaluate and improve medical practice. *New England Journal of Medicine* **319**(18): 1197–1202.

Rotter, T., L. Kinsman, E. James, A. Machotta and E. W. Steyerberg (2012). The quality of the evidence base for clinical pathway effectiveness: room for improvement in the design of evaluation trials. *BMC Medical Research Methodology* **12**(1): 80.

Runciman, W. B., T. D. Hunt, N. A. Hannaford, P. D. Hibbert, J. I. Westbrook, E. W. Coiera, R. O. Day, D. M. Hindmarsh, E. A. McGlynn and J. Braithwaite (2012). CareTrack: assessing the appropriateness of health care delivery in Australia. *Medical Journal of Australia* **197**(10): 549.

Salas, E., H. B. King and M. A. Rosen (2012). Improving teamwork and safety: toward a practical systems approach, a commentary on Deneckere *et al.* *Social Science and Medicine* **75**(6): 986–989.

Salas, E. and G. Klein (2001). Expertise and naturalistic decision making: an overview. In: *Linking Expertise and Naturalistic Decision Making.* Hillsdale, NJ, Lawrence Erlbaum, pp 3–8.

Sim, I. and M. A. Hlatky (1996). Growing pains of meta-analysis. *BMJ* **313**(7059): 702–703.

Taylor, W. J., A. Wong, R. J. Siegert and H. K. McNaughton (2006). Effectiveness of a clinical pathway for acute stroke care in a district general hospital: an audit. *BMC Health Services Research* **6**(1): 16.

Van Houdt, S., J. Heyrman, K. Vanhaecht, W. Sermeus and J. De Lepeleire (2013). Care pathways across the primary-hospital care continuum: using the multi-level framework in explaining care coordination. *BMC Health Services Research* **13**(1): 1–12.

Weng, C., S. W. Tu, I. Sim and R. Richesson (2010). Formal representation of eligibility criteria: a literature review. Journal of Biomedical Informatics **43**(3): 451–467.

World Health Organization (2009). *WHO Guidelines for Safe Surgery.* Geneva, World Health Organization Press.

Wyatt, J. (1991). Information for clinicians: use and sources of medical knowledge. *Lancet* **338**(8779): 1368–1373.

Chapter 16

Aboumater, H. J., L. E. Winner, R. O. Davis, P. B. Trovitch, M. M. Berg, K. M. Violette, W. A. Messersmith, K. K. Maylor and C. U. Lehmann (2008). No time to waste: decreasing patient wait times for chemotherapy administration using automated prioritization in an oncology pharmacy system. *American Journal of Managed Care* **14**(5): 309–316.

Blackwood, B., F. Alderdice, K. Burns, C. Cardwell, G. Lavery and P. O'Halloran (2011). Use of weaning protocols for reducing duration of mechanical ventilation in critically ill adult patients: Cochrane systematic review and meta-analysis. *BMJ* **342**: c7237–c7237.

Boord, J. B., M. Sharifi, R. A. Greevy, M. R. Griffin, V. K. Lee, T. A. Webb, M. E. May, L. R. Waitman, A. K. May and R. A. Miller (2007). Computer-based insulin infusion protocol improves glycemia control over manual protocol. *Journal of the American Medical Informatics Association* **14**(3): 278–287.

Boxwala, A. A., M. Peleg, S. Tu, O. Ogunyemi, Q. T. Zeng, D. Wang, V. L. Patel, R. A. Greenes and E. H. Shortliffe (2004). GLIF3: a representation format for sharable computer-interpretable clinical practice guidelines. *Journal of Biomedical Informatics* **37**(3): 147–161.

Cimino, J. J. (2008). Infobuttons: anticipatory passive decision support. *AMIA Annual Symposium Proceedings* (**November 6**): 1203–1204.

Coiera, E. (2011). Why system inertia makes health reform so hard. *BMJ* **343**(7813): 27–29.

Coiera, E. and S. Lewis (1998). *Information Management System for a Dynamic System and Method Thereof.* US5802542 A. Washington, DC, United States Patent Office.

Damiani, G., L. Pinnarelli, S. C. Colosimo, R. Almiento, L. Sicuro, R. Galasso, L. Sommella and W. Ricciardi (2010). The effectiveness of computerized clinical guidelines in the process of care: a systematic review. *BMC Health Services Research* **10**(1): 2.

De Clercq, P., K. Kaiser and A. Hasman (2008). Computer-interpretable guideline formalisms. *Studies in Health Technology and Informatics* **139**: 22–43.

De Dombal, F., V. Dallos and W. McAdam (1991). Can computer aided teaching packages improve clinical care in patients with acute abdominal pain? *BMJ* **302**(6791): 1495.

Eccles, M., E. McColl, N. Steen, N. Rousseau, J. Grimshaw, D. Parkin and I. Purves (2002). Effect of computerised evidence based guidelines on management of asthma and angina in primary care: cluster randomised controlled trial. *BMJ* **325**: 941–946.

Feder, G., C. Griffiths, C. Highton, S. Eldridge, M. Spence and L. Southgate (1995). Do clinical guidelines introduced with practice based education improve care of asthmatic and diabetic patients? A randomised controlled trial in general practices in east London. *BMJ* **311**(7018): 1473.

Fox, J. and S. Das (2000). *Safe and Sound: Artificial Intelligence in Hazardous Applications.* Cambridge, MA, AAAI Press, co-published by MIT Press.

Fox, J., N. Johns, A. Rahmanzadeh and R. Thomson (1996). PROforma: a method and language for specifying clinical guidelines and protocols. in Medical Informatics Europe '96. Brender, J., J. P. Christensen, R. Scherrer and P. McNair (eds.). *Studies in Health Technology and Informatics.* Amsterdam, IOS Press. **34**: 516–520.

Fuchsberger, C., J. Hunter and P. McCue (2005). Testing Asbru guidelines and protocols for neonatal intensive care. In: Miksch, S., J. Hunter and E. Keravnou, editors. *Artificial Intelligence in Medicine.* Berlin, Springer, pp 101–110.

Haas, C. F. and P. S. Loik (2012). Ventilator discontinuation protocols. *Respiratory Care* **57**(10): 1649–1662.

Henderson, S., R. Crapo, C. J. Wallace, T. East, A. Morris and R. Gardner (1991). Performance of computerized protocols for the management of arterial oxygenation in an intensive care unit. *International Journal of Clinical Monitoring and Computing* **8**(4): 271–280.

Heselmans, A., S. Van de Velde, P. Donceel, B. Aertgeerts and D. Ramaekers (2009). Effectiveness of electronic guideline-based implementation systems in ambulatory care settings: a systematic review. *Implementation Science* **4**(1): 82.

Humber, M., H. Butterworth, J. Fox and R. Thomson (2001). Medical decision support via the Internet: PROforma and Solo. *Studies in Health Technology and Informatics* **84**(1): 464–468.

Isern, D. and A. Moreno (2008). Computer-based execution of clinical guidelines: a review. *International Journal of Medical Informatics* **77**(12): 787–808.

Jousimaa, J., M. Mäkelä, I. Kunnamo, G. MacLennan and J. M. Grimshaw (2002). Primary care guidelines on consultation practices: the effectiveness of computerized versus paper-based versions. *International Journal of Technology Assessment in Health Care* **18**(3): 586–596.

Lobach, D. F. and W. E. Hammond (1997). Computerized decision support based on a clinical practice guideline improves compliance with care standards. *American Journal of Medicine* **102**(1): 89–98.

Majidi, F., J. P. Enterline, B. Ashley, M. E. Fowler, L. L. Ogorzalek, R. Gaudette, G. Stuart, M. Fulton and D. Ettinger (1993). Chemotherapy and treatment scheduling: the Johns Hopkins Oncology Center Outpatient Department. In: *Proceedings of the Annual Symposium on Computer Application in Medical Care*. Washington, D.C., American Medical Informatics Association.

McKinley, B. A., F. A. Moore, R. M. Sailors, C. S. Cocanour, A. Marquez, R. K. Wright, A. S. Tonnesen, C. J. Wallace, A. H. Morris and T. D. East (2001). Computerized decision support for mechanical ventilation of trauma induced ARDS: results of a randomized clinical trial. *Journal of Trauma: Injury, Infection, and Critical Care* **50**(3): 415–425.

Miksch, S., Y. Shahar and P. Johnson (1997). Asbru: a task-specific, intention-based, and time-oriented language for representing skeletal plans. In: *Proceedings of the 7th Workshop on Knowledge Engineering: Methods and Languages (KEML-97)*, Milton Keynes, United Kingdom, The Open University.

Musen, M. A. (1998). Domain ontologies in software engineering: use of Protege with the EON architecture. *Methods of Information in Medicine Methodik der Information in der Medizin* **37**(4): 540–550.

Musen, M. A., S. W. Tu, A. K. Das and Y. Shahar (1996). EON: A component-based approach to automation of protocol-directed therapy. *Journal of the American Medical Informatics Association* **3**(6): 367–388.

Naeem, U. and J. Bigham (2009). Activity recognition in the home using a hierarchal framework with object usage data. *Journal of Ambient Intelligence and Smart Environments* **1**(4): 335–350.

Noy, N. F., R. W. Fergerson and M. A. Musen (2000). The knowledge model of Protege-2000: combining interoperability and flexibility. In: Dieng, R. and O. Corby, editors. *Knowledge Engineering and Knowledge Management: Methods, Models, and Tools*. Berlin, Springer, pp 17–32.

Peleg, M., S. Tu, J. Bury, P. Ciccarese, J. Fox, R. A. Greenes, R. Hall, P. D. Johnson, N. Jones and A. Kumar (2003). Comparing computer-interpretable guideline models: a case-study approach. *Journal of the American Medical Informatics Association* **10**(1): 52–68.

Rood, E., R. J. Bosman, J. I. Van der Spoel, P. Taylor and D. F. Zandstra (2005). Use of a computerized guideline for glucose regulation in the intensive care unit improved both guideline adherence and glucose regulation. *Journal of the American Medical Informatics Association* **12**(2): 172–180.

Samwald, M., K. Fehre, J. De Bruin and K.-P. Adlassnig (2012). The Arden Syntax standard for clinical decision support: experiences and directions. *Journal of Biomedical Informatics* **45**(4): 711–718.

Santibáñez, P., R. Aristizabal, M. L. Puterman, V. S. Chow, W. Huang, C. Kollmannsberger, T. Nordin, N. Runzer and S. Tyldesley (2012). Operations research methods improve chemotherapy patient appointment scheduling. *Joint Commission Journal on Quality and Patient Safety* **38**(12): 541.

Seitinger, A., K. Fehre, K.-P. Adlassnig, A. Rappelsberger, E. Wurm, E. Aberer and M. Binder (2013). An Arden-Syntax–based clinical decision support framework for medical guidelines: Lyme borreliosis as an example. *Studies in Health Technology and Informatics* **198**: 125–132.

Seyfang, A., S. Miksch and M. Marcos (2002). Combining diagnosis and treatment using Asbru. *International Journal of Medical Informatics* **68**(1): 49–57.

Shiffman, R. N., Y. Liaw, C. A. Brandt and G. J. Corb (1999). Computer-based guideline implementation systems: a systematic review of functionality and effectiveness. *Journal of the American Medical Informatics Association* **6**(2): 104–114.

Shojania, K. G., D. Yokoe, R. Platt, J. Fiskio, N. Ma'Luf and D. W. Bates (1998). Reducing vancomycin use utilizing a computer guideline results of a randomized controlled trial. *Journal of the American Medical Informatics Association* **5**(6): 554–562.

Smart, S. and I. Purves (2001). The Problems of large-scale knowledge authoring and the PRODIGY solutions. In: *Proceedings of the AMIA Symposium*. Washington, D.C., American Medical Informatics Association.

Sutton, D. R. and J. Fox (2003). The syntax and semantics of the PRO*forma* guideline modeling language. *Journal of the American Medical Informatics Association* **10**(5): 433–443.

Sutton, D. R., P. Taylor and K. Earle (2006). Evaluation of PRO*forma* as a language for implementing medical guidelines in a practical context. *BMC Medical Informatics and Decision Making* **6**(1): 20.

Thomsen, G. E., D. Pope, T. D. East, A. H. Morris, A. T. Kinder, D. A. Carlson, G. L. Smith, C. J. Wallace, J. F. Orme Jr. and T. P. Clemmer (1993). Clinical performance of a rule-based decision support system for mechanical ventilation of ARDS patients. In: *Proceedings of the Annual Symposium on Computer Application in Medical Care.* Washington, D.C., American Medical Informatics Association.

Tu, S. W., J. R. Campbell, J. Glasgow, M. A. Nyman, R. McClure, J. McClay, C. Parker, K. M. Hrabak, D. Berg and T. Weida (2007). The SAGE guideline model: achievements and overview. *Journal of the American Medical Informatics Association* **14**(5): 589–598.

Tudorache, T., C. Nyulas, N. F. Noy and M. A. Musen (2013). WebProtégé: A collaborative ontology editor and knowledge acquisition tool for the web. *Semantic Web* **4**(1): 89–99.

Tural, C., L. Ruiz, C. Holtzer, J. Schapiro, P. Viciana, J. González, P. Domingo, C. Boucher, C. Rey-Joly and B. Clotet (2002). Clinical utility of HIV-1 genotyping and expert advice: the Havana trial. *AIDS* **16**(2): 209–218.

Vetterlein, T., H. Mandl and K.-P. Adlassnig (2010). Fuzzy Arden Syntax: a fuzzy programming language for medicine. *Artificial Intelligence in Medicine* **49**(1): 1–10.

Wang, D., M. Peleg, S. W. Tu, A. A. Boxwala, R. A. Greenes, V. L. Patel and E. H. Shortliffe (2002). Representation primitives, process models and patient data in computer-interpretable clinical practice guidelines: a literature review of guideline representation models. *International Journal of Medical Informatics* **68**(1): 59–70.

Chapter 17

Allen, D., E. Gillen and L. Rixson (2009). Systematic review of the effectiveness of integrated care pathways: what works, for whom, in which circumstances? *International Journal of Evidence-Based Healthcare* **7**(2): 61–74.

Ash, J. (1997). Organizational factors that influence information technology diffusion in academic health sciences centers. *Journal of the American Medical Informatics Association* **4**(2): 102–111.

Bastian, H., P. Glasziou and I. Chalmers (2010). Seventy-five trials and eleven systematic reviews a day: how will we ever keep up? *PLoS Medicine* **7**(9): e1000326.

Bax, L., L.-M. Yu, N. Ikeda and K. G. Moons (2007). A systematic comparison of software dedicated to meta-analysis of causal studies. *BMC Medical Research Methodology* **7**(1): 40.

Cabana, M. D., C. S. Rand, N. R. Powe, A. W. Wu, M. H. Wilson, P.-A. C. Abboud and H. R. Rubin (1999). Why don't physicians follow clinical practice guidelines? A framework for improvement. *JAMA* **282**(15): 1458–1465.

Chung, G. and E. Coiera (2007). A study of structured clinical abstracts and the semantic classification of sentences. In: *Proceedings of the Workshop on BioNLP 2007: Biological, Translational, and Clinical Language Processing*. Prague, Czech Republic, Association for Computational Linguistics.

Chung, G. and E. Coiera (2008). Are decision trees a feasible knowledge representation to guide extraction of critical information from randomized controlled trial reports? *BMC Medical Informatics and Decision Making* **8**(1): 48.

Cohen, A. M., K. Ambert and M. McDonagh (2012). Studying the potential impact of automated document classification on scheduling a systematic review update. *BMC Medical Informatics and Decision Making* **12**: 33.

Coiera, E. (1992). Intermediate depth representations. *Artificial Intelligence in Medicine* **4**(6): 431–445.

Coiera, E. (1996). Artificial intelligence in medicine: the challenges ahead. *Journal of the American Medical Informatics Association* **3**(6): 363–366.

Coiera, E. (1998). Information epidemics, economics, and immunity on the Internet. *BMJ* **317**(7171): 1469–1470.

Coiera, E. (2001). Maximising the uptake of evidence into clinical practice: an information economics approach. *Medical Journal of Australia* **174**(9): 467–470.

Coiera, E., M. Walther, K. Nguyen and N. H. Lovell (2005). Architecture for knowledge-based and federated search of online clinical evidence. *Journal of Medical Internet Research* **7**(5): e52.

Dick, T. (1833). *On the Improvement of Society by the Diffusion of Knowledge*. Glasgow, Scotland, William Collins and Co.

Egger, M., G. D. Smith, M. Schneider and C. Minder (1997). Bias in meta-analysis detected by a simple, graphical test. *BMJ* **315**(7109): 629–634.

Elhadad, N., M.-Y. Kan, J. L. Klavans and K. McKeown (2005). Customization in a unified framework for summarizing medical literature. *Artificial Intelligence in Medicine* **33**(2): 179–198.

Elliott, J. H., T. Turner, O. Clavisi, J. Thomas, J. P. Higgins, C. Mavergames and R. L. Gruen (2014). Living systematic reviews: an emerging opportunity to narrow the evidence-practice gap. *PLoS Medicine* **11**(2): e1001603.

Feder, G., C. Griffiths, C. Highton, S. Eldridge, M. Spence and L. Southgate (1995). Do clinical guidelines introduced with practice based education improve care of asthmatic and diabetic patients? A randomised controlled trial in general practices in east London. *BMJ* **311**(7018): 1473.

Gosling, A., J. Westbrook and J. Braithwaite (2003a). Clinical team functioning and IT innovation: a study of the diffusion of a point-of-care online evidence system. *Journal of the American Medical Informatics Association* **10**(3): 246–253.

Gosling, A., J. Westbrook and E. Coiera (2003b). Variation in the use of online clinical evidence: a qualitative analysis. *International Journal of Medical Informatics* **69**(1): 1–16.

Grant, R. W., K. E. Lutfey, E. Gerstenberger, C. L. Link, L. D. Marceau and J. B. McKinlay (2009). The decision to intensify therapy in patients with type 2 diabetes: results from an experiment using a clinical case vignette. *Journal of the American Board of Family Medicine* **22**(5): 513–520.

Greenwood, J., J. Sullivan, K. Spence and M. McDonald (2000). Nursing scripts and the organizational influences on critical thinking: report of a study of neonatal nurses' clinical reasoning. *Journal of Advanced Nursing* **31**(5): 1106–1114.

Grilli, R. and J. Lomas (1994). Evaluating the message: the relationship between compliance rate and the subject of a practice guideline. *Medical Care* **32**(3): 202–213.

Hersh, W. R. and D. H. Hickam (1998). How well do physicians use electronic information retrieval systems? A framework for investigation and systematic review. *JAMA* **280**(15): 1347–1352.

Hofer, T., J. Zemencuk and R. Hayward (2004). When there is too much to do. *Journal of General Internal Medicine* **19**(6): 646–653.

Howell, J. M. and K. Boies (2004). Champions of technological innovation: the influence of contextual knowledge, role orientation, idea generation, and idea promotion on champion emergence. *Leadership Quarterly* **15**(1): 123–143.

Jaidee, W., D. Moher and M. Laopaiboon (2010). Time to update and quantitative changes in the results of Cochrane pregnancy and childbirth reviews. *PLoS One* **5**(7): e11553.

Kaplan, B. (1997). Addressing organizational issues into the evaluation of medical systems. *Journal of the American Medical Informatics Association* **4**(2): 94–101.

Kiritchenko, S., B. de Bruijn, S. Carini, J. Martin and I. Sim (2010). ExaCT: automatic extraction of clinical trial characteristics from journal publications. *BMC Medical Informatics and Decision Making* **10:** 56.

Lewis, S. and M. Clarke (2001). Forest plots: trying to see the wood and the trees. *BMJ* **322**(7300): 1479.

Magrabi, F., J. I. Westbrook, E. W. Coiera and A. S. Gosling (2004). Clinicians' assessments of the usefulness of online evidence to answer clinical questions. *Medinfo* **11**(1): 297–300.

Manias, E. and A. Street (2000). Legitimation of nurses' knowledge through policies and protocols in clinical practice. *Journal of Advanced Nursing* **32**(6): 1467–1475.

Martin, J. and American Management Association (1995). *The Great Transition: Using the Seven Disciplines of Enterprise Engineering to Align People, Technology, and Strategy.* New York, Amacom.

Pluye, P., R. M. Grad, J. Johnson-Lafleur, V. Granikov, M. Shulha, B. Marlow and I. L. M. Ricarte (2013). Number needed to benefit from information (NNBI): proposal from a mixed methods research study with practicing family physicians. *Annals of Family Medicine* **11**(6): 559–567.

Pratt, W. and I. Sim (1995). Physician's information customizer (PIC): using a shareable user model to filter the medical literature. In: *International Conference on Medical Informatics (MEDINFO'95).* Vancouver, Canada: 1447–51.

Reiter, E. (2010). Natural language generation. In: Clark, A., C. Fox and S. Lappin, editors. *The Handbook of Computational Linguistics and Natural Language Processing.* Oxford, Wiley-Blackwell.

Rennels, G. D., E. H. Shortliffe, F. E. Stockdale and P. L. Miller (1987). A computational model of reasoning from the clinical literature. *Computer Methods and Programs in Biomedicine* **24**(2): 139–149.

Retsas, A. (2000). Barriers to using research evidence in nursing practice. *Journal of Advanced Nursing* **31**(3): 599–606.

Rosenberg, M. S., D. C. Adams and J. Gurevitch (2000). *MetaWin: Statistical Software for Meta-Analysis With Resampling Tests.* Sunderland, MA, Sinauer Associates.

Shiffman, R. N., G. Michel, A. Essaihi and E. Thornquist (2004). Bridging the guideline implementation gap: a systematic, document-centered approach to guideline implementation. *Journal of the American Medical Informatics Association* **11**(5): 418–426.

Shojania, K. G., M. Sampson, M. T. Ansari, J. Ji, S. Doucette and D. Moher (2007). How quickly do systematic reviews go out of date? A survival analysis. *Annals of Internal Medicine* **147**(4): 224–233.

Sim, I. and D. E. Detmer (2005). Beyond trial registration: a global trial bank for clinical trial reporting. *PLoS Medicine* **2**(11): e365.

Smith, R. and I. Chalmers (2001). Britain's gift: a 'Medline' of synthesised evidence. *BMJ* **323**(7327): 1437–1438.

Tange, H. J., H. C. Schouten, A. D. Kester and A. Hasman (1998). The granularity of medical narratives and its effect on the speed and completeness of information retrieval. *Journal of the American Medical Informatics Association* **5**(6): 571–582.

Toth, B., J. Gray and A. Brice (2005). The number needed to read: a new measure of journal value. *Health Information and Libraries Journal* **22**(2): 81–82.

Tsafnat, G. and E. Coiera (2009). Computational reasoning across multiple models. *Journal of the American Medical Informatics Association* **16**(6): 768–774.

Tsafnat, G., A. Dunn, P. Glasziou and E. Coiera (2013). The automation of systematic reviews. *BMJ* **346**: f139.

Tsafnat, G., P. P. Glasziou, M. K. Choong, A. Dunn, F. Galgani and E. Coiera (2014). Systematic review automation technologies. *Systematic Reviews* **3**(1): 74.

Tu, S. W., M. G. Kahn, M. A. Musen, L. Fagan and J. C. Ferguson (1989). Episodic skeletal-plan refinement based on temporal data. *Communications of the ACM* **32**(12): 1439–1455.

Utterback, J. M. (1996). *Mastering the Dynamics of Innovation.* Cambridge, MA, Harvard Business Press.

Wallace, B., C. H. Schmid, J. Lau and T. A. Trikalinos (2009). Meta-Analyst: software for meta-analysis of binary, continuous and diagnostic data. *BMC Medical Research Methodology* **9**(1): 80.

Wallace, B., K. Small, C. Brodley, J. Lau and T. Trikalinos (2012). Deploying an interactive machine learning system in an evidence-based practice center: abstract. In: *Proceedings of the 2nd ACM SIGHIT Symposium on International Health Informatics.* New York, Association for Computing Machinery.

Westbrook, J., A. S. Gosling and E. Coiera (2004). Do clinicians use online evidence to support patient care? A study of 55,000 clinicians. *Journal of the American Medical Informatics Association* **11**(2): 113–120.

Zamora, J., V. Abraira, A. Muriel, K. Khan and A. Coomarasamy (2006). Meta-DiSc: a software for meta-analysis of test accuracy data. *BMC Medical Research Methodology* **6**(1): 31.

Chapter 18

Bhasale, A., G. Miller, S. Reid and H. Britt (1998). Analysing potential harm in Australian general practice: an incident monitoring study. *Medical Journal of Australia* **169**(2): 173–176.

Boden, D. (1994). *The Business of Talk: Organizations in Action.* Cambridge, United Kingdom, Polity Press.

Caldwell, B. S., S.-T. Uang and L. H. Taha (1995). Appropriateness of communications media use in organizations: situation requirements and media characteristics. *Behaviour and Information Technology* **14**(4): 199–207.

Clark, H. H. and S. E. Brennan (1991). Grounding in communication. *Perspectives on Socially Shared Cognition* **13**(1991): 127–149.

Coiera, E. (2000). When conversation is better than computation. *Journal of the American Medical Informatics Association* **7**(3): 277–286.

Coiera, E. and V. Tombs (1998). Communication behaviours in a hospital setting: an observational study. *BMJ* **316**: 673–677.

Coiera, E., R. Jayasuriya, J. Hardy, A. Bannan and M. Thorpe (2002). Communication loads on clinicians in the emergency department. *Medical Journal of Australia* **176**(9): 415–418.

Covell, D. G., G. C. Uman and P. R. Manning (1985). Information needs in office practice: are they being met? *Annals of Internal Medicine* **103**(4): 596–599.

Cunillera, T., E. Camara, M. Laine and A. Rodriguez-Fornells (2010). Speech segmentation is facilitated by visual cues. *Quarterly Journal of Experimental Psychology* **63**(2): 260–274.

Fitzpatrick, K. and E. Vineski (1993). The role of cordless phones in improving patient care. *Physician Assistant* **17**(6): 87.

Friedman, R. H. (1998). Automated telephone conversations to assess health behavior and deliver behavioral interventions. *Journal of Medical Systems* **22**(2): 95–102.

Grajales, III, F. J., S. Sheps, K. Ho, H. Novak-Lauscher, G. Eysenbach and G. Eysenbach (2014). Social media: a review and tutorial of applications in medicine and health care. *Journal of Medical Internet Research* **16**(2): e13.

Houston, T. K., D. Z. Sands, M. W. Jenckes and D. E. Ford (2004). Experiences of patients who were early adopters of electronic communication with their physician: satisfaction, benefits, and concerns. *American Journal of Managed Care* **10**(9): 601–608.

King, A. C., R. Friedman, B. Marcus, C. Castro, M. Napolitano, D. Ahn and L. Baker (2007). Ongoing physical activity advice by humans versus computers: the Community Health Advice by Telephone (CHAT) trial. *Health Psychology* **26**(6): 718.

Lang, G. S. and K. J. Dickie (1978). *The Practice Oriented Medical Record.* Germantown, MD, Aspen Systems Corp.

Mooney, K. H., S. L. Beck, R. H. Friedman and R. Farzanfar (2002). Telephone-linked care for cancer symptom monitoring. *Cancer Practice* **10**(3): 147–154.

Patterson, P. D., A. J. Pfeiffer, M. D. Weaver, D. Krackhardt, R. M. Arnold, D. M. Yealy and J. R. Lave (2013). Network analysis of team communication in a busy emergency department. *BMC Health Services Research* **13**(1): 1–12.

Ramsay, J., A. Barabesi and J. Preece (1996). Informal communication is about sharing objects and media. *Interacting with Computers* **8**(3): 277–283.

Rice, R. E. (1992). Task analyzability, use of new media, and effectiveness: a multi-site exploration of media richness. *Organization Science* **3**(4): 475–500.

Robert, L. P. and A. R. Dennis (2005). Paradox of richness: a cognitive model of media choice. *IEEE Transactions on Professional Communication* **48**(1): 10–21.

Roter, D. L., S. Larson, D. Z. Sands, D. E. Ford and T. Houston (2008). Can e-mail messages between patients and physicians be patient-centered? *Health Communication* **23**(1): 80–86.

Safran, C., D. Z. Sands and D. M. Rind (1999). Online medical records: a decade of experience. *Methods of Information in Medicine* **38**(4/5): 308–312.

Spencer, R., E. Coiera and P. Logan (2004). Variation in communication loads on clinical staff in the emergency department. *Annals of Emergency Medicine* **44**(3): 268–273.

Tamblyn, R., M. Abrahamowicz and W. Dauphinee (2004). Electrons in flight: e-mail between doctors and patients. *Perspectives* (April 22): 1705–1707.

Tang, P. C., M. A. Jaworski, C. A. Fellencer, N. Kreider, M. LaRosa and W. Marquardt (1996). Clinician information activities in diverse ambulatory care practices. In: *Proceedings of the AMIA Annual Fall Symposium.* Washington, D.C., American Medical Informatics Association.

Thompson, L. A. and W. C. Ogden (1996). Visible speech improves human language understanding: implications for speech processing systems. In: McKevitt, P., editor. *Integration of Natural Language and Vision Processing.* Berlin, Springer, pp 105–116.

Weigl, M., A. Müller, A. Zupanc and P. Angerer (2009). Participant observation of time allocation, direct patient contact and simultaneous activities in hospital physicians. *BMC Health Services Research* **9**(1): 110.

Weiner, M. and P. Biondich (2006). The influence of information technology on patient-physician relationships. *Journal of General Internal Medicine* **21**(S1): S35–S39.

Westbrook, J. I., A. Ampt, L. Kearney and M. I. Rob (2008). All in a day's work: an observational study to quantify how and with whom doctors on hospital wards spend their time. *Medical Journal of Australia* **188**(9): 506.

Westbrook, J. I., E. Coiera, W. Dunsmuir, B. Brown, N. Kelk, R. Paoloni and C. Tran (2010). The impact of interruptions on clinical task completion. *Quality and Safety in Health Care* **19**(4): 284–289.

Westbrook, J. I., C. Duffield, L. Li and N. J. Creswick (2011). How much time do nurses have for patients? A longitudinal study quantifying hospital nurses' patterns of task time distribution and interactions with health professionals. *BMC Health Services Research* **11**(1): 319.

Westbrook, J. I., A. Woods, M. I. Rob, W. T. M. Dunsmuir and R. Day (2010). Association of interruptions with increased risk and severity of medication administration errors. *Archives of Internal Medicine* **170**(8): 683–690.

Whittaker, S. (1995). Rethinking video as a technology for interpersonal communications: theory and design implications. *International Journal of Human-Computer Studies* **42**(5): 501–529.

Wilson, R., W. B. Runciman, R. W. Gibberd, B. Harrison, L. Newby and J. Hamilton (1995). The Quality in Australian Health Care Study. *Medical Journal of Australia* **163**(9): 458–471.

Young, M., D. Sparrow, D. Gottlieb, A. Selim and R. Friedman (2001). A telephone-linked computer system for COPD care. *Chest* **119**(5): 1565–1575.

Chapter 19

Babbage, C. (1833). *On the Economy of Machinery and Manufactures.* London, Charles Knight.

Barrows, Jr., R. C. and J. Ezzard (2011). Technical architecture of ONC-approved plans for statewide health information exchange. In: *AMIA Annual Symposium Proceedings.* Washington, D.C., American Medical Informatics Association.

Bergmann, J., O. J. Bott, D. P. Pretschner and R. Haux (2007). An e-consent–based shared EHR system architecture for integrated healthcare networks. *International Journal of Medical Informatics* **76**(2): 130–136.

Berners-Lee, T., J. Hendler and O. Lassila (2001). The semantic web. *Scientific American* **284**(5): 28–37.

Blobel, B., K. Engel and P. Pharow (2006). Semantic interoperability: HL7 version 3 compared to advanced architecture standards. *Methods of Information in Medicine* **45**(4): 343–353.

Coiera, E. (2009). Building a national health IT system from the middle out. *Journal of the American Medical Informatics Association* **16**(3): 271–273.

Coiera, E. and R. Clarke (2004). e-Consent: the design and implementation of consumer consent mechanisms in an electronic environment. *Journal of the American Medical Informatics Association* **11**(2): 129–140.

Dolin, R. H., L. Alschuler, C. Beebe, P. V. Biron, S. L. Boyer, D. Essin, E. Kimber, T. Lincoln and J. E. Mattison (2001). The HL7 clinical document architecture. *Journal of the American Medical Informatics Association* **8**(6): 552–569.

El Emam, K., E. Jonker, L. Arbuckle and B. Malin (2011). A systematic review of re-identification attacks on health data. *PLoS One* **6**(12): e28071.

Feigenbaum, L., I. Herman, T. Hongsermeier, E. Neumann and S. Stephens (2007). The semantic web in action. *Scientific American* **297**(6): 90–97.

Fontaine, P., S. E. Ross, T. Zink and L. M. Schilling (2010). Systematic review of health information exchange in primary care practices. *Journal of the American Board of Family Medicine* **23**(5): 655–670.

Ford, D. V., K. H. Jones, J.-P. Verplancke, R. A. Lyons, G. John, G. Brown, C. J. Brooks, S. Thompson, O. Bodger and T. Couch (2009). The SAIL Databank: building a national architecture for e-health research and evaluation. *BMC Health Services Research* **9**(1): 157.

Greenhalgh, T., K. Stramer, T. Bratan, E. Byrne, Y. Mohammad and J. Russell (2008). Introduction of shared electronic records: multi-site case study using diffusion of innovation theory. *BMJ* **337:** a1786.

Greenhalgh, T., K. Stramer, T. Bratan, E. Byrne, J. Russell and H. W. W. Potts (2010). Adoption and non-adoption of a shared electronic summary record in England: a mixed-method case study. *BMJ* **340:** c3111.

Harris, P. A., R. Taylor, R. Thielke, J. Payne, N. Gonzalez and J. G. Conde (2009). Research electronic data capture (REDCap): a metadata-driven methodology and workflow process for providing translational research informatics support. *Journal of Biomedical Informatics* **42**(2): 377–381.

Heinze, O., M. Birkle, L. Köster and B. Bergh (2011). Architecture of a consent management suite and integration into IHE-based regional health information networks. *BMC Medical Informatics and Decision Making* **11**(1): 58.

HL7 (Health Level 7). (2014). *FHIR Documentation Index.* Retrieved 14 June 2014, from http://www.hl7.org/implement/standards/fhir/index.html.

Kalra, D., T. Beale and S. Heard (2005). The openEHR foundation. *Studies in Health Technology and Informatics* **115:** 153–173.

Knoppers, B. M., E. S. Dove, J.-E. Litton and J. Nietfeld (2012). Questioning the limits of genomic privacy. *American Journal of Human Genetics* **91**(3): 577.

Kuperman, G. J. (2011). Health-information exchange: why are we doing it, and what are we doing? *Journal of the American Medical Informatics Association* **18**(5): 678–682.

Kushida, C. A., D. A. Nichols, R. Jadrnicek, R. Miller, J. K. Walsh and K. Griffin (2012). Strategies for de-identification and anonymization of electronic health record data for use in multicenter research studies. *Medical Care* **50**(Jul): S82–S101.

Lawton, L. S. (1993). *Integrated Digital Networks.* Wilmslow, United Kingdom, Sigma Press.

Mandl, K. D. and I. S. Kohane (2009). No small change for the health information economy. *New England Journal of Medicine* **360**(13): 1278–1281.

Mandl, K. D., J. C. Mandel, S. N. Murphy, *et al.* (2012). The SMART Platform: early experience enabling substitutable applications for electronic health records. *Journal of the American Medical Informatics Association*: JAMIA **19**(4): 597–603.

Mandl, K. D., I. S. Kohane, D. McFadden, G. M. Weber, M. Natter, J. Mandel, S. Schneeweiss, S. Weiler, J. G. Klann and J. Bickel (2014). Scalable collaborative infrastructure for a learning healthcare system (SCILHS): architecture. *Journal of the American Medical Informatics Association* **21**(4): 615–620.

McMurry, A. J., C. A. Gilbert, B. Y. Reis, H. C. Chueh, I. S. Kohane and K. D. Mandl (2007). A self-scaling, distributed information architecture for public health, research, and clinical care. *Journal of the American Medical Informatics Association* **14**(4): 527–533.

Morella, C. (2006). *ANSI's World Standards Day Awards.* www.ansi.org/meetings_events/ All_awards/Ronald_Brown_Award.aspx?menuid=8.

Obitko, M. (2007). *Semantic Web Architecture.* Retrieved 15 June 2014, from http://obitko. com/tutorials/ontologies-semantic-web/semantic-web-architecture.html.

Pirnejad, H., Z. Niazkhani, M. Berg and R. Bal (2008). Intra-organizational communication in healthcare. *Methods of Information in Medicine* **47**(4): 336–345.

Safran, C., M. Bloomrosen, W. E. Hammond, S. Labkoff, S. Markel-Fox, P. C. Tang and D. E. Detmer (2007). Toward a national framework for the secondary use of health data: an American Medical Informatics Association White Paper. *Journal of the American Medical Informatics Association* **14**(1): 1–9.

Schadow, G. and C. N. Mead (2006). The HL7 reference information model under scrutiny. *Studies in Health Technology and Informatics* **124**: 151–156.

Shadbolt, N., W. Hall and T. Berners-Lee (2006). The semantic web revisited. *IEEE Intelligent Systems* **21**(3): 96–101.

Smith, B. and W. Ceusters (2006). HL7 RIM: an incoherent standard. *Studies in Health Technology and Informatics* **124**: 133–138.

Tanenbaum, A. S. (2003). *Computer Networks,* 4th edition. Upper Saddle River, NJ, Prentice Hall.

Chapter 20

Aarts, J. W. M. (2012). *Personalized Fertility Care in the Internet Era.* Radboud University, Nijmegen. The Netherlands.

Ahn, Y.-Y., J. P. Bagrow and S. Lehmann (2010). Link communities reveal multiscale complexity in networks. *Nature* **466**(7307): 761–764.

Aiello, L. M., A. Barrat, R. Schifanella, C. Cattuto, B. Markines and F. Menczer (2012). Friendship prediction and homophily in social media. *ACM Transactions on the Web (TWEB)* **6**(2): 9.

Aral, S. and D. Walker (2012). Identifying influential and susceptible members of social networks. *Science* **337**(6092): 337–341.

Australian Medical Association (2012). *Social Media and the Medical Profession: A Guide to Online Professionalism for Medical Practitioners and Medical Students.* Retrieved 23 September 2014, from https://ama.com.au/submission-draftsocial-media-policy.

Badaly, D. (2013). Peer similarity and influence for weight-related outcomes in adolescence: a meta-analytic review. *Clinical Psychology Review* **33**(8): 1218–1236.

Banerjee, A. K., S. Okun, I. R. Edwards, P. Wicks, M. Y. Smith, S. J. Mayall, B. Flamion, C. Cleeland and E. Basch (2013). Patient-reported outcome measures in safety event reporting: PROSPER consortium guidance. *Drug Safety* **36**(12): 1129–1149.

Barabási, A.-L. (2007). Network medicine: from obesity to the diseasome. *New England Journal of Medicine* **357**(4): 404–407.

Bardach, N. S., R. Asteria-Peñaloza, W. J. Boscardin and R. A. Dudley (2013). The relationship between commercial website ratings and traditional hospital performance measures in the USA. *BMJ Quality and Safety* **22**(3): 194–202.

Bargh, J. A. and K. Y. A. McKenna (2004). The Internet and social life. *Annual Review of Psychology* **55**(1): 573–590.

Beaudoin, C. E. and C.-C. Tao (2008). Modeling the impact of online cancer resources on supporters of cancer patients. *New Media and Society* **10**(2): 321–344.

Bond, R. M., C. J. Fariss, J. J. Jones, A. D. I. Kramer, C. Marlow, J. E. Settle and J. H. Fowler (2012). A 61-million-person experiment in social influence and political mobilization. *Nature* **489**(7415): 295–298.

Brabham, D. C. (2008). Crowdsourcing as a model for problem solving: an introduction and cases. Convergence: *International Journal of Research into New Media Technologies* **14**(1): 75–90.

Briones, R., X. Nan, K. Madden and L. Waks (2012). When vaccines go viral: an analysis of HPV vaccine coverage on YouTube. *Health Communication* **27**(5): 478–485.

Broadhead, R. S., D. D. Heckathorn, D. L. Weakliem, D. L. Anthony, H. Madray, R. J. Mills and J. Hughes (1998). Harnessing peer networks as an instrument for AIDS prevention: results from a peer-driven intervention. *Public Health Reports* **113**(Suppl 1): 42.

Brown, G. D. and W. J. Matthews (2011). Decision by sampling and memory distinctiveness: range effects from rank-based models of judgment and choice. *Frontiers in Psychology* **2**: 299.

Burke, M. A. and F. Heiland (2007). Social dynamics of obesity. *Economic Inquiry* **45**(3): 571–591.

Butcher, L. (2010). Oncologists using Twitter to advance cancer knowledge. *Oncology Times* **32**(1): 8.

Butler, D. (2013). When Google got flu wrong. *Nature* **494**(7436): 155–156.

Centola, D. (2010). The spread of behavior in an online social network experiment. *Science* **329**(5996): 1194–1197.

Centola, D. (2011). An experimental study of homophily in the adoption of health behavior. *Science* **334**(6060): 1269–1272.

Chew, C. and G. Eysenbach (2010). Pandemics in the age of Twitter: content analysis of tweets during the 2009 H1N1 outbreak. *PLoS One* **5**(11): e14118.

Chretien, K. C., J. Azar and T. Kind (2011). Physicians on Twitter. *JAMA* **305**(6): 566–568.

Christakis, N. A. and J. H. Fowler (2007). The spread of obesity in a large social network over 32 years. *New England Journal of Medicine* **357**(4): 370–379.

Christakis, N. A. and J. H. Fowler (2008). The collective dynamics of smoking in a large social network. *New England Journal of Medicine* **358**(21): 2249–2258.

Christakis, N. A. and J. H. Fowler (2012). Social contagion theory: examining dynamic social networks and human behavior. *Statistics in Medicine* **32**(4): 556.

Christakis, N. A. and J. H. Fowler (2014). Friendship and natural selection. *Proceedings of the National Academy of Sciences* **111**(Supplement 3): 10796–10801.

Clauson, K. A., H. H. Polen, M. N. K. Boulos and J. H. Dzenowagis (2008). Scope, completeness, and accuracy of drug information in Wikipedia. *Annals of Pharmacotherapy* **42**(12): 1814–1821.

Cohen-Cole, E. and J. M. Fletcher (2008). Is obesity contagious? Social networks vs. environmental factors in the obesity epidemic. *Journal of Health Economics* **27**(5): 1382–1387.

Coiera, E. (2004). Four rules for the reinvention of healthcare. *BMJ* **328**(7449): 1197–1199.

Coiera, E. (2013). Social networks, social media, and social diseases. *BMJ* **346**(7912): 22 (f3007).

Collier, N., N. T. Son and M. N. T. Ngoc (2010). OMG U got flu? Analysis of shared health messages for bio-surveillance. Paper presented at the Fourth International Symposium on Semantic Mining in Biomedicine (SMBM), Hinxton, United Kingdom.

Copello, A., J. Orford, R. Hodgson, G. Tober and C. Barrett (2002). Social behaviour and network therapy: basic principles and early experiences. *Addictive Behaviors* **27**(3): 345–366.

Creswick, N. and J. I. Westbrook (2010). Social network analysis of medication advice-seeking interactions among staff in an Australian hospital. *International Journal of Medical Informatics* **79**(6): e116–e125.

Cunningham, F. C., G. Ranmuthugala, J. Plumb, A. Georgiou, J. I. Westbrook and J. Braithwaite (2012a). Health professional networks as a vector for improving healthcare quality and safety: a systematic review. *BMJ Quality and Safety* **21**(3): 239–249.

Cunningham, S. A., E. Vaquera, C. C. Maturo and K. Venkat Narayan (2012b). Is there evidence that friends influence body weight? A systematic review of empirical research. *Social Science and Medicine* **75**(7): 1175–1183.

Dale, J., S. Williams and V. Bowyer (2012). What is the effect of peer support on diabetes outcomes in adults? A systematic review. *Diabetic Medicine* **29**(11): 1361–1377.

de la Haye, K., G. Robins, P. Mohr and C. Wilson (2010). Obesity-related behaviors in adolescent friendship networks. *Social Networks* **32**(3): 161–167.

de La Haye, K., G. Robins, P. Mohr and C. Wilson (2011a). Homophily and contagion as explanations for weight similarities among adolescent friends. *Journal of Adolescent Health* **49**(4): 421–427.

de La Haye, K., G. Robins, P. Mohr and C. Wilson (2011b). How physical activity shapes, and is shaped by, adolescent friendships. *Social Science and Medicine* **73**(5): 719–728.

Dunbar, R. (1996). *Grooming, Gossip, and the Evolution of Language*. Cambridge, MA, Harvard University Press.

Dunn, A. G., R. O. Day, K. D. Mandl and E. Coiera (2012a). Learning from hackers: open-source clinical trials. *Science Translational Medicine* **4**(132): 132–135.

Dunn, A. G., B. Gallego and E. Coiera (2012b). Industry influenced evidence production in collaborative research communities: a network analysis. *Journal of Clinical Epidemiology* **65**(5): 535–543.

Ellen, J. M. (2009). Social networks research and challenges to causal inference. *Journal of Adolescent Health* **45**(2): 109–110.

Ellison, N. B., C. Steinfield and C. Lampe (2007). The benefits of Facebook 'friends': social capital and college students' use of online social network sites. *Journal of Computer-Mediated Communication* **12**(4): 1143–1168.

Eysenbach, G. (2008a). Medicine 2.0: social networking, collaboration, participation, apomediation, and openness. *Journal of Medical Internet Research* **10**(3): e22.

Eysenbach, G. (2008b). The impact of the Internet on cancer outcomes. *CA: A Cancer Journal for Clinicians* **53**(6): 356–371.

Eysenbach, G. (2009). Infodemiology and infoveillance: framework for an emerging set of public health informatics methods to analyze search, communication and publication behavior on the Internet. *Journal of Medical Internet Research* **11**(1): e11.

Fletcher, A., C. Bonell and A. Sorhaindo (2011). You are what your friends eat: systematic review of social network analyses of young people's eating behaviours and bodyweight. *Journal of Epidemiology and Community Heath* **65**(6): 548–555.

Fowler, J. H. and N. A. Christakis (2008). Dynamic spread of happiness in a large social network: longitudinal analysis over 20 years in the Framingham Heart Study. *BMJ* **337**: a2338.

Fowler, J. H., J. E. Settle and N. A. Christakis (2011). Correlated genotypes in friendship networks. *Proceedings of the National Academy of Sciences* **108**(5): 1993–1997.

Funk, K. L., V. J. Stevens, L. J. Appel, A. Bauck, P. J. Brantley, C. M. Champagne, J. Coughlin, A. T. Dalcin, J. Harvey-Berino and J. F. Hollis (2010). Associations of Internet website use with weight change in a long-term weight loss maintenance program. *Journal of Medical Internet Research* **12**(3): e29.

Gallant, M. P. (2003). The influence of social support on chronic illness self-management: a review and directions for research. *Health Education and Behavior* **30**(2): 170–195.

Glass, R. J., L. M. Glass, W. E. Beyeler and H. J. Min (2006). Targeted social distancing design for pandemic influenza. *Emerging Infectious Diseases* **12**(11): 1671–1681.

Gold, B. C., S. Burke, S. Pintauro, P. Buzzell and J. Harvey-Berino (2007). Weight loss on the Web: a pilot study comparing a structured behavioral intervention to a commercial program. *Obesity (Silver Spring)* **15**(1): 155–155.

Grajales, III, F. J., S. Sheps, K. Ho, H. Novak-Lauscher, G. Eysenbach and G. Eysenbach (2014). Social media: a review and tutorial of applications in medicine and health care. *Journal of Medical Internet Research* **16**(2): e13.

Granovetter, M. S. (1973). The strength of weak ties. *American Journal of Sociology* **78**(6): 1360–1380.

Greaves, F., U. Pape, D. King and et al. (2012). Associations between Web-based patient ratings and objective measures of hospital quality. *Archives of Internal Medicine* **172**(5): 435–436.

Greaves, F., D. Ramirez-Cano, C. Millett, A. Darzi and L. Donaldson (2013). Harnessing the cloud of patient experience: using social media to detect poor quality healthcare. *BMJ Quality and Safety* **22**(3): 251–255.

Harvey-Berino, J., S. Pintauro, P. Buzzell and E. C. Gold (2004). Effect of Internet support on the long-term maintenance of weight loss. *Obesity Research* **12**(2): 320–329.

Haythornthwaite, C. (2005). Social networks and Internet connectivity effects. *Information, Community and Society* **8**(2): 125–147.

Heaney, C. A. and B. A. Israel (2002). Social networks and social support. In: Glanz, K., B. K. Rimer and K. Viswanath, editors. *Health Behavior and Health Education: Theory, Research, and Practice.* San Francisco, CA, Jossey-Bass, vol **3, pp** 185–209.

Hwang, K. O., A. J. Ottenbacher, A. P. Green, M. R. Cannon-Diehl, O. Richardson, E. V. Bernstam and E. J. Thomas (2010). Social support in an Internet weight loss community. *International Journal of Medical Informatics* **79**(1): 5–13.

Iedema, R., S. Allen, K. Britton and T. H. Gallagher (2012). What do patients and relatives know about problems and failures in care? *BMJ Quality and Safety* **21**(3): 198–205.

Indes, J. E., L. Gates, E. L. Mitchell and B. E. Muhs (2013). Social media in vascular surgery. *Journal of Vascular Surgery* **57**(4): 1159–1162.

Iyengar, R., C. Van den Bulte and T. W. Valente (2011). Opinion leadership and social contagion in new product diffusion. *Marketing Science* **30**(2): 195–212.

Kaplan, A. M. and M. Haenlein (2010). Users of the world, unite! The challenges and opportunities of social media. *Business Horizons* **53**(1): 59–68.

Kaplan, R. M. and S. L. Hartwell (1987). Differential effects of social support and social network on physiological and social outcomes in men and women with type II diabetes mellitus. *Health Psychology* **6**(5): 387.

Kawrykow, A., G. Roumanis, A. Kam, D. Kwak, C. Leung, C. Wu, E. Zarour, L. Sarmenta, M. Blanchette and J. Waldispühl (2012). Phylo: a citizen science approach for improving multiple sequence alignment. *PLoS One* **7**(3): e31362.

Lau, A. Y. S. and E. W. Coiera (2008). Impact of Web searching and social feedback on consumer decision making: a prospective online experiment. *Journal of Medical Internet Research* **10**(1): e2.

Lau, A. Y., A. G. Dunn, N. Mortimer, A. Gallagher, J. Proudfoot, A. Andrews, S.-T. Liaw, J. Crimmins, A. Arguel and E. Coiera (2013a). Social and self-reflective use of a Web-based personally controlled health management system. *Journal of Medical Internet Research* **15**(9): e211.

Lau, A. Y. S., E. Gabarron, L. Fernandez-Luque and M. Armayones (2012). Social media in health – what are the safety concerns for health consumers? *Health Information Management Journal* **41**(2): 30–35.

Lau, A. Y. S., A. Parker, J. Early, G. Sacks, F. Anvari and E. Coiera (2012b). Comparative usage of a Web-based personally controlled health management system and normal support: a case study in IVF. *Electronic Journal of Health Informatics* **7**(2): e12.

Lau, A. Y. S., J. Proudfoot, A. Andrews, S. T. Liaw, J. Crimmins, A. Arguel and E. Coiera (2013b). Which bundles of features in a Web-based personally controlled health management are associated with consumer help-seeking behaviors for physical and emotional wellbeing? *Journal of Medical Internet Research* **15**(5): e79.

Lau, A., K. Siek, L. Fernandez-Luque, H. Tange, P. Chhanabhai, S. Li, P. Elkin, A. Arjabi, L. Walczowski and C. Ang (2011). The role of social media for patients and consumer health. *International Medical Informatics Association (IMIA) Yearbook* **6**(1): 131–138.

Lau, A. Y. S., V. Sintchenko, J. Crimmins, F. Magrabi, B. Gallego and E. Coiera (2012c). Impact of a Web-based personally controlled health management system on influenza vaccination and health services utilization rates: a randomized controlled trial. *Journal of the American Medical Informatics Association* **19**(5): 719–727.

Leskovec, J., K. J. Lang, A. Dasgupta and M. W. Mahoney (2009). Community structure in large networks: natural cluster sizes and the absence of large well-defined clusters. *Internet Mathematics* **6**(1): 29–123.

Li, J. S., T. A. Barnett, E. Goodman, R. C. Wasserman and A. R. Kemper (2013). Approaches to the prevention and management of childhood obesity: the role of social networks and the use of social media and related electronic technologies a scientific statement from the American Heart Association. *Circulation* **127**(2): 260–267.

Litt, M. D., R. M. Kadden, E. Kabela-Cormier and N. M. Petry (2009). Changing network support for drinking: Network Support Project 2-year follow-up. *Journal of Consulting and Clinical Psychology* **77**(2): 229.

Maher, C. A., L. K. Lewis, K. Ferrar, S. Marshall, I. De Bourdeaudhuij and C. Vandelanotte (2014). Are health behavior change interventions that use online social networks effective? A systematic review. *Journal of Medical Internet Research* **16**(2): e40.

Maltby, J., A. M. Wood, I. Vlaev, M. J. Taylor and G. D. Brown (2012). Contextual effects on the perceived health benefits of exercise: the exercise rank hypothesis. *Journal of Sport and Exercise Psychology* **34**(6): 828–841.

Mascia, D. and A. Cicchetti (2011). Physician social capital and the reported adoption of evidence-based medicine: exploring the role of structural holes. *Social Science and Medicine* **72**(5): 798–805.

McLaughlin, M., Y. Nam, J. Gould, C. Pade, K. A. Meeske, K. S. Ruccione and J. Fulk (2012). A videosharing social networking intervention for young adult cancer survivors. *Computers in Human Behavior* **28**(2): 631–641.

McLuhan, M. (1964). *Understanding Media: The Extensions of Man.* New York, Mentor.

Melrose, K. L., G. D. Brown and A. M. Wood (2013). Am I abnormal? Relative rank and social norm effects in judgments of anxiety and depression symptom severity. *Journal of Behavioral Decision Making* **26**(2): 174–184.

Merchant, R. M., S. Elmer and N. Lurie (2011). Integrating social media into emergency-preparedness efforts. *New England Journal of Medicine* **365**(4): 289–291.

Napolitano, M. A., S. Hayes, G. G. Bennett, A. K. Ives and G. D. Foster (2013). Using Facebook and text messaging to deliver a weight loss program to college students. *Obesity (Silver Spring)* **21**(1): 25–31.

Neiger, B. L., R. Thackeray, S. A. Van Wagenen, C. L. Hanson, J. H. West, M. D. Barnes and M. C. Fagen (2012). Use of social media in health promotion: purposes, key performance indicators, and evaluation metrics. *Health Promotion Practice* **13**(2): 159–164.

Newman, M. E. (2006). Modularity and community structure in networks. *Proceedings of the National Academy of Sciences of the United States of America* **103**(23): 8577–8582.

Pachucki, M. A., P. F. Jacques and N. A. Christakis (2011). Social network concordance in food choice among spouses, friends, and siblings. *American Journal of Public Health* **101**(11): 2170.

Palla, G., I. Derényi, I. Farkas and T. Vicsek (2005). Uncovering the overlapping community structure of complex networks in nature and society. *Nature* **435**(7043): 814–818.

Parks, M. R. and K. Floyd (1996). Making friends in cyberspace. *Journal of Computer Mediated Communication* **1**(4): 80–97.

Patterson, P. D., A. J. Pfeiffer, M. D. Weaver, D. Krackhardt, R. M. Arnold, D. M. Yealy and J. R. Lave (2013). Network analysis of team communication in a busy emergency department. *BMC Health Services Research* **13**(1): 1–12.

Pullen, C. H., P. A. Hageman, L. Boeckner, S. N. Walker and M. K. Oberdorfer (2008). Feasibility of Internet-delivered weight loss interventions among rural women ages 50–69. *Journal of Geriatric Physical Therapy* **31**(3): 105–112.

Ranmuthugala, G., J. Plumb, F. Cunningham, A. Georgiou, J. Westbrook and J. Braithwaite (2011). How and why are communities of practice established in the healthcare sector? A systematic review of the literature. *BMC Health Services Research* **11**(1): 273.

Rathi, V., K. Dzara, C. P. Gross, I. Hrynaszkiewicz, S. Joffe, H. M. Krumholz, K. M. Strait and J. S. Ross (2012). Sharing of clinical trial data among trialists: a cross sectional survey. *BMJ* **345:** e7570.

Rector, L. H. (2008). Comparison of Wikipedia and other encyclopedias for accuracy, breadth, and depth in historical articles. *Reference Services Review* **36**(1): 7–22.

Barlow, J., D. Singh, S. Bayer and R. Curry (2007). A systematic review of the benefits of home telecare for frail elderly people and those with long-term conditions. *Journal of Telemedicine and Telecare* **13**(4): 172–179.

Bensink, M., D. Hailey and R. Wootton (2007). A systematic review of successes and failures in home telehealth. Part 2. Final quality rating results. *Journal of Telemedicine and Telecare* **13**(Suppl 3): 10–14.

Börve, A., A. Holst, A. Gente-Lidholm, R. Molina-Martinez and J. Paoli (2012). Use of the mobile phone multimedia messaging service for teledermatology. *Journal of Telemedicine and Telecare* **18**(5): 292–296.

Boulos, M. N. K., L. Hetherington and S. Wheeler (2007). Second Life: an overview of the potential of 3-D virtual worlds in medical and health education. *Health Information and Libraries Journal* **24**(4): 233–245.

Bowles, B. A. and R. Teale (1994). Communications services in support of collaborative health care. *BT Technology Journal* **12**(3): 29–44.

Braithwaite, J. and E. Coiera (2010). Beyond patient safety Flatland. *Journal of the Royal Society of Medicine* **103**(6): 219–225.

Bunn, F., G. Byrne and S. Kendall (2005). The effects of telephone consultation and triage on healthcare use and patient satisfaction: a systematic review. *British Journal of General Practice* **55**(521): 956–961.

Callen, J., J. McIntosh and J. Li (2010). Accuracy of medication documentation in hospital discharge summaries: a retrospective analysis of medication transcription errors in manual and electronic discharge summaries. *International Journal of Medical Informatics* **79**(1): 58–64.

Clarke, M., A. Shah and U. Sharma (2011). Systematic review of studies on telemonitoring of patients with congestive heart failure: a meta-analysis. *Journal of Telemedicine and Telecare* **17**(1): 7–14.

Coiera, E. (2000). When conversation is better than computation. *Journal of the American Medical Informatics Association* **7**(3): 277–286.

Coiera, E. (2014). Communication spaces. *Journal of the American Medical Informatics Association* **21**(3): 414–422.

Coiera, E., Y. Wang, F. Magrabi, O. P. Concha, B. Gallego and W. Runciman (2014). Predicting the cumulative risk of death during hospitalization by modeling weekend, weekday and diurnal mortality risks. *BMC Health Services Research* **14**(1): 226.

Cole-Lewis, H. and T. Kershaw (2010). Text messaging as a tool for behavior change in disease prevention and management. *Epidemiologic Reviews* **32**(1): 56–69.

Concha, O. P., B. Gallego, K. Hillman, G. P. Delaney and E. Coiera (2014). Do variations in hospital mortality patterns after weekend admission reflect reduced quality of care or different patient cohorts? A population-based study. *BMJ Quality and Safety* **23**(3): 215–222.

Darkins, A., S. Kendall, E. Edmonson, M. Young and P. Stressel (2014). Reduced cost and mortality using home telehealth to promote self-management of complex chronic conditions: a retrospective matched cohort study of 4,999 veteran patients. *Telemedicine and e-Health* 2014 May 19. [Epub ahead of print]

Della Mea, V., S. Forti, F. Puglisi, P. Bellutta, P. Dalla Palma, F. Mauri, C. Beltrami and N. Finato (1996). Telepathology using Internet multimedia electronic mail: remote consultation on gastrointestinal pathology. *Journal of Telemedicine and Telecare* **2**(1): 28–34.

DelliFraine, J. L. and K. H. Dansky (2008). Home-based telehealth: a review and meta-analysis. *Journal of Telemedicine and Telecare* **14**(2): 62–66.

Doyle, P. and B. Hayes-Roth (1998). Agents in annotated worlds. In: *Proceedings of the Second International Conference on Autonomous Agents*. Minneapolis, MN, USA, pp 173–180.

Dunbar, P. J., D. Madigan, L. A. Grohskopf, D. Revere, J. Woodward, J. Minstrell, P. A. Frick, J. M. Simoni and T. M. Hooton (2003). A two-way messaging system to enhance antiretroviral adherence. *Journal of the American Medical Informatics Association* **10**(1): 11–15.

Ekeland, A. G., A. Bowes and S. Flottorp (2010). Effectiveness of telemedicine: a systematic review of reviews. *International Journal of Medical Informatics* **79**(11): 736–771.

Feiner, S., B. Macintyre and D. Seligmann (1993). Knowledge-based augmented reality. *Communications of the ACM* **36**(7): 53–62.

Franken, E. and K. Berbaum (1996). Subspecialty radiology consultation by interactive telemedicine. *Journal of Telemedicine and Telecare* **2**(1): 35–41.

Free, C., G. Phillips, L. Galli, L. Watson, L. Felix, P. Edwards, V. Patel and A. Haines (2013). The effectiveness of mobile-health technology-based health behaviour change or disease management interventions for health care consumers: a systematic review. *PLoS Medicine* **10**(1): e1001362.

Gordon, L., D. Bird, B. Oldenburg, R. Friedman, A. Russell and P. Scuffham (2014). A cost-effectiveness analysis of a telephone-linked care intervention for individuals with type 2 diabetes. *Diabetes Research and Clinical Practice* **104**(1): 103–111.

Hailey, D., R. Roine and A. Ohinmaa (2002). Systematic review of evidence for the benefits of telemedicine. *Journal of Telemedicine and Telecare* **8**(Suppl 1): 1–7.

Harris, M., B. O'Toole and A. Giles (2002). Communication across the divide: a trial of structured communication between general practice and emergency departments. *Australian Family Physician* **31**(2): 197.

Henderson, C., M. Knapp, J.-L. Fernández, J. Beecham, S. P. Hirani, M. Cartwright, L. Rixon, M. Beynon, A. Rogers and P. Bower (2013). Cost effectiveness of telehealth for patients with long term conditions (Whole Systems Demonstrator telehealth questionnaire study): nested economic evaluation in a pragmatic, cluster randomised controlled trial. *BMJ* **346**: f1035.

Hersh, W., M. Helfand, J. Wallace, D. Kraemer, P. Patterson, S. Shapiro and M. Greenlick (2002). A systematic review of the efficacy of telemedicine for making diagnostic and management decisions. *Journal of Telemedicine and Telecare* **8**(4): 197–209.

Hersh, W. R., D. H. Hickam, S. M. Severance, T. L. Dana, K. P. Krages and M. Helfand (2006). Diagnosis, access and outcomes: update of a systematic review of telemedicine services. *Journal of Telemedicine and Telecare* **12**(Suppl 2): 3–31.

Houston, T. K., D. Z. Sands, M. W. Jenckes and D. E. Ford (2004). Experiences of patients who were early adopters of electronic communication with their physician: satisfaction, benefits, and concerns. *American Journal of Managed Care* **10**(9): 601–608.

Istepanian, R. S., E. Jovanov and Y. Zhang (2004). Guest editorial introduction to the special section on m-health: beyond seamless mobility and global wireless health-care connectivity. *IEEE Transactions on Information Technology in Biomedicine* **8**(4): 405–414.

Jacques, P. S., D. J. France, M. Pilla, E. Lai and M. S. Higgins (2006). Evaluation of a hands-free wireless communication device in the perioperative environment. *Telemedicine Journal and e-Health* **12**(1): 42–49.

Jensen, A. M. D., M. M. Jensen, A. S. Korsager, M. Ong, F. Magrabi and E. Coiera (2011). Using virtual worlds to train healthcare workers: a case study using Second Life to improve the safety of inpatient transfers. electronic *Journal of Health Informatics* **7**(1): e7.

Johansson, T. and C. Wild (2010). Telemedicine in acute stroke management: systematic review. *International Journal of Technology Assessment in Health Care* **26**(02): 149–155.

Kairy, D., P. Lehoux, C. Vincent and M. Visintin (2009). A systematic review of clinical outcomes, clinical process, healthcare utilization and costs associated with telerehabilitation. *Disability and Rehabilitation* **31**(6): 427–447.

Kim, Y., A. H. Chen, E. Keith, H. F. Yee Jr. and M. B. Kushel (2009). Not perfect, but better: primary care providers' experiences with electronic referrals in a safety net health system. *Journal of General Internal Medicine* **24**(5): 614–619.

KleinJan, G., A. Bunschoten, O. Brouwer, N. van den Berg, R. Valdés-Olmos and F. van Leeuwen (2013). Multimodal imaging in radioguided surgery. *Clinical and Translational Imaging* **1**(6): 433–444.

Knowles, E., J. Munro, A. O'Cathain and J. Nicholl (2006). Equity of access to health care: evidence from NHS Direct in the UK. *Journal of Telemedicine and Telecare* **12**(5): 262–265.

Kraai, I. H., M. Luttik, R. M. de Jong, T. Jaarsma and H. Hillege (2011). Heart failure patients monitored with telemedicine: patient satisfaction: a review of the literature. *Journal of Cardiac Failure* **17**(8): 684–690.

Krishna, S., E. Balas, S. Boren and N. Maglaveras (2002). Patient acceptance of educational voice messages: a review of controlled clinical studies. *Methods of Information in Medicine* **41**(5): 360–369.

Krishna, S., S. A. Boren and E. A. Balas (2009). Healthcare via cell phones: a systematic review. *Telemedicine and e-Health* **15**(3): 231–240.

Kuperman, G. J., D. F. Sittig, M. M. Shabot and J. Teich (1999). Clinical decision support for hospital and critical care. *Journal of Healthcare Information Management* **13**: 81–96.

Kuruzovich, J., C. M. Angst, S. Faraj and R. Agarwal (2008). Wireless communication role in patient response time: a study of vocera integration with a nurse call system. *Computers Informatics Nursing* **26**(3): 159–166.

Lattimer, V., S. George, F. Thompson, E. Thomas, M. Mullee, J. Turnbull, H. Smith, M. Moore, H. Bond and A. Glasper (1998). Safety and effectiveness of nurse telephone consultation in out of hours primary care: randomised controlled trial. *BMJ* **317**(7165): 1054–1059.

Lattimer, V., F. Sassi, S. George, M. Moore, J. Turnbull, M. Mullee and H. Smith (2000). Cost analysis of nurse telephone consultation in out of hours primary care: evidence from a randomised controlled trial. *BMJ* **320**(7241): 1053–1057.

Leirer, V. O., D. G. Morrow, E. D. Tanke and G. M. Pariante (1991). Elders' nonadherence: its assessment and medication reminding by voice mail. *Gerontologist* **31**(4): 514–520.

Leong, S. L., D. Gingrich, P. R. Lewis, D. T. Mauger and J. H. George (2005). Enhancing doctor-patient communication using email: a pilot study. *Journal of the American Board of Family Practice* **18**(3): 180–188.

Lester, R. T., P. Ritvo, E. J. Mills, A. Kariri, S. Karanja, M. H. Chung, W. Jack, J. Habyarimana, M. Sadatsafavi and M. Najafzadeh (2010). Effects of a mobile phone short message service on antiretroviral treatment adherence in Kenya (WelTel Kenya1): a randomised trial. *Lancet* **376**(9755): 1838–1845.

Liang, W.-Y., C.-Y. Hsu, C.-R. Lai, D. M.-T. Ho and I.-J. Chiang (2008). Low-cost telepathology system for intraoperative frozen-section consultation: our experience and review of the literature. *Human Pathology* **39**(1): 56–62.

Mair, F. and P. Whitten (2000). Systematic review of studies of patient satisfaction with telemedicine. *BMJ* **320**(7248): 1517–1520.

McLaren, P. (1994). Telepsychiatry in the USA. *Journal of Telemedicine and Telecare* **1**(2): 121–122.

Melzer, S. M. and S. R. Poole (1999). Computerized pediatric telephone triage and advice programs at children's hospitals: operating and financial characteristics. *Archives of Pediatrics and Adolescent Medicine* **153**(8): 858–863.

Mistry, H. (2012). Systematic review of studies of the cost-effectiveness of telemedicine and telecare: changes in the economic evidence over twenty years. *Journal of Telemedicine and Telecare* **18**(1): 1–6.

Motamedi, S. M., J. Posadas-Calleja, S. Straus, D. W. Bates, D. L. Lorenzetti, B. Baylis, J. Gilmour, S. Kimpton and W. A. Ghali (2011). The efficacy of computer-enabled discharge communication interventions: a systematic review. *BMJ Quality and Safety* **20**(5): 403–415.

Munro, J., J. Nicholl, A. O'Cathain and E. Knowles (2000). Impact of NHS Direct on demand for immediate care: observational study. *BMJ* **321**(7254): 150–153.

Munro, J., F. Sampson and J. Nicholl (2005). The impact of NHS Direct on the demand for out-of-hours primary and emergency care. *British Journal of General Practice* **55**(519): 790–792.

Nilsson, S. and B. Johansson (2007). Fun and usable: augmented reality instructions in a hospital setting. In: *Proceedings of the 19th Australasian Conference on Computer–Human Interaction: Entertaining User Interfaces.* Adelaide, Australia, Association for Computing Machinery.

North, F., O. Odunukan and P. Varkey (2011). The value of telephone triage for patients with appendicitis. *Journal of Telemedicine and Telecare* **17**(8): 417–420.

Nymo, B. J. (1993). Telemedicine. *Telektronikk* **89**(1): 4–11.

O'Leary, K. J., D. M. Liebovitz, J. Feinglass, D. T. Liss, D. B. Evans, N. Kulkarni, M. P. Landler and D. W. Baker (2009). Creating a better discharge summary: improvement in quality and timeliness using an electronic discharge summary. *Journal of Hospital Medicine* **4**(4): 219–225.

Okur, A., S.-A. Ahmadi, A. Bigdelou, T. Wendler and N. Navab (2011). MR in OR: first analysis of AR/VR visualization in 100 intra-operative Freehand SPECT acquisitions. In: *Tenth IEEE International Symposium on Mixed and Augmented Reality (ISMAR).* Basel, Switzerland, Institute of Electrical and Electronics Engineers.

Patel, P. B. and D. R. Vinson (2013). Physician e-mail and telephone contact after emergency department visit improves patient satisfaction: a crossover trial. *Annals of Emergency Medicine* **61**(6): 631–637.

Pendleton, D., T. Schofield, P. Tate and P. Havelock (1984). *The Consultation: An Approach to Learning and Teaching.* Oxford, Oxford University Press.

Piccolo, D., H. P. Soyer, W. Burgdorf, R. Talamini, K. Peris, L. Bugatti, V. Canzonieri, L. Cerroni, S. Chimenti and G. De Rosa (2002). Concordance between telepathologic diagnosis and conventional histopathologic diagnosis: a multiobserver store-and-forward study on 20 skin specimens. *Archives of Dermatology* **138**(1): 53–58.

Piper, A. M., R. Campbell and J. D. Hollan (2010). Exploring the accessibility and appeal of surface computing for older adult health care support. In: *Proceedings of the 28th International Conference on Human Factors in Computing Systems.* Atlanta, GA, USA, Association for Computing Machinery.

Richards, J. D. and T. Harris (2011). Beam me up Scotty! Impact of personal wireless communication devices in the emergency department. *Emergency Medicine Journal* **28**(2): 29–32.

Richardson, J. E. and J. S. Ash (2010). The effects of hands-free communication device systems: communication changes in hospital organizations. *Journal of the American Medical Informatics Association* **17**(1): 91–98.

Rind, D. M., C. Safran, R. S. Phillips, Q. Wang, D. R. Calkins, T. L. Delbanco, H. L. Bleich and W. V. Slack (1994). Effect of computer-based alerts on the treatment and outcomes of hospitalized patients. *Archives of Internal Medicine* **154**(13): 1511.

Rogers, E. M. (1995). *Diffusion of Innovations.* New York, Free Press.

Roter, D. L., S. Larson, D. Z. Sands, D. E. Ford and T. Houston (2008). Can e-mail messages between patients and physicians be patient-centered? *Health Communication* **23**(1): 80–86.

Scholl, J. and K. Groth (2012). Of organization, device and context: interruptions from mobile communication in highly specialized care. *Interacting with Computers* **24**(5): 358–373.

Seto, E. (2008). Cost comparison between telemonitoring and usual care of heart failure: a systematic review. *Telemedicine and e-Health* **14**(7): 679–686.

Shuhaiber, J. H. (2004). Augmented reality in surgery. *Archives of Surgery* **139**(2): 170–174.

Solvoll, T., J. Scholl and G. Hartvigsen (2013). Physicians interrupted by mobile devices in hospitals: understanding the interaction between devices, roles, and duties. *Journal of Medical Internet Research* **15**(3): e56.

Steventon, A., M. Bardsley, J. Billings, J. Dixon, H. Doll, S. Hirani, M. Cartwright, L. Rixon, M. Knapp and C. Henderson (2012). Effect of telehealth on use of secondary care and mortality: findings from the Whole System Demonstrator cluster randomised trial. *BMJ* **344:** e3874.

Tachakra, S., X. Wang, R. S. Istepanian and Y. Song (2003). Mobile e-health: the unwired evolution of telemedicine. *Telemedicine Journal and E-health* **9**(3): 247–257.

Terenzi, G. and A. Terenzi (2014). Risk Management in Hospitals Using Augmented Reality: The ANGELS Project. Augmented Reality and Risk Management in Hospitals. Rome.

Thrall, J. H. (2007). Teleradiology. Part II. Limitations, risks, and opportunities. *Radiology* **244**(2): 325–328.

Udsen, F. W., O. Hejlesen and L. H. Ehlers (2014). A systematic review of the cost and cost-effectiveness of telehealth for patients suffering from chronic obstructive pulmonary disease. *Journal of Telemedicine and Telecare* *20(4)*: 212–220.

Van der Heijden, J., N. De Keizer, J. Bos, P. Spuls and L. Witkamp (2011). Teledermatology applied following patient selection by general practitioners in daily practice improves efficiency and quality of care at lower cost. *British Journal of Dermatology* 165(5): 1058–1065.

Vervloet, M., A. J. Linn, J. C. van Weert, D. H. De Bakker, M. L. Bouvy and L. Van Dijk (2012). The effectiveness of interventions using electronic reminders to improve adherence to chronic medication: a systematic review of the literature. *Journal of the American Medical Informatics Association* 19(5): 696–704.

Wamala, D., A. Katamba and O. Dworak (2011). Feasibility and diagnostic accuracy of Internet-based dynamic telepathology between Uganda and Germany. *Journal of Telemedicine and Telecare* 17(5): 222–225.

Warshaw, E. M., Y. J. Hillman, N. L. Greer, E. M. Hagel, R. MacDonald, I. R. Rutks and T. J. Wilt (2011). Teledermatology for diagnosis and management of skin conditions: a systematic review. *Journal of the American Academy of Dermatology* 64(4): 759–772. e721.

Weiner, M. and P. Biondich (2006). The influence of information technology on patient–physician relationships. *Journal of General Internal Medicine* 21(Suppl 1): S35–S39.

Westbrook, J. I., E. W. Coiera, M. Brear, S. Stapleton, M. I. Rob, M. Murphy and P. Cregan (2008). Impact of an ultrabroadband emergency department telemedicine system on the care of acutely ill patients and clinicians' work. *Medical Journal of Australia* 188(12): 704–708.

Whitten, P. S., F. S. Mair, A. Haycox, C. R. May, T. L. Williams and S. Hellmich (2002). Systematic review of cost effectiveness studies of telemedicine interventions. *BMJ* 324(7351): 1434–1437.

Williams, E. D., D. Bird, A. W. Forbes, A. Russell, S. Ash, R. Friedman, P. A. Scuffham and B. Oldenburg (2012). Randomised controlled trial of an automated, interactive telephone intervention (TLC Diabetes) to improve type 2 diabetes management: baseline findings and six-month outcomes. *BMC Public Health* 12(1): 602.

Williams, T. L., C. R. May and A. Esmail (2001). Limitations of patient satisfaction studies in telehealthcare: a systematic review of the literature. *Telemedicine Journal and e-Health* 7(4): 293–316.

Wobbrock, J. O., M. R. Morris and A. D. Wilson (2009). User-defined gestures for surface computing. In: *Proceedings of the 27th International Conference on Human Factors in Computing Systems.* Boston, MA, USA, Association for Computing Machinery.

Wootton, R. (2001). Telemedicine. *BMJ* 323(7312): 557–560.

Wu, R. C., K. Tran, V. Lo, K. J. O'Leary, D. Morra, S. D. Quan and L. Perrier (2012). Effects of clinical communication interventions in hospitals: a systematic review of information and communication technology adoptions for improved communication between clinicians. *International Journal of Medical Informatics* 81(11): 723–732.

Ye, J., G. Rust, Y. Fry-Johnson and H. Strothers (2010). E-mail in patient–provider communication: a systematic review. *Patient Education and Counseling* 80(2): 266–273.

Young, L. B., P. S. Chan, X. Lu, B. K. Nallamothu, C. Sasson and P. M. Cram (2011). Impact of telemedicine intensive care unit coverage on patient outcomes: a systematic review and meta-analysis. *Archives of Internal Medicine* 171(6): 498–506.

Chapter 22

Board of Directors of the American Medical Informatics Association (1994). Standards for medical identifiers, codes, and messages needed to create an efficient computer-stored medical record. *Journal of the American Medical Informatics Association* **1**(1): 1–7.

Feinstein, A. R. (1988). ICD, POR, and DRG: unsolved scientific problems in the nosology of clinical medicine. *Archives of Internal Medicine* **148**(10): 2269–2274.

Friedman, C., L. Shagina, Y. Lussier and G. Hripcsak (2004). Automated encoding of clinical documents based on natural language processing. *Journal of the American Medical Informatics Association* **11**(5): 392–402.

Glowinski, A., E. Coiera and M. O'Neil (1991). The role of domain models in maintaining consistency of large medical knowledge bases. In: AIME 91: *Proceedings of the Third Conference on Artificial Intelligence in Medicine, Maastricht, June 24–27, 1991.* Berlin, Springer, pp 72–81.

Gregory, J., J. Mattison and C. Linde (1995). Naming notes: transitions from free text to structured entry. *Methods of Information in Medicine* **34**(1–2): 57–67.

Hohnloser, J., F. Puerner and H. Soltanian (1996). Improving coded data entry by an electronic patient record system. *Methods of Information in Medicine* **35**(2): 108–111.

Hohnloser, J. H., F. Pürner and P. Kadlec (1995). Coding medical concepts: a controlled experiment with a computerised coding tool. *International Journal of Clinical Monitoring and Computing* **12**(3): 141–145.

Oesterlen, F. (1855). *Medical Logic*, (English Translation). London: Sydenham Society.

Rector, A., W. Nowlan and A. Glowinski (1993). Goals for concept representation in the GALEN project. In: *Proceedings of the Annual Symposium on Computer Application in Medical Care*, American Medical Informatics Association.

Rosch, E. (1988). Principles of categorization. In: Rosch, E. and B. B. Lloyd, editors. *Readings in Cognitive Science.* Los Altos, CA, Morgan Kaufmann, pp 312–322.

Simborg, D. W. (2011). There is no neutral position on fraud! *Journal of the American Medical Informatics Association* **18**(5): 675–677.

Wisniewski, E. J. and D. L. Medin (1994). On the interaction of theory and data in concept learning. *Cognitive Science* **18**(2): 221–281.

Chapter 23

American Medical Association (2007). *Current Procedural Terminology: CPT.* Chicago, American Medical Association.

Averill, R. F., R. L. Mullin, B. A. Steinbeck, N. I. Goldfield and T. M. Grant (2001). Development of the ICD-10 procedure coding system (ICD-10-PCS). *Topics in Health Information Management* **21**(3): 54–88.

Baker, J. J. (2001). Medicare payment system for hospital inpatients: diagnosis-related groups. *Journal of Health Care Finance* **28**(3): 1–13.

Bos, L. (2006). SNOMED-CT: The advanced terminology and coding system for eHealth. *Studies in Health Technology and Informatics* **121**: 279–290.

Campbell, K. E., D. E. Oliver, K. A. Spackman and E. H. Shortliffe (1998). Representing thoughts, words, and things in the UMLS. *Journal of the American Medical Informatics Association* **5**(5): 421–431.

Chute, C. G. (2000). Clinical classification and terminology some history and current observations. *Journal of the American Medical Informatics Association* **7**(3): 298–303.

Cornet, R. and N. de Keizer (2008). Forty years of SNOMED: a literature review. *BMC Medical Informatics and Decision Making* **8**(Suppl 1): S2.

Cote, R. A. and S. Robboy (1980). Progress in medical information management: Systematized Nomenclature of Medicine (SNOMED). *JAMA* **243**(8): 756–762.

Elkin, P. L., S. H. Brown, C. S. Husser, B. A. Bauer, D. Wahner-Roedler, S. T. Rosenbloom and T. Speroff (2006). Evaluation of the content coverage of SNOMED CT: ability of SNOMED clinical terms to represent clinical problem lists. *Mayo Clinic Proceedings* **81**(6): 741–748.

Feinstein, A. R. (1988). ICD, POR, and DRG: unsolved scientific problems in the nosology of clinical medicine. *Archives of Internal Medicine* **148**(10): 2269–2274.

Fetter, R. B., Y. Shin, J. L. Freeman, R. F. Averill and J. D. Thompson (1980). Case mix definition by diagnosis-related groups. *Medical Care* **18**(2 Suppl): iii, 1–53.

Gersenovic, M. (1995). The ICD family of classifications. *Methods of Information in Medicine* **34**(1–2): 172–175.

Humphreys, B. L. and D. A. Lindberg (1989). Building the unified medical language system. *Proceedings of the Annual Symposium on Computer Application in Medical Care.* Washington, D.C., USA. 475–480.

Humphreys, B. L., D. A. Lindberg, H. M. Schoolman and G. O. Barnett (1998). The unified medical language system: an informatics research collaboration. *Journal of the American Medical Informatics Association* **5**(1): 1–11.

Langlotz, C. P. (2006). RadLex: a new method for indexing online educational materials1. *Radiographics* **26**(6): 1595–1597.

McDonald, C. J., S. M. Huff, J. G. Suico, G. Hill, D. Leavelle, R. Aller, A. Forrey, K. Mercer, G. DeMoor and J. Hook (2003). LOINC, a universal standard for identifying laboratory observations: a 5-year update. *Clinical Chemistry* **49**(4): 624–633.

National E-health Transition Authority, Clinical Terminology Overview (2012). http://www.nehta.gov.au/media-centre/nehta-publications/brochures/277-clinical-terminology-factsheet, downloaded 21/11/14.

Nelson, S. J., K. Zeng, J. Kilbourne, T. Powell and R. Moore (2011). Normalized names for clinical drugs: RxNorm at 6 years. *Journal of the American Medical Informatics Association* **18**(4): 441–448.

O'Neil, M., C. Payne and J. Read (1995). Read Codes Version 3: a user led terminology. *Methods of Information in Medicine* **34**(1–2): 187–192.

Oesterlen, F. (1855). *Medical Logic*, (English Translation). London: Sydenham Society.

Rector, A. L., W. D. Solomon, W. A. Nowlan, T. Rush, P. Zanstra and W. Claassen (1995). A terminology server for medical language and medical information systems. *Methods of Information in Medicine* **34**(1-2): 147–157.

Regier, D., W. Narrow, E. Kuhl and D. Kupfer (2009). The conceptual development of DSM-V. *American Journal of Psychiatry* **166**(6): 645–650.

Rothwell, D. J. (1995). SNOMED-based knowledge representation. *Methods of Information in Medicine* **34**(1–2): 209–213.

Sable, J. H., S. Nash and A. Wang (2001). Culling a clinical terminology: a systematic approach to identifying problematic content. In: *Proceedings of the AMIA Symposium*. Washington, D.C., USA, American Medical Informatics Association. 578–582.

Sampalli, T., M. Shepherd, J. Duffy and R. Fox (2010). An evaluation of SNOMED CT in the domain of complex chronic conditions. *International Journal of Integrated Care* **10**: e038.

Schulz, E. B., J. W. Barrett and C. Price (1998). Read code quality assurance from simple syntax to semantic stability. *Journal of the American Medical Informatics Association* **5**(4): 337–346.

Soler, J.-K., I. Okkes, M. Wood and H. Lamberts (2008). The coming of age of ICPC: celebrating the 21st birthday of the International Classification of Primary Care. *Family Practice* **25**(4): 312–317.

Spackman, K. A., K. E. Campbell and R. Cã (1997). SNOMED RT: a reference terminology for health care. In: *Proceedings of the AMIA Annual Fall Symposium*. American Medical Informatics Association.

Stearns, M. Q., C. Price, K. A. Spackman and A. Y. Wang (2001). SNOMED clinical terms: overview of the development process and project status. In: *Proceedings of the AMIA Symposium*. Washington, D.C., American Medical Informatics Association. 662–666.

World Health Organization (2011). ICD-10: *International Statistical Classification of Diseases and Related Health Problems – 10th revision edition 2010 Instruction Manual*. Geneva, World Health Organization.

Chapter 24

Afantenos, S., V. Karkaletsis and P. Stamatopoulos (2005). Summarization from medical documents: a survey. *Artificial Intelligence in Medicine* **33**(2): 157–177.

Aronson, A. R. (2001). Effective mapping of biomedical text to the UMLS Metathesaurus: the MetaMap program. In: *Proceedings of the AMIA Symposium*. Washington, D.C., USA, American Medical Informatics Association. 17–21.

Austin, P. C., P. A. Daly and J. V. Tu (2002). A multicenter study of the coding accuracy of hospital discharge administrative data for patients admitted to cardiac care units in Ontario. *American Heart Journal* **144**(2): 290–296.

Burns, E., E. Rigby, R. Mamidanna, A. Bottle, P. Aylin, P. Ziprin and O. Faiz (2012). Systematic review of discharge coding accuracy. *Journal of Public Health* **34**(1): 138–148.

Ceusters, W., B. Smith, A. Kumar and C. Dhaen (2004). Ontology-based error detection in SNOMED-CT. Proceedings of the 11th World Congress on Medical Informatics. Fieschi, M., E. Coiera and Y. J. Li (eds.). *Studies in Health Technology and Informatics* Volume **107**(1): 482–486.

Chen, L., H. Liu and C. Friedman (2005). Gene name ambiguity of eukaryotic nomenclatures. *Bioinformatics* **21**(2): 248–256.

Chung, G. Y. and E. Coiera (2007). A study of structured clinical abstracts and the semantic classification of sentences. In: *Proceedings of the Workshop on BioNLP 2007: Biological,*

Translational, and Clinical Language Processing. Prague, Czech Republic, Association for Computational Linguistics.

Cimino, J. (1994). Controlled medical vocabulary construction: methods from the Canongroup. *Journal of the American Medical Informatics Association* **1**(3): 296–297.

Evans, D., J. Cimino, W. Hersh, S. Huff and D. Bell (1994). Toward a medical-concept representation language. *Journal of the American Medical Informatics Association* **1**(3): 207–217.

Feinstein, A. R. (1967). *Clinical Judgment*. Baltimore, Williams & Wilkins.

Glowinski, A. J. (1994). Integrating guidelines and the clinical record: the role of semantically constrained terminologies. In: Gordon, J. C. and P. Christensen, editors. *Health Telematics For Clinical Guidelines and Protocols*. Amsterdam, IOS Press.

Goble, C. A., A. Glowinski and K. G. Jeffery (1993a). Semantic constraints in a medical information system. In: *Advances in Databases*. Berlin, Springer, pp 40–57.

Goble, C. A., A. J. Glowinski, W. Nowlan and A. L. Rector (1993b). A descriptive semantic formalism for medicine. In: *Proceedings of the Ninth IEEE International Conference on Data Engineering*. Vienna, Austria. 624–631.

Goldberg, A. E. (2006). *Constructions at Work: The Nature of Generalization in Language*. Oxford, Oxford University Press.

Heinsohn, J., D. Kudenko, B. Nebel and H.-J. Profitlich (1994). An empirical analysis of terminological representation systems. *Artificial Intelligence* **68**(2): 367–397.

Henderson, T., J. Shepheard and V. Sundararajan (2006). Quality of diagnosis and procedure coding in ICD-10 administrative data. *Medical Care* **44**(11): 1011–1019.

Hersh, W., S. Price and L. Donohoe (2000). Assessing thesaurus-based query expansion using the UMLS Metathesaurus. In: *Proceedings of the AMIA Symposium*, American Medical Informatics Association.

Hogarth, R. M. (1986). Generalization in decision research: the role of formal models. *IEEE Transactions on Systems, Man and Cybernetics* **16**(3): 439–449.

Hüske-Kraus, D. (2003). Text generation in clinical medicine: a review. *Methods of Information in Medicine* **42**(1): 51–60.

Lorence, D. P. and I. A. Ibrahim (2002). Benchmarking variation in coding accuracy across the United States. *Journal of Health Care Finance* **29**(4): 29–42.

Mollá, D. and J. L. Vicedo (2007). Question answering in restricted domains: an overview. *Computational Linguistics* **33**(1): 41–61.

Monk, R. (1990). *Ludwig Wittgenstein: The Duty of Genius*. London, Vintage.

Norman, D. A. (1993). Cognition in the head and in the world: an introduction to the special issue on situated action. *Cognitive Science* **17**(1): 1–6.

Ong, M., F. Magrabi and E. Coiera (2010). Automated categorisation of clinical incident reports using statistical text classification. *Quality and Safety in Health Care* **19**: 1–7.

Ong, M., F. Magrabi and E. Coiera (2012). Automated identification of extreme-risk events in clinical incident reports. *Journal of the American Medical Informatics Association* **19**(e1): e110–e118.

Romano, P. S. and D. H. Mark (1994). Bias in the coding of hospital discharge data and its implications for quality assessment. *Medical Care* **32**(1): 81–90.

Rosch, E. (1988). Principles of categorization. In: Rosch, E. and B. B. Lloyd, editors. *Readings in Cognitive Science*. Los Altos, CA, Morgan Kaufmann, pp 312–322.

Rosse, C., A. Kumar, J. L. Mejino Jr., D. L. Cook, L. T. Detwiler and B. Smith (2005). A strategy for improving and integrating biomedical ontologies. In: *AMIA Annual Symposium Proceedings*. Washington, D.C., American Medical Informatics Association.

Sintchenko, V., S. Anthony, X.-H. Phan, F. Lin and E. W. Coiera (2010). A PubMed-wide associational study of infectious diseases. *PLoS One* **5**(3): e9535.

Tatonetti, N. P., G. H. Fernald and R. B. Altman (2012). A novel signal detection algorithm for identifying hidden drug-drug interactions in adverse event reports. *Journal of the American Medical Informatics Association* **19**(1): 79–85.

Tsafnat, G., A. Dunn, P. Glasziou and E. Coiera (2013). The automation of systematic reviews. *BMJ* **346:** f139.

Tuttle, M. S. and S. J. Nelson (1994). The role of the UMLS in 'storing'and 'sharing'across systems. *International Journal of Bio-medical Computing* **34**(1): 207–237.

Wittgenstein, L. (1953). *Philosophical Investigations*. New York, Macmillan.

Chapter 25

Agency for Healthcare Research and Quality. *Patient Safety Indicators Overview: AHRQ Quality Indicators*. Rockville, MD, Agency for Healthcare Research and Quality. Retrieved 25 September 2014, from http://www.qualityindicators.ahrq.gov/Modules/psi_resources.aspx.

Ahmad, F., H. A. Skinner, D. E. Stewart and W. Levinson (2010). Perspectives of family physicians on computer-assisted health-risk assessments. *Journal of Medical Internet Research* **12**(2): e12.

Ammenwerth, E., P. Schnell-Inderst, C. Machan and U. Siebert (2008). The effect of electronic prescribing on medication errors and adverse drug events: a systematic review. *Journal of the American Medical Informatics Association* **15**(5): 585–600.

Balas, E. A., S. Krishna, R. A. Kretschmer, T. R. Cheek, D. F. Lobach and S. A. Boren (2004). Computerized knowledge management in diabetes care. *Medical Care* **42**(6): 610–621.

Bannister, F., P. McCabe and D. Remenyi (2001). How much did we really pay for that? The awkward problem of information technology costs. *Electronic Journal of Information Systems Evaluation* **5**(1): 1–20.

Barnett, G. O., J. J. Cimino, J. A. Hupp and E. P. Hoffer (1987). DXplain: an evolving diagnostic decision-support system. *JAMA* **258**(1): 67–74.

Bassi, J. and F. Lau (2013). Measuring value for money: a scoping review on economic evaluation of health information systems. *Journal of the American Medical Informatics Association* **20**(4): 792–801.

Bates, D., D. Cullen, N. Laird, L. Peterson, S. Small, D. Servi, G. Laffel, B. Sweitzer, B. Shea, R. Hallisey, M. Vander Vliet, R. Nemeskal and L. Leape (1995). Incidence of adverse drug events and potential adverse drug events: implications for prevention. *JAMA* **274**(1): 29–34.

Bates, D. W., L. L. Leape, D. J. Cullen, N. Laird, L. A. Petersen, J. M. Teich, E. Burdick, M. Hickey, S. Kleefield and B. Shea (1998). Effect of computerized physician order entry and a team intervention on prevention of serious medication errors. *JAMA* **280**(15): 1311–1316.

Bates, D. W., J. M. Teich, J. Lee, D. Seger, G. J. Kuperman, N. Ma'Luf, D. Boyle and L. Leape (1999). The impact of computerized physician order entry on medication error prevention. *Journal of the American Medical Informatics Association* **6**(4): 313–321.

Bayoumi, I., M. A. Balas, S. M. Handler, L. Dolovich, B. Hutchison and A. Holbrook (2014). The effectiveness of computerized drug-lab alerts: a systematic review and meta-analysis. *International Journal of Medical Informatics* **83**(6): 406–415.

Birkmeyer, J. D., C. M. Birkmeyer, D. E. Wennberg and M. Young (2000). *Leapfrog Patient Safety Standards: The Potential Benefits of Universal Adoption.* Washington, DC, The Leapfrog Group.

Bizovi, K. E., B. E. Beckley, M. C. McDade, A. L. Adams, R. A. Lowe, A. D. Zechnich and J. R. Hedges (2002). The effect of computer-assisted prescription writing on emergency department prescription errors. *Academic Emergency Medicine* **9**(11): 1168–1175.

Bond, W. F., L. M. Schwartz, K. R. Weaver, D. Levick, M. Giuliano and M. L. Graber (2012). Differential diagnosis generators: an evaluation of currently available computer programs. *Journal of General Internal Medicine* **27**(2): 213–219.

Chaudhry, B., J. Wang, S. Wu, M. Maglione, W. Mojica, E. Roth, S. C. Morton and P. G. Shekelle (2006). Systematic review: impact of health information technology on quality, efficiency, and costs of medical care. *Annals of Internal Medicine* **144**(10): 742–752.

Cimino, J. J. (2008). Infobuttons: anticipatory passive decision support. In: *AMIA Annual Symposium Proceedings.* American Medical Informatics Association. Washington, D.C. 1203–1204.

Cimino, J. J., G. Elhanan and Q. Zeng (1997). Supporting infobuttons with terminological knowledge. In: *Proceedings of the AMIA Annual Fall Symposium.* Nashville, TN, American Medical Informatics Association.

Coiera, E. (1990). Monitoring diseases with empirical and model-generated histories. *Artificial Intelligence in Medicine* **2**(3): 135–147.

Coiera, E. (1994). Question the assumptions. In: Barahona, P. and J. Christensen, editors. *Knowledge and Decisions in Health Telematics: The Next Decade.* Amsterdam, IOS Press, vol 12, pp 61–66.

Coiera, E., J. I. Westbrook and K. Rogers (2008). Clinical decision velocity is increased when meta-search filters enhance an evidence retrieval system. *Journal of American Medical Informatics Association* **15**(5): 638–646.

Cushman, R. (1997). Serious technology assessment for health care information technology. *Journal of the American Medical Informatics Association* **4**(4): 259–265.

Dean, J. C. and C. C. Ilvento (2006). Improved cancer detection using computer-aided detection with diagnostic and screening mammography: prospective study of 104 cancers. *AJR American Journal of Roentgenology* **187**(1): 20–28.

Dexheimer, J. W., T. R. Talbot, D. L. Sanders, S. T. Rosenbloom and D. Aronsky (2008). Prompting clinicians about preventive care measures: a systematic review of randomized controlled trials. *Journal of the American Medical Informatics Association* **15**(3): 311–320.

Dexter, F., R. H. Epstein, J. D. Lee and J. Ledolter (2009). Automatic updating of times remaining in surgical cases using bayesian analysis of historical case duration data and instant messaging updates from anesthesia providers. *Anesthesia and Analgesia* **108**(3): 929–940.

Doi, K. (2005). Current status and future potential of computer-aided diagnosis in medical imaging. *British Journal of Radiology* **78**(Suppl 1): s3–s19.

Dunn, A. G., M.-S. Ong, J. I. Westbrook, F. Magrabi, E. Coiera and W. Wobcke (2011). A simulation framework for mapping risks in clinical processes: the case of in-patient transfers. *Journal of the American Medical Informatics Association* **18**(3): 259–266.

Edwards, G., P. Compton, R. Malor, A. Srinivasan and L. Lazarus (1993). PEIRS: a pathologist-maintained expert system for the interpretation of chemical pathology reports. *Pathology* **25**(1): 27–34.

Elson, R. B., J. G. Faughnan and D. P. Connelly (1997). An industrial process view of information delivery to support clinical decision making implications for systems design and process measures. *Journal of the American Medical Informatics Association* **4**(4): 266–278.

Emery, J., H. Morris, R. Goodchild, T. Fanshawe, A. Prevost, M. Bobrow and A.-L. Kinmonth (2007). The GRAIDS Trial: a cluster randomised controlled trial of computer decision support for the management of familial cancer risk in primary care. *British Journal of Cancer* **97**(4): 486–493.

Emery, J., R. Walton, M. Murphy, J. Austoker, P. Yudkin, C. Chapman, A. Coulson, D. Glasspool and J. Fox (2000). Computer support for interpreting family histories of breast and ovarian cancer in primary care: comparative study with simulated cases. *BMJ* **321**(7252): 28–32.

Eslami, S., N. F. de Keizer and A. Abu-Hanna (2008). The impact of computerized physician medication order entry in hospitalized patients: a systematic review. *International Journal of Medical Informatics* **77**(6): 365–376.

Evans, R. W. (1996). A critical perspective on the tools to support clinical decision making. *Transfusion* **36**(8): 671–673.

Fenton, J. J., S. H. Taplin, P. A. Carney, L. Abraham, E. A. Sickles, C. D'Orsi, E. A. Berns, G. Cutter, R. E. Hendrick, W. E. Barlow and J. G. Elmore (2007). Influence of computer-aided detection on performance of screening mammography. *New England Journal of Medicine* **356**(14): 1399–1409.

Fry, J. P. and R. A. Neff (2009). Periodic prompts and reminders in health promotion and health behavior interventions: systematic review. *Journal of Medical Internet Research* **11**(2): e16.

Furuya, H., T. Morimoto and Y. Ogawa (2013). Relationship between the use of an electronic commercial prescribing system and medical errors and medication errors in a teaching hospital. *Tokai Journal of Experimental and Clinical Medicine* **38**(1): 33.

Garg, A. X., N. K. Adhikari, H. McDonald, M. P. Rosas-Arellano, P. Devereaux, J. Beyene, J. Sam and R. B. Haynes (2005). Effects of computerized clinical decision support systems on practitioner performance and patient outcomes. *JAMA* **293**(10): 1223–1238.

Glasspool, D., J. Fox, F. Castillo and V. Monaghan (2003). Interactive decision support for medical planning. In: *Proceedings, 9th Conference on Artificial Intelligence in Medicine in Europe*, AIME 2003, Protaras, Cyprus, 2003. Lecture Notes in Computer Science, Vol. 2780 Springer. 335–339.

Gospodarevskaya, E. and J. I. Westbrook (2014). Call for discussion about the framework for categorizing economic evaluations of health information systems and assessing their quality. *Journal of the American Medical Informatics Association* **21**: 190–191.

Harpole, L. H., R. Khorasani, J. Fiskio, G. J. Kuperman and D. W. Bates (1997). Automated evidence-based critiquing of orders for abdominal radiographs: impact on utilization and appropriateness. *Journal of the American Medical Informatics Association* **4**(6): 511–521.

Heathfield, H., D. Pitty and R. Hanka (1998). Evaluating information technology in health care: barriers and challenges. *BMJ* **316**(7149): 1959.

Hillman, K., J. Chen, M. Cretikos, R. Bellomo, D. Brown, G. Doig, S. Finfer, A. Flabouris and M. S. Investigators (2005). Introduction of the medical emergency team (MET) system: a cluster-randomised controlled trial. *Lancet* **365**(9477): 2091–2097.

Jaspers, M. W., M. Smeulers, H. Vermeulen and L. W. Peute (2011). Effects of clinical decision-support systems on practitioner performance and patient outcomes: a synthesis of high-quality systematic review findings. *Journal of the American Medical Informatics Association* **18**(3): 327–334.

Johnson, K. B. and M. J. Feldman (1995). Medical informatics and pediatrics: decision-support systems. *Archives of Pediatrics and Adolescent Medicine* **149**(12): 1371.

Kaplan, R. S. and D. P. Norton (1996). Using the balanced scorecard as a strategic management system. *Harvard Business Review* **74**(1): 75–85.

Kaushal, R. and D. W. Bates (2001). Computerized physician order entry (CPOE) with clinical decision support systems (CDSSs). In: *Making Health Care Safer: A Critical Analysis of Patient Safety Practices.* Rockville, MD, Agency for Healthcare Research and Quality, p 58.

Kawamoto, K., C. A. Houlihan, E. A. Balas and D. F. Lobach (2005). Improving clinical practice using decision support systems: a systematic review of randomised controlled trials to identify system features critical to success. *BMJ* **330**: 765–768.

Kheterpal, S., R. Gupta, J. M. Blum, K. K. Tremper, M. O'Reilly and P. E. Kazanjian (2007). Electronic reminders improve procedure documentation compliance and professional fee reimbursement. *Anesthesia and Analgesia* **104**(3): 592–597.

Kohn, L. T., J. M. Corrigan and M. S. Donaldson (2001). *Crossing the Quality Chasm: A New Health System for the 21st Century.* Washington, DC, Committee on Quality of Health Care in America, Institute of Medicine.

Kuperman, G. J., A. Bobb, T. H. Payne, A. J. Avery, T. K. Gandhi, G. Burns, D. C. Classen and D. W. Bates (2007). Medication-related clinical decision support in computerized provider order entry systems: a review. *Journal of the American Medical Informatics Association* **14**(1): 29–40.

Kuperman, G. J., D. F. Sittig, M. M. Shabot and J. Teich (1999). Clinical decision support for hospital and critical care. *Journal of Healthcare Information Management* **13**: 81–96.

Lau, A. Y. S., V. Sintchenko, J. Crimmins, F. Magrabi, B. Gallego and E. Coiera (2012). Impact of a Web-based personally controlled health management system on influenza vaccination and health services utilization rates: a randomized controlled trial. *Journal of the American Medical Informatics Association* **19**(5): 719–727.

Lepage, E., R. Gardner, R. Laub and O. Golubjatnikov (1992). Improving blood transfusion practice: role of a computerized hospital information system. *Transfusion* **32**(3): 253–259.

Mathe, J., J. Sztipanovits, M. Levy, E. K. Jackson and W. Schulte (2012). Cancer treatment planning: formal methods to the rescue. Paper presented at the 4th International Workshop on Software Engineering in Health Care (SEHC 2012), Zurich, Switzerland.

McDonald, C. J., S. L. Hui, D. M. Smith, W. M. Tierney, S. J. Cohen, M. Weinberger and G. P. McCabe (1984). Reminders to physicians from an introspective computer medical record: a two-year randomized trial. *Annals of Internal Medicine* **100**(1): 130–138.

McGreevey, III, J. D. (2013). Order sets in electronic health records: principles of good practice. *Chest* **143**(1): 228–235.

Monane, M., D. M. Matthias, B. A. Nagle and M. A. Kelly (1998). Improving prescribing patterns for the elderly through an online drug utilization review intervention: a system linking the physician, pharmacist, and computer. *JAMA* **280**(14): 1249–1252.

Morton, M. J., D. H. Whaley, K. R. Brandt and K. K. Amrami (2006). Screening mammograms: interpretation with computer-aided detection: prospective evaluation. *Radiology* **239**(2): 375–383.

Müller, H., N. Michoux, D. Bandon and A. Geissbuhler (2004). A review of content-based image retrieval systems in medical applications: clinical benefits and future directions. *International Journal of Medical Informatics* **73**(1): 1–23.

O'Connor, A., A. Rostom, V. Fiset, J. Tetroe, V. Entwistle and H. Llewellyn-Thomas (1999). Decision aids for patients facing health treatment or screening decisions: systematic review. *BMJ* **319**(7212): 731–734.

Ong, M., F. Magrabi, G. Jones and E. Coiera (2012). Last orders: follow-up of tests ordered on the day of hospital discharge. *Archives of Internal Medicine* **172**(17): 1347–1349.

O'Reilly, M., A. Talsma, S. VanRiper, S. Kheterpal and R. Burney (2006). An anesthesia information system designed to provide physician-specific feedback improves timely administration of prophylactic antibiotics. *Anesthesia and Analgesia* **103**(4): 908–912.

Overhage, J. M., W. M. Tierney and C. J. McDonald (1996). Computer reminders to implement preventive care guidelines for hospitalized patients. *Archives of Internal Medicine* **156**(14): 1551.

Poihonen, J. and J. M. Leventhal (1999). Medication-management issues at the point of care. *Journal of Healthcare Information Management* **13**: 43–52.

Protti, D. (2002). A proposal to use a balanced scorecard to evaluate Information for Health: an information strategy for the modern NHS (1998–2005). *Computers in Biology and Medicine* **32**(3): 221–236.

Randolph, A. G., R. B. Haynes, J. C. Wyatt, D. J. Cook and G. H. Guyatt (1999). Users' guides to the medical literature: XVIII. How to use an article evaluating the clinical impact of a computer-based clinical decision support system. *JAMA* **282**(1): 67–74.

Raschke, R. A., B. Gollihare, T. A. Wunderlich, J. R. Guidry, A. I. Leibowitz, J. C. Peirce, L. Lemelson, M. A. Heisler and C. Susong (1998). A computer alert system to prevent injury from adverse drug events: development and evaluation in a community teaching hospital. *JAMA* **280**(15): 1317–1320.

Rind, D. M., C. Safran, R. S. Phillips, Q. Wang, D. R. Calkins, T. L. Delbanco, H. L. Bleich and W. V. Slack (1994). Effect of computer-based alerts on the treatment and outcomes of hospitalized patients. *Archives of Internal Medicine* **154**(13): 1511.

Sandberg, W. S., E. H. Sandberg, A. R. Seim, S. Anupama, J. M. Ehrenfeld, S. F. Spring and J. L. Walsh (2008). Real-time checking of electronic anesthesia records for documentation errors and automatically text messaging clinicians improves quality of documentation. *Anesthesia and Analgesia* **106**(1): 192–201.

Shojania, K. G., D. Yokoe, R. Platt, J. Fiskio, N. Ma'Luf and D. W. Bates (1998). Reducing vancomycin use utilizing a computer guideline results of a randomized controlled trial. *Journal of the American Medical Informatics Association* **5**(6): 554–562.

Shu, K., D. Boyle, C. Spurr, J. Horsky, H. Heiman, P. O'Connor, J. Lepore and D. W. Bates (2001). Comparison of time spent writing orders on paper with computerized physician order entry. *Studies in Health Technology and Informatics* **84**(2): 1207–1211.

Singh, H. and M. S. Vij (2010). Eight recommendations for policies for communicating abnormal test results. *Joint Commission Journal on Quality and Patient Safety* **36**(5): 226–232.

Sintchenko, V., J. R. Iredell and G. L. Gilbert (2007). Pathogen profiling for disease management and surveillance. *Nature Reviews Microbiology* **5**(6): 464–470.

Sklarin, N. T., S. Granovsky, E. M. O'Reilly and A. D. Zelenetz (2011). Electronic chemotherapy order entry: a major cancer center's implementation. *Journal of Oncology Practice* **7**(4): 213–218.

Snow, M. G., R. J. Fallat, W. R. Tyler and S. P. Hsu (1988). Pulmonary consult: concept to application of an expert system. *Journal of Clinical Engineering* **13**(3): 201–206.

Spyropoulos, C. D. (2000). AI planning and scheduling in the medical hospital environment. *Artificial Intelligence in Medicine* **20**(2): 101–111.

Stern, M., K. Williams, D. Eddy and R. Kahn (2008). Validation of prediction of diabetes by the Archimedes model and comparison with other predicting models. *Diabetes Care* **31**(8): 1670–1671.

Stivaros, S., A. Gledson, G. Nenadic, X. Zeng, J. Keane and A. Jackson (2010). Decision support systems for clinical radiological practice: towards the next generation. *British Journal of Radiology* **83**(995): 904.

Subbe, C., R. Davies, E. Williams, P. Rutherford and L. Gemmell (2003). Effect of introducing the Modified Early Warning score on clinical outcomes, cardio-pulmonary arrests and intensive care utilisation in acute medical admissions. *Anaesthesia* **58**(8): 797–802.

Teich, J. M., P. R. Merchia, J. L. Schmiz, G. J. Kuperman, C. D. Spurr and D. W. Bates (2000). Effects of computerized physician order entry on prescribing practices. *Archives of Internal Medicine* **160**(18): 2741–2747.

Tennant, R., M. A. Mohammed, J. J. Coleman and U. Martin (2007). Monitoring patients using control charts: a systematic review. *International Journal for Quality in Health Care* **19**(4): 187–194.

Than, M. P. and D. F. Flaws (2009). Communicating diagnostic uncertainties to patients: the problems of explaining unclear diagnosis and risk. *Evidence-Based Medicine* **14**(3): 66–67.

Thomas, K. W., C. S. Dayton and M. W. Peterson (1999). Evaluation of Internet-based clinical decision support systems. *Journal of Medical Internet Research* **1**(2): e6.

Thor, J., J. Lundberg, J. Ask, J. Olsson, C. Carli, K. P. Härenstam and M. Brommels (2007). Application of statistical process control in healthcare improvement: systematic review. *Quality and Safety in Health Care* **16**(5): 387–399.

Tierney, W. M., M. E. Miller, J. M. Overhage and C. J. McDonald (1993). Physician inpatient order writing on microcomputer workstations: effects on resource utilization. *JAMA* **269**(3): 379–383.

Tsafnat, G., A. Dunn, P. Glasziou and E. Coiera (2013). The automation of systematic reviews. *BMJ* **346**: f139.

Van Grembergen, W. and R. Van Bruggen (1997). Measuring and improving corporate information technology through the balanced scorecard. In: *Proceedings of the European Conference on the Evaluation of Information Technology*, Delft, The Netherlands.

Venkatesh, V., M. G. Morris, G. B. Davis and F. D. Davis (2003). User acceptance of information technology: toward a unified view. *MIS Quarterly* **27**(3): 425–478.

Walton, R., S. Dovey, E. Harvey and N. Freemantle (1999). Computer support for determining drug dose: systematic review and meta-analysis. *BMJ* **318**(7189): 984–990.

Welch, B. M. and K. Kawamoto (2013). Clinical decision support for genetically guided personalized medicine: a systematic review. *Journal of the American Medical Informatics Association* **20**(2): 388–400.

Wells, S., S. Furness, N. Rafter, E. Horn, R. Whittaker, A. Stewart, K. Moodabe, P. Roseman, V. Selak, D. Bramley and R. Jackson (2008). Integrated electronic decision support increases cardiovascular disease risk assessment four fold in routine primary care practice. *European Journal of Cardiovascular Prevention and Rehabilitation* **15**(2): 173–178.

Westbrook, J. I., M. T. Baysari, L. Li, R. Burke, K. L. Richardson and R. O. Day (2013). The safety of electronic prescribing: manifestations, mechanisms, and rates of system-related errors associated with two commercial systems in hospitals. *Journal of the American Medical Informatics Association* **20**(d6): 1159–1167.

Westbrook, J. I., E. W. Coiera and A. S. Gosling (2005). Do online information retrieval systems help experienced clinicians answer clinical questions? *Journal of the American Medical Informatics Association* **12**(3): 315–321.

Westbrook, J. I., M. Reckmann, L. Li, W. B. Runciman, R. Burke, C. Lo, M. T. Baysari, J. Braithwaite and R. O. Day (2012). Effects of two commercial electronic prescribing systems on prescribing error rates in hospital in-patients: a before and after study. *PLoS Medicine* 9(1): e1001164

Interlude – artificial intelligence in medicine

Clancey, W. J. and E. H. Shortliffe (1984). *Readings in Medical Artificial Intelligence: The First Decade*. Boston, MA, USA, Addison-Wesley Longman.

Durinck, J., E. Coiera, R. Baud, L. Console, J. Cruz, P. Frutiger, P. Hucklenbroich, A. Rickards and K. Spitzer (1994). The role of knowledge based systems in clinical practice. In: *Knowledge and Decisions in Health Telematics: The Next Decade*. Amsterdam, IOS Press, pp 199–203.

Genesereth, M. R. and N. J. Nilsson (1987). *Logical Foundations of Artificial Intelligence*. Los Altos, CA, Morgan Kaufmann.

Ledley, R. S. and L. B. Lusted (1959). Reasoning foundations of medical diagnosis. *Science* **130**(3366): 9–21.

Miller, P. L. (1988). *Selected Topics in Medical Artificial Intelligence*. New York, Springer.

Shortliffe, E. H. (1987). Computer programs to support clinical decision making. *JAMA* **258**(1): 61–66.

Steels, L. and R. A. Brooks (1995). *The Artificial Life Route to Artificial Intelligence: Building Embodied, Situated Agents*. Lawrence Erlbaum Associates, Inc., Hillsdale, NJ.

Szolovits, P. (1982). *Artificial Intelligence in Medicine.* American Association for the Advancement of Science selected symposium. Boulder, CO, Westview Press.

Chapter 26

Bourlard, H. and C. J. Wellekens (1990). Links between Markov models and multilayer perceptrons. *IEEE Transactions on Pattern Analysis and Machine Intelligence* **12**(12): 1167–1178.

Coiera, E. (1990). Monitoring diseases with empirical and model-generated histories. *Artificial Intelligence in Medicine* **2**(3): 135–147.

Coiera, E. (1992). The qualitative representation of physical systems. *Knowledge Engineering Review* **7**(01): 55–77.

Cooper, G. F. (1988). *Computer-Based Medical Diagnosis Using Belief Networks and Bounded Probabilities.* In: *Selected Topics in Medical Artificial Intelligence Computers and Medicine.* Miller, P. L. (ed). New York: Springer-Verlag, 85–98.

Eddy, D. M. and L. Schlessinger (2003). Validation of the Archimedes diabetes model. *Diabetes Care* **26**(11): 3102–3110.

Gallego, B., A. G. Dunn and E. Coiera (2013). Role of electronic health records in comparative effectiveness research. *Journal of Comparative Effectiveness Research* **2**(6): 529–532.

Garrett, S. M., G. M. Coghill, A. Srinivasan and R. D. King (2007). Learning qualitative models of physical and biological systems. In: *Computational Discovery of Scientific Knowledge.* Berlin: Springer-Verlag, pp 248–272.

Hart, A. and J. Wyatt (1989). Connectionist models in medicine: an investigation of their potential. In: *AIME 89: Proceedings of the Second European Conference on Artificial Intelligence in Medicine, London, August 29th–31st 1989.* Berlin, Springer, pp 115–124.

Hornik, K., M. Stinchcombe and H. White (1989). Multilayer feedforward networks are universal approximators. *Neural Networks* **2**(5): 359–366.

Ironi, L., M. Stefanelli and G. Lanzola (1990). Qualitative models in medical diagnosis. *Artificial Intelligence in Medicine* **2**(2): 85–101.

Kohonen, T. (1988). An introduction to neural computing. *Neural Networks* **1**(1): 3–16.

Kuipers, B. and J. P. Kassirer (1984). Causal reasoning in medicine: analysis of a protocol. *Cognitive Science* **8**(4): 363–385.

Meadows, D. H. (2008). *Thinking in Systems: A Primer.* White River Junction, VT, Chelsea Green Publishing.

Nikoonahad, M. and D. Liu (1990). Medical ultrasound imaging using neural networks. *Electronics Letters* **26**(8): 545–546.

Pietka, E. (1989). Neural nets for ECG classification. In: *Images of the Twenty-First Century. Proceedings of the Annual International Conference of the IEEE Engineering in Medicine and Biology Society.* Seattle: Institute of Electrical and Electronics Engineers, 1989.

Riesbeck, C. K. and R. C. Schank (2013). *Inside Case-Based Reasoning.* Psychology Press.

Sebald, A. (1989). Use of neural networks for detection of artifacts in arterial pressure waveforms. In: *Images of the Twenty-First Century. Proceedings of the Annual*

International Conference of the IEEE Engineering in Medicine and Biology Society. Seattle: Institute of Electrical and Electronics Engineers, 1989,

Uckun, S. (1991). Model-based reasoning in biomedicine. *Critical Reviews in Biomedical Engineering* **19**(4): 261–292.

Uckun, S., B. M. Dawant and D. P. Lindstrom (1993). Model-based diagnosis in intensive care monitoring: the YAQ approach. *Artificial Intelligence in Medicine* **5**(1): 31–48.

Widman, L. E. (1992). A model-based approach to the diagnosis of the cardiac arrhythmias. *Artificial Intelligence in Medicine* **4**(1): 1–19.

Chapter 27

Abston, K. C. *et al.* Inducing practice guidelines from a hospital database. *Proceedings of the AMIA Annual Fall Symposium.* American Medical Informatics Association, Nashville TN, 1997, 168–172.

Bratko, I., I. Mozetič and N. Lavrač (1990). *KARDIO: A Study in Deep and Qualitative Knowledge for Expert Systems.* Cambridge, MA, MIT Press.

Burnham, K. P. and D. R. Anderson (2002). *Model Selection and Multimodel Inference: A Practical Information-Theoretic Approach.* New York, N.Y., Springer.

Compton, P., G. Edwards, B. Kang, L. Lazarus, R. Malor, P. Preston and A. Srinivasan (1992). Ripple Down Rules: turning knowledge acquisition into knowledge maintenance. *Artificial Intelligence in Medicine* **4**(6): 463–475.

Compton, P. and R. Jansen (1990). A philosophical basis for knowledge acquisition. *Knowledge Acquisition* **2**(3): 241–258.

Compton, P., L. Peters, G. Edwards and T. G. Lavers (2006). Experience with Ripple-Down Rules. *Knowledge-Based Systems* **19**(5): 356–362.

Cooke, N. J. (1999). Knowledge elicitation.In: Nickerson, R. S., R. W. Schvaneveldt, S. T. Dumais, D. S. Lindsay, M. T. H. Chi, F. T. Durso, editors. *Handbook of Applied Cognition,* New York, Wiley, pp 479–510.

Cortes, C. and V. Vapnik (1995). Support-vector networks. *Machine Learning* **20**(3): 273–297.

Forestier, G., F. Lalys, L. Riffaud, B. Trelhu and P. Jannin (2012). Classification of surgical processes using dynamic time warping. *Journal of Biomedical Informatics* **45**(2): 255–264.

Gentric, J.-C., B. Trelhu, P. Jannin, L. Riffaud, J.-C. Ferré and J.-Y. Gauvrit (2013). Development of workflow task analysis during cerebral diagnostic angiographies: time-based comparison of junior and senior tasks. *Journal of Neuroradiology* **40**(5): 342–347.

Grünwald, P. D. (2007). *The Minimum Description Length Principle.* Cambridge, MA, MIT Press.

Hau, D. and E. Coiera (1997). Learning qualitative models of dynamic systems. *Machine Learning* **26:** 177–211.

Huang, Z., X. Lu and H. Duan (2013). Latent treatment pattern discovery for clinical processes. *Journal of Medical Systems* **37**(2): 1–10.

Jensen, P. B., L. J. Jensen and S. Brunak (2012). Mining electronic health records: towards better research applications and clinical care. *Nature Reviews Genetics* **13**(6): 395–405.

King, R. D., S. Muggleton, R. A. Lewis and M. Sternberg (1992). Drug design by machine learning: the use of inductive logic programming to model the structure–activity relationships of trimethoprim analogues binding to dihydrofolate reductase. *Proceedings of the National Academy of Sciences of the United States of America* **89**(23): 11322–11326.

Mani, S., C. Aliferis, S. Krishnaswami and T. Kotchen (2007). Learning causal and predictive clinical practice guidelines from data. *Studies in Health Technology and Informatics* **129**(2): 850.

Mans, R., H. Schonenberg, G. Leonardi, S. Panzarasa, A. Cavallini, S. Quaglini and W. van der Aalst (2008). Process mining techniques: an application to stroke care. *Studies in Health Technology and Informatics* **136**: 573.

Mans, R. S., M. H. Schonenberg, M. Song, W. M. P. van der Aalst and P. J. M. Bakker (2009). Application of process mining in healthcare: a case study in a Dutch hospital. In: *Biomedical Engineering Systems and Technologies*, Springer, pp 425–438.

McCoy, A. B., A. Wright, A. Laxmisan, M. J. Ottosen, J. A. McCoy, D. Butten and D. F. Sittig (2012). Development and evaluation of a crowdsourcing methodology for knowledge base construction: identifying relationships between clinical problems and medications. *Journal of the American Medical Informatics Association* **19**(5): 713–718.

Olson, J. R. and H. H. Rueter (1987). Extracting expertise from experts: methods for knowledge acquisition. *Expert Systems* **4**(3): 152–168.

Ong, M.-S., F. Magrabi and E. Coiera (2012). Automated identification of extreme-risk events in clinical incident reports. *Journal of the American Medical Informatics Association* **19**(e1): e110–e118.

Quinlan, J. R. (1986). Induction of decision trees. *Machine Learning* **1**(1): 81–106.

Richards, D. (2009a). A social software/Web 2.0 approach to collaborative knowledge engineering. *Information Sciences* **179**(15): 2515–2523.

Richards, D. (2009b). Two decades of Ripple Down Rules research. *Knowledge Engineering Review* **24**(02): 159–184.

Strauss, A. and J. Corbin (1994). Grounded theory methodology. In: Denzin, N. K. and Y. S. Lincoln, editors. *Handbook of Qualitative Research*. Thousand Oaks, CA, Sage Publications, pp 273–285.

Swanson, D. R. (1986). Fish oil, Raynaud's syndrome, and undiscovered public knowledge. *Perspectives in Biology and Medicine* **30**(1): 7.

Tatonetti, N. P., J. C. Denny, S. N. Murphy, G. H. Fernald, G. Krishnan, V. Castro, P. Yue, P. S. Tsau, I. Kohane and D. M. Roden (2011). Detecting drug interactions from adverse-event reports: interaction between paroxetine and pravastatin increases blood glucose levels. *Clinical Pharmacology and Therapeutics* **90**(1): 133–142.

Toussi, M., J.-B. Lamy, P. Le Toumelin and A. Venot (2009). Using data mining techniques to explore physicians' therapeutic decisions when clinical guidelines do not provide recommendations: methods and example for type 2 diabetes. *BMC Medical Informatics and Decision Making* **9**(1): 28.

Wagholikar, K. B., K. L. MacLaughlin, T. M. Kastner, P. M. Casey, M. Henry, R. A. Greenes, H. Liu and R. Chaudhry (2013). Formative evaluation of the accuracy of a clinical decision support system for cervical cancer screening. *Journal of the American Medical Informatics Association* **20**(4): 749–757.

Wallace, C. S. (2005). *Statistical and Inductive Inference by Minimum Message Length.* Springer-Verlag, New York, Inc. Secaucus, NJ.

Welbank, M. (1990). An overview of knowledge acquisition methods. *Interacting with Computers* **2**(1): 83–91.

Wright, A., A. McCoy, S. Henkin, M. Flaherty and D. Sittig (2013). Validation of an association rule mining-based method to infer associations between medications and problems. *Applied Clinical Informatics* **4**(1): 100–109.

Chapter 28

Atlas, E., R. Nimri, S. Miller, E. A. Grunberg and M. Phillip (2010). MD-Logic Artificial Pancreas System: a pilot study in adults with type 1 diabetes. *Diabetes Care* **33**(5): 1072–1076.

Barlow, J., D. Singh, S. Bayer and R. Curry (2007). A systematic review of the benefits of home telecare for frail elderly people and those with long-term conditions. *Journal of Telemedicine and Telecare* **13**(4): 172–179.

Celler, B. G., N. H. Lovell and D. Chan (1999). The potential impact of home telecare on clinical practice. *Medical Journal of Australia* **171**(10): 518–521.

Coiera, E. W. (1990). Monitoring diseases with empirical and model-generated histories. *Artificial Intelligence in Medicine* **2**(3): 135–147.

Cooper, J. B., R. S. Newbower and R. J. Kitz (1984). An analysis of major errors and equipment failures in anesthesia management: considerations for prevention and detection. *Anesthesiology* **60**(1): 34–42.

Evans, R. S., K. G. Kuttler, K. J. Simpson, *et al.* (2014). *Journal of the American Medical Informatics Association* doi:10.1136/amiajnl-2014-002816.

Fagan, L. M., E. H. Shortliffe and B. G. Buchanan (1984). Computer-based medical decision making: from MYCIN to VM. In: Clancey, J. and Shortliffe E. H., editors. *Readings in Medical Artificial Intelligence: The First Decade.* Reading, MA, Addison-Wesley, pp 241–255.

Gardner, R. M. (1981). Direct blood pressure measurement: dynamic response requirements. *Anesthesiology* **54**(3): 227–236.

Gravenstein, J. S., A. K. Ream, N. T. Smith and R. S. Newbower (1987). *The Automated Anesthesia Record and Alarm Systems.* Boston, Butterworth-Heinemann.

Greenwald, S. D., R. S. Patil and R. G. Mark (1990). Improved detection and classification of arrhythmias in noise-corrupted electrocardiograms using contextual information. In: *Computers in Cardiology 1990, Proceedings.* Chicago: Institute of Electrical and Electronics Engineers.

Harris, E. K., B. K. Cooil, G. Shakarji and G. Z. Williams (1980). On the use of statistical models of within-person variation in long-term studies of healthy individuals. *Clinical Chemistry* **26**(3): 383–391.

Hillman K, J. Chen, M. Cretikos, R. Bellomo, D. Brown, G. Doig, S. Finfer A. Flabouris and MERIT study investigators (2005). Introduction of the medical emergency team (MET) system: a cluster-randomised controlled trial. *Lancet* **365**(9477): 2091–2097.

Johannigman, J. A., P. Muskat, S. Barnes, K. Davis and R. D. Branson (2008). Autonomous control of ventilation. *Journal of Trauma–Injury, Infection, and Critical Care* **64**(4 Suppl): S302–S320.

Koski, E. M., A. Mäkivirta, T. Sukuvaara and A. Kari (1990). Frequency and reliability of alarms in the monitoring of cardiac postoperative patients. *International Journal of Clinical Monitoring and Computing* **7**(2): 129–133.

Lellouche, F., J. Mancebo, P. Jolliet, J. Roeseler, F. Schortgen, M. Dojat, B. Cabello, L. Bouadma, P. Rodriguez and S. Maggiore (2006). A multicenter randomized trial of computer-driven protocolized weaning from mechanical ventilation. *American Journal of Respiratory and Critical Care Medicine* **174**(8): 894–900.

Mohammed, M., P. Worthington and W. Woodall (2008). Plotting basic control charts: tutorial notes for healthcare practitioners. *Quality and Safety in Health Care* **17**(2): 137–145.

Muravchick, S., J. E. Caldwell, R. H. Epstein, M. Galati, W. J. Levy, M. O'Reilly, J. S. Plagenhoef, M. Rehman, D. L. Reich and M. M. Vigoda (2008). Anesthesia information management system implementation: a practical guide. *Anesthesia and Analgesia* **107**(5): 1598–1608.

Nii, H. P. (1986). The blackboard model of problem solving and the evolution of blackboard architectures. *AI Magazine* **7**(2): 38.

Parasuraman, R. and D. H. Manzey (2010). Complacency and bias in human use of automation: an attentional integration. *Human Factors* **52**(3): 381–410.

Rampil, I. (1987). Intelligent detection of artifact. In: Gravenstein, R. N. J., A. Ream and N. T. Smith, editors. *The Automated Anesthesia Record and Alarm Systems.* Boston, Butterworth-Heinemann, pp 175–190.

Schmidt, P. E., P. Meredith, D. R. Prytherch, D. Watson, V. Watson, R. M. Killen, P. Greengross, M. A. Mohammed and G. B. Smith (2014). Impact of introducing an electronic physiological surveillance system on hospital mortality. *BMJ Quality & Safety* doi:10.1136/bmjqs-2014-003073.

Skitka, L. (1999). Does automation bias decision-making? *International Journal of Human–Computer Studies* **51**: 991–1006.

Skitka, L., K. Mosier, M. Burdick and B. Rosenblatt (2000). Automation bias and errors: are crews better than individuals. *International Journal of Aviation Psychology* **10**(1): 85–97.

Subbe, C., R. Davies, E. Williams, P. Rutherford and L. Gemmell (2003). Effect of introducing the Modified Early Warning score on clinical outcomes, cardio-pulmonary arrests and intensive care utilisation in acute medical admissions. *Anaesthesia* **58**(8): 797–802.

Sweller, J., P. Ayres and S. Kalyuga (2011). *Cognitive Load Theory.* New York: Springer.

Sykes, M. (1987). Essential monitoring. *British Journal of Anaesthesia* **59**(7): 901–912.

Tennant, R., M. A. Mohammed, J. J. Coleman and U. Martin (2007). Monitoring patients using control charts: a systematic review. *International Journal for Quality in Health Care* **19**(4): 187–194.

Thor, J., J. Lundberg, J. Ask, J. Olsson, C. Carli, K. P. Härenstam and M. Brommels (2007). Application of statistical process control in healthcare improvement: systematic review. *Quality and Safety in Health Care* **16**(5): 387–399.

Wickens, C., J. Hollands, R. Parasuraman and S. Banbury (2012). *Engineering Psychology and Human Performance.* Upper Saddle River, NJ, Pearson.

Chapter 29

Berger, M., R. Shiau and J. M. Weintraub (2006). Review of syndromic surveillance: implications for waterborne disease detection. *Journal of Epidemiology and Community Health* **60**(6): 543–550.

Bravata, D. M., K. M. McDonald, W. M. Smith, C. Rydzak, H. Szeto, D. L. Buckeridge, C. Haberland and D. K. Owens (2004). Systematic review: surveillance systems for early detection of bioterrorism-related diseases. *Annals of Internal Medicine* **140**(11): 910–922.

Cooper, D., G. Smith, F. Chinemana, C. Joseph, P. Loveridge, P. Sebastionpillai, E. Gerard and M. Zambon (2008). Linking syndromic surveillance with virological self-sampling. *Epidemiology and Infection* **136**(02): 222–224.

Dunn, A., F. Bourgeois, S. Murthy, K. Mandl, R. Day and E. Coiera (2012a). The role and impact of research agendas on the comparative-effectiveness research among antihyperlipidemics. *Clinical Pharmacology and Therapeutics* **91**(4): 685–691.

Dunn, A. G., B. Gallego and E. Coiera (2012b). Industry influenced evidence production in collaborative research communities: a network analysis. *Journal of Clinical Epidemiology* **65**(5): 535–543.

Effler, P., M. Ching-Lee, A. Bogard, M.-C. Ieong, T. Nekomoto and D. Jernigan (1999). Statewide system of electronic notifiable disease reporting from clinical laboratories: comparing automated reporting with conventional methods. *JAMA* **282**(19): 1845–1850.

Franz, D. R., P. B. Jahrling, A. M. Friedlander, D. J. McClain, D. L. Hoover, W. R. Bryne, J. A. Pavlin, G. W. Christopher and E. M. Eitzen (1997). Clinical recognition and management of patients exposed to biological warfare agents. *JAMA* **278**(5): 399–411.

Gallego, B. (2010). *Temporal and Spatial Clustering of Bacterial Genotypes: Infectious Disease Informatics*. Springer, pp 359–371.

Gallego, B., V. Sintchenko, Q. Wang, L. Hiley, G. L. Gilbert and E. Coiera (2009). Biosurveillance of emerging biothreats using scalable genotype clustering. *Journal of Biomedical Informatics* **42**(1): 66–73.

Kahn, M., S. Steib, V. Fraser and W. Dunagan (1993). An expert system for culture-based infection control surveillance. In: *Proceedings of the Annual Symposium on Computer Application in Medical Care*. Washington, D.C., American Medical Informatics Association.

Keller, M., M. Blench, H. Tolentino, C. C. Freifeld, K. D. Mandl, A. Mawudeku, G. Eysenbach and J. S. Brownstein (2009). Use of unstructured event-based reports for global infectious disease surveillance. *Emerging Infectious Diseases* **15**(5): 689.

Kermack, M. and A. Mckendrick (1927). Contributions to the mathematical theory of epidemics. Part I. *Proceedings of the Royal Society of London. Series A, Mathematical and Physical Sciences.* **138**(834): 55–83.

Kulldorff, M., *et al.* (2007). Multivariate scan statistics for disease surveillance. *Statistics in Medicine* **26**(8): 1824–1833.

Lowndes, C. M. and K. A. Fenton (2004). Surveillance systems for STIs in the European Union: facing a changing epidemiology. *Sexually Transmitted Infections* **80**(4): 264–271.

McCann, E. (2014). WHO credits mHealth app with helping Nigeria get rid of Ebola. *mHealthNews*. http://www.mhealthnews.com/news/who-credits-mhealth-app-helping-nigeria-get-rid-ebola.

Merchant, R. M., S. Elmer and N. Lurie (2011). Integrating social media into emergency preparedness efforts. *New England Journal of Medicine* **365**(4): 289–291.

M'ikanatha, N. M., R. Lynfield, C. A. Van Beneden and H. De Valk (2008). *Infectious Disease Surveillance*. Chichester, United Kingdom, John Wiley & Sons.

Panackal, A. A., N. M. M'ikanatha, F.-C. Tsui, J. McMahon, M. M. Wagner, B. W. Dixon, J. Zubieta, M. Phelan, S. Mirza and J. Morgan (2002). Automatic electronic laboratory-based reporting of notifiable infectious diseases at a large health system. *Emerging Infectious Diseases* **8**(7): 685–691.

Rushworth, R., S. Bell, G. Rubin, R. Hunter and M. Ferson (1991). Improving surveillance of infectious diseases in New South Wales. *Medical Journal of Australia* **154**(12): 828–831.

Salathé, M., C. C. Freifeld, S. R. Mekaru, A. F. Tomasulo and J. S. Brownstein (2013). Influenza A (H7N9) and the importance of digital epidemiology. *New England Journal of Medicine* **369**(5): 401–404.

Sintchenko, V., G. Gilbert, E. Coiera and D. Dwyer (2002). Treat or test first? Decision analysis of empirical antiviral treatment of influenza virus infection versus treatment based on rapid test results. *Journal of Clinical Virology* **25**(1): 15–21.

Thackeray, R., B. Neiger, A. Smith and S. Van Wagenen (2012). Adoption and use of social media among public health departments. *BMC Public Health* **12**(1): 242.

Wagner, M. M., V. Dato, J. N. Dowling and M. Allswede (2003). Representative threats for research in public health surveillance. *Journal of Biomedical Informatics* **36**(3): 177–188.

Wagner, M. M., A. W. Moore and R. M. Aryel (2011). *Handbook of Biosurveillance*. London, Academic Press.

Wallinga, J. and P. Teunis (2004). Different epidemic curves for severe acute respiratory syndrome reveal similar impacts of control measures. *American Journal of Epidemiology* **160**(6): 509–516.

Waterer, G. W., V. S. Baselski and R. G. Wunderink (2001). *Legionella* and community-acquired pneumonia: a review of current diagnostic tests from a clinician's viewpoint. *American Journal of Medicine* **110**(1): 41–48.

Weber, S. G. and D. Pitrak (2003). Accuracy of a local surveillance system for early detection of emerging infectious disease. *JAMA* **290**(5): 596–598.

Wein, L. M., D. L. Craft and E. H. Kaplan (2003). Emergency response to an anthrax attack. *Proceedings of the National Academy of Sciences of the United States of America* **100**(7): 4346–4351.

World Health Organization (2002). *The Importance of Pharmacovigilance*. Geneva, World Health Organization.

Yates, D. and S. Paquette (2011). Emergency knowledge management and social media technologies: a case study of the 2010 Haitian earthquake. *International Journal of Information Management* **31**(1): 6–13.

Chapter 30

Barabási, A.-L. (2007). Network medicine: from obesity to the 'diseasome'. *New England Journal of Medicine* **357**(4): 404–407.

Gibson, D. G., G. A. Benders, C. Andrews-Pfannkoch, E. A. Denisova, H. Baden-Tillson, J. Zaveri, T. B. Stockwell, A. Brownley, D. W. Thomas and M. A. Algire (2008). Complete chemical synthesis, assembly, and cloning of a *Mycoplasma genitalium* genome. *Science* **319**(5867): 1215–1220.

Hecker, M., S. Lambeck, S. Toepfer, E. Van Someren and R. Guthke (2009). Gene regulatory network inference: data integration in dynamic models: a review. *Biosystems* **96**(1): 86–103.

Ito, T., T. Chiba, R. Ozawa, M. Yoshida, M. Hattori and Y. Sakaki (2001). A comprehensive two-hybrid analysis to explore the yeast protein interactome. *Proceedings of the National Academy of Sciences of the United States of America* **98**(8): 4569–4574.

Kahn, S. D. (2011). On the future of genomic data. *Science* **331**(6018): 728–729.

Mardis, E. R. (2008). The impact of next-generation sequencing technology on genetics. *Trends in Genetics* **24**(3): 133–141.

Metzker, M. L. (2010). Sequencing technologies: the next generation. *Nature Reviews Genetics* **11**(1): 31–46.

Pevzner, P. and R. Shamir (2011). *Bioinformatics for Biologists.* Cambridge, Cambridge University Press.

Saris, C. G., S. Horvath, P. W. van Vught, M. A. van Es, H. M. Blauw, T. F. Fuller, P. Langfelder, J. DeYoung, J. H. Wokke and J. H. Veldink (2009). Weighted gene co-expression network analysis of the peripheral blood from amyotrophic lateral sclerosis patients. *BMC Genomics* **10**(1): 405.

Schatz, M. C., B. Langmead and S. L. Salzberg (2010). Cloud computing and the DNA data race. *Nature Biotechnology* **28**(7): 691.

Scheibye-Alsing, K., S. Hoffmann, A. Frankel, P. Jensen, P. F. Stadler, Y. Mang, N. Tommerup, M. J. Gilchrist, A.-B. Nygård and S. Cirera (2009). Sequence assembly. *Computational Biology and Chemistry* **33**(2): 121–136.

Shendure, J. and H. Ji (2008). Next-generation DNA sequencing. *Nature Biotechnology* **26**(10): 1135-1145.

Takahashi, K., N. Ishikawa, Y. Sadamoto, H. Sasamoto, S. Ohta, A. Shiozawa, F. Miyoshi, Y. Naito, Y. Nakayama and M. Tomita (2003). E-cell 2: multi-platform E-cell simulation system. *Bioinformatics* **19**(13): 1727–1729.

Chapter 31

Alizadeh, A. A., M. B. Eisen, R. E. Davis, C. Ma, I. S. Lossos, A. Rosenwald, J. C. Boldrick, H. Sabet, T. Tran and X. Yu (2000). Distinct types of diffuse large B-cell lymphoma identified by gene expression profiling. *Nature* **403**(6769): 503–511.

Ashburner, M., C. A. Ball, J. A. Blake, D. Botstein, H. Butler, J. M. Cherry, A. P. Davis, K. Dolinski, S. S. Dwight and J. T. Eppig (2000). Gene Ontology: tool for the unification of biology: the Gene Ontology Consortium. *Nature Genetics* **25**(1): 25–29.

Ashley, E. A., A. J. Butte, M. T. Wheeler, R. Chen, T. E. Klein, F. E. Dewey, J. T. Dudley, K. E. Ormond, A. Pavlovic, A. A. Morgan, D. Pushkarev, N. F. Neff, L. Hudgins, L. Gong, L. M. Hodges, D. S. Berlin, C. F. Thorn, K. Sangkuhl, J. M. Hebert, M. Woon, H. Sagreiya, R. Whaley, J. W. Knowles, M. F. Chou, J. V. Thakuria, A. M. Rosenbaum, A. W.

Zaranek, G. M. Church, H. T. Greely, S. R. Quake and R. B. Altman (2010). Clinical assessment incorporating a personal genome. *Lancet* **375**(9725): 1525–1535.

Berg, J. S., M. Adams, N. Nassar, C. Bizon, K. Lee, C. P. Schmitt, K. C. Wilhelmsen and J. P. Evans (2012). An informatics approach to analyzing the incidentalome. *Genetics in Medicine* **15**(1): 36–44.

Borriello, S. P. (1999). Science, medicine, and the future: near patient microbiological tests. *BMJ* **319**(7205): 298.

Burke, W. and B. M. Psaty (2007). Personalized medicine in the era of genomics. *JAMA* **298**(14): 1682–1684.

Butte, A. J., P. Tamayo, D. Slonim, T. R. Golub and I. S. Kohane (2000). Discovering functional relationships between RNA expression and chemotherapeutic susceptibility using relevance networks. *Proceedings of the National Academy of Sciences of the United States of America* **97**(22): 12182–12186.

Cavallari, L. H. and N. A. Limdi (2009). Warfarin pharmacogenomics. *Current Opinion in Molecular Therapeutics* **11**(3): 243–251.

Coiera, E. (2012). The true meaning of personalised medicine. *Yearbook of Medical Informatics* **7**(1): 4–6.

Dupuy, A. and R. M. Simon (2007). Critical review of published microarray studies for cancer outcome and guidelines on statistical analysis and reporting. *Journal of the National Cancer Institute* **99**(2): 147–157.

Eggermont, A. M. and C. Robert (2011). New drugs in melanoma: it's a whole new world. *European Journal of Cancer* **47**(14): 2150–2157.

Fischbach, M. A. and C. T. Walsh (2009). Antibiotics for emerging pathogens. *Science* **325**(5944): 1089–1093.

Fortunel, N. O., H. H. Otu, H. H. Ng, J. Chen, X. Mu, T. Chevassut, X. Li, M. Joseph, C. Bailey, J. A. Hatzfeld, A. Hatzfeld, F. Usta, V. B. Vega, P. M. Long, T. A. Libermann and B. Lim (2003). Comment on " 'Stemness': transcriptional profiling of embryonic and adult stem cells" and "a stem cell molecular signature". *Science* **302**(5644): 393; author reply 393.

Gallego, B., A. G. Dunn and E. Coiera (2013). Role of electronic health records in comparative effectiveness research. *Journal of Comparative Effectiveness Research* **2**(6): 529–532.

Golub, T. R., D. K. Slonim, P. Tamayo, C. Huard, M. Gaasenbeek, J. P. Mesirov, H. Coller, M. L. Loh, J. R. Downing and M. A. Caligiuri (1999). Molecular classification of cancer: class discovery and class prediction by gene expression monitoring. *Science* **286**(5439): 531–537.

Griesenbach, U., D. Geddes and E. Alton (2006). Gene therapy progress and prospects: cystic fibrosis. *Gene Therapy* **13**(14): 1061–1067.

Jenks, P. J. (1998). Sequencing microbial genomes: what will it do for microbiology? *Journal of Medical Microbiology* **47**(5): 375–382.

Kohane, I. S., D. R. Masys and R. B. Altman (2006). The incidentalome: a threat to genomic medicine. *JAMA* **296**(2): 212–215.

Lengauer, T. and T. Sing (2006). Bioinformatics-assisted anti-HIV therapy. *Nature Reviews Microbiology* **4**(10): 790–797.

Liberzon, A., A. Subramanian, R. Pinchback, H. Thorvaldsdottir, P. Tamayo and J. P. Mesirov (2011). Molecular signatures database (MSigDB) 3.0. *Bioinformatics* **27**(12): 1739–1740.

Ng, P. C., S. S. Murray, S. Levy and J. C. Venter (2009). An agenda for personalized medicine. *Nature* **461**(7265): 724–726.

Partridge, S. R., G. Tsafnat, E. Coiera and J. R. Iredell (2009). Gene cassettes and cassette arrays in mobile resistance integrons. *FEMS Microbiology Reviews* **33**(4): 757–784.

Pe'er, I., R. Yelensky, D. Altshuler and M. J. Daly (2008). Estimation of the multiple testing burden for genomewide association studies of nearly all common variants. *Genetic Epidemiology* **32**(4): 381–385.

Pleasance, E. D., P. J. Stephens, S. O'Meara, D. J. McBride, A. Meynert, D. Jones, M.-L. Lin, D. Beare, K. W. Lau and C. Greenman (2010). A small-cell lung cancer genome with complex signatures of tobacco exposure. *Nature* **463**(7278): 184–190.

Pruitt, K. D. and D. R. Maglott (2001). RefSeq and LocusLink: NCBI gene-centered resources. *Nucleic Acids Research* **29**(1): 137–140.

Rice, T. K., N. J. Schork and D. Rao (2008). Methods for handling multiple testing. *Advances in Genetics* **60:** 293–308.

Ruano, G. (2004). Quo vadis personalized medicine? *Personalized Medicine* **1**(1): 1–7.

Rubinstein, R. and I. Simon (2005). MILANO: custom annotation of microarray results using automatic literature searches. *BMC Bioinformatics* **6:** 12.

Sintchenko, V., S. Anthony, X.-H. Phan, F. Lin and E. W. Coiera (2010). A PubMed-wide associational study of infectious diseases. *PLoS One* **5**(3): e9535.

Subramanian, A., P. Tamayo, V. K. Mootha, S. Mukherjee, B. L. Ebert, M. A. Gillette, A. Paulovich, S. L. Pomeroy, T. R. Golub, E. S. Lander and J. P. Mesirov (2005). Gene set enrichment analysis: a knowledge-based approach for interpreting genome-wide expression profiles. *Proceedings of the National Acadamy of Science of the United States of America* **102**(43): 15545–15550.

Tsafnat, G., D. Jasch, A. Misra, M. K. Choong, F. P.-Y. Lin and E. Coiera (2014). Gene–disease association with literature based enrichment. *Journal of Biomedical Informatics* **49:** 221–226.

Westbrook, M. J., M. F. Wright, S. L. Van Driest, T. L. McGregor, J. C. Denny, R. L. Zuvich, E. W. Clayton and K. B. Brothers (2012). Mapping the incidentalome: estimating incidental findings generated through clinical pharmacogenomics testing. *Genetics in Medicine* **15**(5): 325–331.

Wood, A. J., D. G. Savage and K. H. Antman (2002). Imatinib mesylate: a new oral targeted therapy. *New England Journal of Medicine* **346**(9): 683–693.

Chapter 32

Ammenwerth, E., P. Schnell-Inderst and A. Hoerbst (2012). The impact of electronic patient portals on patient care: a systematic review of controlled trials. *Journal of Medical Internet Research* **14**(6): e162.

Andrews, G., P. Cuijpers, M. G. Craske, P. McEvoy and N. Titov (2010). Computer therapy for the anxiety and depressive disorders is effective, acceptable and practical health care: a meta-analysis. *PLoS One* **5**(10): e13196.

Balmford, J., R. Borland and P. Benda (2008). Patterns of use of an automated interactive personalized coaching program for smoking cessation. *Journal of Medical Internet Research* **10**(5): e54.

Barry, M. J. and S. Edgman-Levitan (2012). Shared decision making: the pinnacle of patient-centered care. *New England Journal of Medicine* **366**(9): 780–781.

Belkora, J. (2009). Promoting critical reflection in breast cancer decision making. In: Edwards, A. and G. Elwyn, editors. *Shared Decision-Making in Health Care: Achieving Evidence-Based Patient Choice*. Oxford, Oxford University Press, pp 297–204.

Charles, C., A. Gafni and T. Whelan (1997). Shared decision-making in the medical encounter: what does it mean? (or it takes at least two to tango). *Social Science and Medicine* **44**(5): 681–692.

Chrischilles, E. A., J. P. Hourcade, W. Doucette, D. Eichmann, B. Gryzlak, R. Lorentzen, K. Wright, E. Letuchy, M. Mueller and K. Farris (2013). Personal health records: a randomized trial of effects on elder medication safety. *Journal of the American Medical Informatics Association* **21**(4): 679–686.

Coiera, E. (1998). Information epidemics, economics, and immunity on the internet. *BMJ* **317**(7171): 1469–1470.

Coiera, E. (2012). The true meaning of personalised medicine. *Yearbook of Medical Informatics* **7**(1): 4–6.

Coiera, E. and E. Hovenga (2007). Building a sustainable health system. *Methods of Information in Medicine* **46**(Supp1): 11–18.

Coiera, E., A. Lau, G. Tsafnat, V. Sintchenko and F. Magrabi (2009). The changing nature of clinical decision support systems: a focus on consumers, genomics, public health and decision safety. *Yearbook of Medical Informatics,* pp 84–95.

Crawford, M. J., D. Rutter, C. Manley, T. Weaver, K. Bhui, N. Fulop and P. Tyrer (2002). Systematic review of involving patients in the planning and development of health care. *BMJ* **325**(7375): 1263.

Davidson, K., J. Pennebaker, K. Petrie and J. Weinman (1997). Perceptions of health and illness. In: *Virtual Narratives: Illness Representations in On-line Support Groups*. Amsterdam, Harwood Academic Publishers, pp 463–486.

De Choudhury, M., M. R. Morris and R. W. White (2014). Seeking and sharing health information online: comparing search engines and social media. In: *Proceedings of the 32nd Annual ACM Conference on Human Factors in Computing Systems*. Toronto, ON, Canada, Association for Computing Machinery.

Edwards, A. and G. Elwyn, editors (2009). *Shared Decision-Making in Health Care: Achieving Evidence-Based Patient Choice*. Oxford, Oxford University Press.

Elwyn, G., A. M. O'Connor, C. Bennett, R. G. Newcombe, M. Politi, M.-A. Durand, E. Drake, N. Joseph-Williams, S. Khangura and A. Saarimaki (2009). Assessing the quality of decision support technologies using the International Patient Decision Aid Standards instrument (IPDASi). *PLoS One* **4**(3): e4705.

Eysenbach, G. (2000). Consumer health informatics. *BMJ* **320**(7251): 1713–1716.

Eysenbach, G. (2011). CONSORT-EHEALTH: Improving and standardizing evaluation reports of Web-based and mobile health interventions. *Journal of Medical Internet Research* **13**(4): e126.

Eysenbach, G., T. L. Diepgen (1998). Towards quality management of medical information on the Internet: evaluation, labelling, and filtering of information. *BMJ* **317**(7171): 1496–1502.

Eysenbach, G. and C. Köhler (2002). How do consumers search for and appraise health information on the World Wide Web? Qualitative study using focus groups, usability tests, and in-depth interviews. *BMJ* **324**(7337): 573–577.

Eysenbach, G. and P. E. Kummervold (2005). Is cybermedicine killing you? The story of a Cochrane disaster. *Journal of Medical Internet Research* **7**(2): e21.

Giardina, T. D., S. Menon, D. E. Parrish, D. F. Sittig and H. Singh (2013). Patient access to medical records and healthcare outcomes: a systematic review. *Journal of the American Medical Informatics Association* **21**(4): 737–7419.

Glasspool, D., J. Fox, F. Castillo and V. Monaghan (2003). Interactive decision support for medical planning. *Artificial Intelligence in Medicine* **2780**: 335–339.

Grant, R. W., J. S. Wald, J. L. Schnipper, T. K. Gandhi, E. G. Poon, E. J. Orav, D. H. Williams, L. A. Volk and B. Middleton (2008). Practice-linked online personal health records for type 2 diabetes mellitus: a randomized controlled trial. *Archives of Internal Medicine* **168**(16): 1776–1782.

Hedwig, M. and D. Natter (2005). Effects of active information processing on the understanding of risk information. *Applied Cognitive Psychology* **19**(1): 123–135.

Hoffmann, T., F. Légaré, M. Simmons, K. McNamara, K. McCaffery, L. Trevena, B. Hudson, P. Glasziou and C. Del Mar (2014). Shared decision making: what do clinicians need to know and why should they bother? *Medical Journal of Australia* **201**(1): 35–30.

Janis, I. L. and L. Mann (1977). *Decision Making*. New York, Free Press.

Joosten, E. A., L. DeFuentes-Merillas, G. De Weert, T. Sensky, C. Van Der Staak and C. A. de Jong (2008). Systematic review of the effects of shared decision-making on patient satisfaction, treatment adherence and health status. *Psychotherapy and Psychosomatics* **77**(4): 219–226.

Kinnersley, P., A. Edwards, K. Hood, R. Ryan, H. Prout, N. Cadbury, F. MacBeth, P. Butow and C. Butler (2008). Interventions before consultations to help patients address their information needs by encouraging question asking: systematic review. *BMJ* **337**: a485.

Lau, A. and E. W. Coiera (2007). Do people experience cognitive biases while searching for information? *Journal of the American Medical Informatics Association* **14**(5): 599–608.

Lau, A. and E. W. Coiera (2008). Impact of Web searching and social feedback on consumer decision making: a prospective online experiment. *Journal of Medical Internet Research* **10**(1): e2.

Lau, A. and E. W. Coiera (2009). Can cognitive biases during consumer health information searches be reduced to improve decision making? *Journal of the American Medical Informatics Association* **16**(1): 54–65.

Lau, A., T. Kwok and E. Coiera (2010). The influence of crowds on consumer health decisions: an online prospective study. *Studies in Health Technology and Informatics* **160**(1): 33–37.

Lau, A., J. Proudfoot, A. Andrews, S. Liaw, J. Crimmins, A. Arguel and E. Coiera (2013). Which bundles of features in a Web-based personally controlled health management are associated with consumer help-seeking behaviors for physical and emotional wellbeing? *Journal of Medical Internet Research* **15**(5): e79.

Lau, A., K. Siek, L. Fernandez-Luque, H. Tange, P. Chhanabhai, S. Li, P. Elkin, A. Arjabi, L. Walczowski and C. Ang (2011). The role of social media for patients and consumer health. *Yearbook of Medical Informatics* **6**(1): 131–138.

Lau, A., V. Sintchenko, J. Crimmins, F. Magrabi, B. Gallego and E. Coiera (2012). Impact of a web-based personally controlled health management system on influenza vaccination and health services utilization rates: a randomized controlled trial. *Journal of the American Medical Informatics Association* **19**(5): 719–727.

Lieberman, M. A., M. Golant, J. Giese-Davis, A. Winzlenberg, H. Benjamin, K. Humphreys, C. Kronenwetter, S. Russo and D. Spiegel (2003). Electronic support groups for breast carcinoma: a clinical trial of effectiveness. *Cancer* **97**(4): 920–925.

Lorig, K. R., D. D. Laurent, R. A. Deyo, M. E. Marnell, M. A. Minor and P. L. Ritter (2002). Can a back pain e-mail discussion group improve health status and lower health care costs? A randomized study. *Archives of Internal Medicine* **167**(7): 792–796.

Murray, E., J. Burns, T. S. See, R. Lai and I. Nazareth (2005). Interactive health communication applications for people with chronic disease. *Cochrane Database of Systematic Reviews* (**4**): CD004274.

Newell, B. and T. Rakow (2007). The role of experience in decisions from description. *Psychonomic Bulletin and Review* **14**(6): 1133–1139.

O'Connor, A. (1995). Validation of a decisional conflict scale. *Medical Decision Making* **15**(1): 25–30.

O'Connor, A. (2001). Using patient decision aids to promote evidence-based decision making. *ACP Journal Club* **135**(1): A11–A12.

O'Connor, A., E. R. Drake, G. A. Wells, P. Tugwell, A. Laupacis and T. Elmslie (2003). A survey of the decision-making needs of Canadians faced with complex health decisions. *Health Expectations* **6**(2): 97–109.

O'Connor, A., A. Rostom, V. Fiset, J. Tetroe, V. Entwistle and H. Llewellyn-Thomas (1999). Decision aids for patients facing health treatment or screening decisions: systematic review. *BMJ* **319**(7212): 731–734.

Paton, C., M. Hansen, L. Fernandez-Luque and A. Y. S. Lau (2012). Self-tracking, social media and personal health records for patient empowered self-care: contribution of the IMIA Social Media Working Group. *Yearbook of Medical Informatics* **7**(1): 16–24.

Peckham, B. M., W. V. Slack, W. F. Carr, L. J. Van Cura and A. E. Schultz (1967). Computerized data collection in the management of uterine cancer. *Clinical Obstetrics and Gynecology* **10**(4): 1003–1015.

Pirolli, P. (2009). An elementary social information foraging model. In *Proceedings of the SIGCHI Conference on Human Factors in Computing Systems*, pp. 605–614. ACM. Boston.

Pletneva, N. and A. Vargas (2011). D8. 1.1. Requirements for the general public health search. Khresmoi Project public deliverable.

Proudfoot, J., B. Klein, A. Barak, P. Carlbring, P. Cuijpers, A. Lange, L. Ritterband and G. Andersson (2011). Establishing guidelines for executing and reporting Internet intervention research. *Cognitive Behaviour Therapy* **40**(2): 82–97.

Ross, S. E. and C.-T. Lin (2003). The effects of promoting patient access to medical records: a review. *Journal of the American Medical Informatics Association* **10**(2): 129–138.

Ruland, C. M., H. H. Holte, J. Røislien, C. Heaven, G. A. Hamilton, J. Kristiansen, H. Sandbæk, S. O. Kvaløy, L. Hasund and M. C. Ellison (2010). Effects of a computer-supported interactive tailored patient assessment tool on patient care, symptom distress, and patients' need for symptom management support: a randomized clinical trial. *Journal of the American Medical Informatics Association* **17**(4): 403–410.

Sanders, A. R., I. van Weeghel, M. Vogelaar, W. Verheul, R. H. Pieters, N. J. de Wit and J. M. Bensing (2013). Effects of improved patient participation in primary care on health-related outcomes: a systematic review. *Family Practice* **30**(4): 365–378.

Schnipper, J. L., T. K. Gandhi, J. S. Wald, R. W. Grant, E. G. Poon, L. A. Volk, A. Businger, D. H. Williams, E. Siteman and L. Buckel (2012). Effects of an online personal health record on medication accuracy and safety: a cluster-randomized trial. *Journal of the American Medical Informatics Association* **19**(5): 728–734.

Shaw, B. R., F. McTavish, R. Hawkins, D. H. Gustafson and S. Pingree (2000). Experiences of women with breast cancer: exchanging social support over the chess computer network. *Journal of Health Communication* **5**(2): 135–159.

Shepherd, H. L., A. Barratt, L. J. Trevena, K. McGeechan, K. Carey, R. M. Epstein, P. N. Butow, C. B. Del Mar, V. Entwistle and M. H. Tattersall (2011). Three questions that patients can ask to improve the quality of information physicians give about treatment options: a cross-over trial. *Patient Education and Counseling* **84**(3): 379--85.

Slack, W. V., H. B. Kowaloff, R. B. Davis, T. Delbanco, S. E. Locke, C. Safran and H. L. Bleich (2012). Evaluation of computer-based medical histories taken by patients at home. *Journal of the American Medical Informatics Association* **19**(4): 545–548.

Slack, W. V. and C. W. Slack (1977). Talking to a computer about emotional problems: a comparative study. *Psychotherapy: Theory, Research and Practice* **14**(2): 156.

Stacey, D., F. Légaré, N. Col, C. Bennett, M. Barry, K. Eden, M. Holmes-Rovner, H. Llewellyn-Thomas, A. Lyddiatt, R. Thomson, L. Trevena and J. Wu (2014). Decision aids for people facing health treatment or screening decisions. *Cochrane Database of Systematic Reviews* **10**(1): CD001431.

Steinbrook, R. (2008). Personally controlled online health data: the next big thing in medical care? *New England Journal of Medicine* **358**(16): 1653–1656.

Stevens, J. V., L. K. Funk, J. P. Brantley, P. T. Erlinger, H. V. Myers, M. C. Champagne, A. Bauck, D. C. Samuel-Hodge and F. J. Hollis (2008). Design and implementation of an interactive website to support long-term maintenance of weight loss. *Journal of Medical Internet Research* **10**(1): e1.

Swan, M. (2009). Emerging patient-driven health care models: an examination of health social networks, consumer personalized medicine and quantified self-tracking. *International Journal of Environmental Research and Public Health* **6**(2): 492–525.

Tang, P. C., J. S. Ash, D. W. Bates, J. M. Overhage and D. Z. Sands (2006). Personal health records: definitions, benefits, and strategies for overcoming barriers to adoption. *Journal of American Medical Informatics Association* 13(2): 121–126.

van den Berg, M. H., J. W. Schoones and T. P. Vliet Vlieland (2007). Internet-based physical activity interventions: a systematic review of the literature. *Journal of Medical Internet Research* **9**(3): e26.

Wagner, P. J., J. Dias, S. Howard, K. W. Kintziger, M. F. Hudson, Y.-H. Seol and P. Sodomka (2012). Personal health records and hypertension control: a randomized trial. *Journal of the American Medical Informatics Association* **19**(4): 626–634.

Wang, L., J. Wang, M. Wang, Y. Li, Y. Liang and D. Xu (2011). Using Internet search engines to obtain medical information: a comparative study. *Journal of Medical Internet Research* **14**(3): e74–e74.

Wantland, D. J., C. J. Portillo, W. L. Holzemer, R. Slaughter and E. M. McGhee (2004). The effectiveness of Web-based vs. non-Web-based interventions: a meta-analysis of behavioral change outcomes. *Journal of Medical Internet Research* **6**(4): e40.

Webb, L. T., J. Joseph, L. Yardley and S. Michie (2010). Using the Internet to promote health behavior change: a systematic review and meta-analysis of the impact of theoretical basis, use of behavior change techniques, and mode of delivery on efficacy. *Journal of Medical Internet Research* **12**(1): e4.

Index

Pages followed by f indicate figures; those followed by t indicate tables.